365 Ultimate Quinoa Recipes

(365 Ultimate Quinoa Recipes - Volume 1)

Doris Lamont

Copyright: Published in the United States by Doris Lamont/ © DORIS LAMONT

Published on December, 07 2020

All rights reserved. No part of this publication may be reproduced, stored in retrieval system, copied in any form or by any means, electronic, mechanical, photocopying, recording or otherwise transmitted without written permission from the publisher. Please do not participate in or encourage piracy of this material in any way. You must not circulate this book in any format. DORIS LAMONT does not control or direct users' actions and is not responsible for the information or content shared, harm and/or actions of the book readers.

In accordance with the U.S. Copyright Act of 1976, the scanning, uploading and electronic sharing of any part of this book without the permission of the publisher constitute unlawful piracy and theft of the author's intellectual property. If you would like to use material from the book (other than just simply for reviewing the book), prior permission must be obtained by contacting the author at author@slushierecipes.com

Thank you for your support of the author's rights.

Content

365 AWESOME QUINOA RECIPES 9

1. Healthy Chocolate Quinoa Cupcakes 9
2. Refried Beans & Quinoa Burger Patties 9
3. "Baraka Restaurant" Quinoa & Caramelized Squash And Carrots Salad 10
4. A SHRIMP AND QUINOA PAELLA ... 10
5. Acorn Squash Stuffed With Quinoa, Golden Raisins, Walnuts & Sage 11
6. Addictive Quinoa Salad 12
7. African Squash And Peanut Stew With Coconut Milk And Quinoa 13
8. All Week Long Toasted Almond Quinoa And Arugula Salad 13
9. Almond, Peach And Quinoa Crumble 14
10. Apple Cinnamon Quinoa Porridge 14
11. Apple And Red Quinoa Salad 14
12. Apple Cinnamon Breakfast Quinoa 15
13. Asian Style Red Quinoa Salad With Tofu . 15
14. Asparagus, Avocado, And Caramelized Onion Quinoa 16
15. Autumn Harvest Quinoa Muffins 16
16. Autumnal Quinoa Salad 17
17. Avocado & Kale Quinoa Salad 18
18. BBQ Quinoa Burgers 18
19. Baked Broccoli And Carrot Quinoa Patties 18
20. Baked Quinoa Pudding With Persimmon And Pistachios 19
21. Baked Quinoa With Roasted Butternut Squash & Gruyère 20
22. Baked Quinoa Pork Meatballs 20
23. Baked Turkey Quinoa Spinach Meatballs . 21
24. Balsamic Mushroom Quinoa 21
25. Banana Bread Granola With Quinoa And Cocoa Nibs 22
26. Beet Salad With Apple, Quinoa, Kale And Walnuts 22
27. Better Than Central Market's Chipotle Quinoa 23
28. Black Bean And Quinoa Enchiladas 23
29. Black Bean And Quinoa Veggie Burgers .. 24
30. Black Bean, Quinoa And Citrus Salad [v] [veg] [gf] 25
31. Black Quinoa Salad With Grilled Vegetables, Basil, Feta And Pine Nuts 25
32. Black Quinoa Salad With Kidney Beans ... 26
33. Blueberry White Chocolate Granola With A Quinoa Crunch! 26
34. Braised Collard Rolls With Lamb And Quinoa 27
35. Breakfast Quinoa 28
36. Breakfast Quinoa Bowl 28
37. Breakfast Quinoa With Oats And Chia Seeds 28
38. Breakfast Quinoa 29
39. Brown Butter Broccoli Over Quinoa And Feta 29
40. Buffalo Style Quinoa Chili 30
41. California Pizza Kitchen Style Quinoa & Arugula Salad 30
42. Cauliflower Cheddar Quinoa Fritters 31
43. Chard And Quinoa Crustless Tart 31
44. Chayote, Avocado And Macadamia Quinoa With Coconut Lime Vinaigrette 32
45. Cheesy Greek Style Baked Quinoa 33
46. Cherry Tomato Quinoa Caprese 33
47. Chicken & Quinoa Stuffed Peppers 33
48. Chicken Quinoa 34
49. Chipotle Peach Quinoa Salad 34
50. Chocolate Quinoa Crackers 35
51. Chopped Parsley Salad With Quinoa, Comte + Pumpkin Seeds 35
52. Cilantro And Lime Quinoa 35
53. Cinnamon French Toast Breakfast Quinoa 36
54. Cinnamon Maple Quinoa With Roasted Apples, Dried Fruit And Toasted Almonds 36
55. Coconut Quinoa Crunch Yogurt Parfait With Gingered Maple Syrup 37
56. Coconut Quinoa Porridge With Berry Compote 37
57. Coconut Quinoa Pudding 38
58. Coconut Quinoa And Warm Broccoli Bowl With Ginger Lemongrass Dressing 39
59. Coconut Ginger Quinoa With Carrots And Shrimp 39
60. Colca Cañon Quinoa Soup 40
61. Colorful Rice Cooker Blueberry Morning Quinoa 40
62. Corn Salad With Tomatoes, Avocado,

Quinoa And Feta 41
63. Cranberry Almond Quinoa Pilaf 41
64. Cranberry Smoothie Quinoa Pudding 41
65. Creamy Quinoa Custard Pie Layered With Bananas And Date Toffee 42
66. Creamy Quinoa Onion Soup 42
67. Crispy Quinoa Chocolate Bars 43
68. Crispy Quinoa And Mustard Green Cakes 43
69. Crispy Shrimp & Red Quinoa Patties 44
70. Crockpot Chicken Quinoa Soup 45
71. Curried Quinoa With Cherries And Roasted Chickpeas 45
72. Curried Quinoa With Spinach And Avocado 46
73. Curried Red Quinoa, Peas And Paneer Salad 46
74. Curried Eggplant & Sweet Onion With Quinoa 47
75. Curry Quinoa Pilaf With Roasted Butternut Squash And Raisin Mix 47
76. Dark Chocolate Cherry Quinoa Bark 48
77. Double Chocolate Quinoa Brownies 49
78. Double Corn, Quinoa & Cheddar Muffins 49
79. Earthy Quinoa "Tabbouleh" 49
80. Easy Greek Quinoa Salad With Shrimp 50
81. Easy Quinoa Sweet Porridge 51
82. Easy Scallion, Green Pea And Lemon Quinoa Pilaf With Sesame Seeds 51
83. Eat Your Peas & Carrots Quinoa Pasta (with Bacon!) 51
84. Edamame And Quinoa Salad 52
85. Epic Quinoa Kale Salad With Orange Miso Dressing & Teriyaki Cashews 52
86. Everything Bagel Quinoa Cakes With Smoked Salmon And Crème Fraîche 53
87. Everything I Want To Eat Quinoa And Lentil Salad 54
88. Flax And Quinoa Seed Bread (LC, GF) 55
89. Flourless Quinoa Chocolate Cake 55
90. Fresh Stuffed Red Pepper Shells With Pearl Couscous, Forbidden Rice, Kamut Or Red Quinoa 56
91. Fried Quinoa, Apples, Beets & Herbs 57
92. Garden Herbed Quinoa 57
93. Garden Tomato, Ceci And Black Pepper Feta Quinoa 57
94. Garlic Roasted Vegetables And Quinoa 58
95. Georgian Quinoa Salad With Eggplant & Sour Cherries 58
96. Golden Quinoa Cakes With Salsa Fresca .. 60
97. Gourmet Vegetarian Pâté With Walnuts And Quinoa 61
98. Greek Quinoa Salad 62
99. Greek Salad And Parsley Tabbouleh With Quinoa 62
100. Green Quinoa Patties 63
101. Grilled Avocado Halves With Cumin Spiced Quinoa And Black Bean Salad 63
102. Grilled Pineapple And Red Curry Quinoa 64
103. Guacamole Quinoa 64
104. Harissa Steak & Eggs With Quinoa Tabbouleh Hash 65
105. Harvest Quinoa And Mixed Veggie Salad 65
106. Heirloom Tomato, Basil And Goat Cheese "Pie" (With A Rice, Millet, And Quinoa Crust) .66
107. Heirloom Tomato Avocado Quinoa Lettuce Wraps 66
108. Herb, Feta, And Quinoa Filled Frittata 67
109. Herbed Quinoa Salad With Roasted Shrimp 67
110. Herbed Yellow Cherry Tomato, White Lima Bean And Black Quinoa Medley 68
111. Holiday Pomegranate Quinoa Salad 69
112. Holy Shitake Quinoa Sushi 69
113. How To Cook Quinoa 69
114. Hungarian Stuffed Reds With Red Quinoa 70
115. Italian Tuna, Quinoa And White Bean Salad 71
116. KOSHERMOMS RECIPE: BABY QUINOA SALAD WITH ROASTED VEGETABLES 71
117. Kale & Quinoa Salad 71
118. Kale And Quinoa Salad 72
119. Kale And Tomato Quinoa Bowl With Lemon Mint Vinaigrette 73
120. Lemon Cranberry Quinoa Salad 73
121. Lemon Herb Quinoa With Hemp Seeds, Spring Peas, And Basil 74
122. Lemon Tri Color Quinoa Tabbouleh 74
123. Lemon Quinoa With Fresh Pesto 75
124. Lemony Quinoa Broccoli Salad 75

125. Lemony Quinoa Salad With Summer Vegetables 76
126. Lemony Shrimp And Quinoa 76
127. Light Chicken Quinoa Divan 77
128. Loaded Quinoa Veggie Sliders 77
129. Maple Mulberry Quinoa Oatmeal Bowl 78
130. Maple Quinoa Granola 78
131. Mediterranean Toasted Quinoa Salad ~ Chickpeas, Roasted Red Peppers & Herbs 79
132. Mediterranean Vegetable Bowls With Quinoa, Toasted Chickpeas, And Harissa Tahini 80
133. Millet And Quinoa Summer Squash Salad 81
134. Miso Masala Kabocha & Cauliflower Quinoa Salad 81
135. Miso Quinoa Pilaf With Grilled Cucumber, Eggplant, And Soy Dressing 82
136. Moroccan Quinoa & Chickpea Salad With Dried Fruit 83
137. Moroccan Tilapia With Red Pepper, Lemon And Quinoa 83
138. Mung Bean, Lentil, And Quinoa Salad Stuffed Avocado 84
139. Mushroom Quinoa Soup 84
140. Mushrooms & Quinoa 85
141. My Favorite Quinoa Breakfast Hash 85
142. Nectarine Quinoa 86
143. Nectarine Quinoa Salad 86
144. No Bake Quinoa Breakfast Bar 87
145. Nutty Cherry Lentil Quinoa Salad 87
146. Nutty Quinoa Salmon Burgers 88
147. Oats And Quinoa Breakfast Bars 88
148. Okra And Tomato Quinoa 89
149. Olive Oil Fried Chicken With Pesto Quinoa And Heirloom Tomatoes 89
150. One Pot Corn, Tomato & Quinoa Pilaf ... 90
151. Orange Basil Quinoa Salad 90
152. Orange And Strawberry Quinoa Salad 91
153. Oven Roasted Brussels Sprouts With Bacon, Chestnuts & Quinoa 91
154. Overnight Toasted Oat And Quinoa Bowl 92
155. Paula Shoyer's Chocolate Quinoa Cake 92
156. Perfect Long Grain Brown Rice With Black Or Red Quinoa 93
157. Peruvian Quinoa Lettuce Roll Ups 94
158. Peruvian Tri Color Quinoa Salad 94

159. Pesto Quinoa Veggie Bowl 95
160. Pesto Quinoa Pilaf 95
161. Pickled Shrimp With Tzatzki Quinoa 96
162. Poblano Stuffed Quinoa With Honey Lime Vinaigrette 97
163. Pork With Peaches & Quinoa 97
164. Preserved Lemon Quinoa 98
165. Quinoa "Fried Rice" 98
166. Quinoa & Mango Salad With Lemony Ginger Dressing 99
167. Quinoa & Pine Nut Salad 99
168. Quinoa & Roasted Sweet Potato Superfood Salad 100
169. Quinoa & Bulgur Salad With Spinach, Chards, Radishes, Soft Boiled Eggs And Cappe 100
170. Quinoa 'Mac' And Cauliflower Chard Cheese Sauce 101
171. Quinoa (Sort Of) Diane 101
172. Quinoa Black Bean Burgers 102
173. Quinoa Black Bean Summer Salad With Tahini Dressing 103
174. Quinoa Burritos 103
175. Quinoa Confetti Salad 104
176. Quinoa Cookies With Coconut & Chocolate Chunks 104
177. Quinoa Couscous Salad 105
178. Quinoa Cranberry Chocolate Chip Cookies 105
179. Quinoa Crepes 106
180. Quinoa Crisps 106
181. Quinoa Croquettes 106
182. Quinoa Crêpes With Blackberry And Plum Compote 107
183. Quinoa Eetch (Red Quinoa Tabouli) 107
184. Quinoa Fried Rice Recipe 108
185. Quinoa Fried Rice With Tomatoes 108
186. Quinoa Granola 109
187. Quinoa Lettuce Wraps 109
188. Quinoa Minestrone With Kale Pesto 110
189. Quinoa Patties 110
190. Quinoa Pilaf 111
191. Quinoa Pilaf With Citrus Soy Dressing .. 111
192. Quinoa Pilaf With Curry Powder 112
193. Quinoa Pilau 112
194. Quinoa Pizza Dough 113
195. Quinoa Pizza With Tomato And

- Mushrooms 113
- 196. Quinoa Ranch Casserole 114
- 197. Quinoa Salad With Strawberries, Goat Cheese & Crispy Kale 114
- 198. Quinoa Salad With Currants, Pistachios, Red Onion And Mint 114
- 199. Quinoa Salad With Feta, Blood Oranges And Mint 115
- 200. Quinoa Salad With Roasted Tomatoes And Fried Leeks 115
- 201. Quinoa Salad With Spinach, Strawberries And Goat Cheese 116
- 202. Quinoa Salad With Tangerine Balsamic Tofu And Cinnamon Vinaigrette 116
- 203. Quinoa Salad With Toasted Pine Nuts, Raisins And Lime 117
- 204. Quinoa Salad With Roasted Grapes 117
- 205. Quinoa Salsa Egg Muffins 118
- 206. Quinoa Shakshuka With Feta And Kale . 118
- 207. Quinoa Soup 119
- 208. Quinoa Spinach Salad With Peanut Ginger Dressing 119
- 209. Quinoa Springtime Salad 119
- 210. Quinoa Stuffed Bell Peppers 120
- 211. Quinoa Stuffed Grape Leaves 120
- 212. Quinoa Stuffed Peppers 121
- 213. Quinoa Stuffed Squash 122
- 214. Quinoa Stuffed With Everything Good .. 123
- 215. Quinoa Tabbouleh 123
- 216. Quinoa Tabbouleh Chickpea Burger With Beet Ketchup & Roasted Peaches 124
- 217. Quinoa Tabbouleh Stuffing With Roasted Squash And Mushrooms 124
- 218. Quinoa Tabbouleh With Kale 125
- 219. Quinoa Tabouli 125
- 220. Quinoa And Apple Muffins 126
- 221. Quinoa And Carrot Tabbouleh Salad 126
- 222. Quinoa And Chickpea Flour Falafel With Romesco Sauce 127
- 223. Quinoa And Corn Patties 128
- 224. Quinoa And Edamame Salad With Basil, Mint, And Lemon 128
- 225. Quinoa And Farro Salad With Pickled Fennel 129
- 226. Quinoa And Grilled Marinated Vegetable Salad 130
- 227. Quinoa And Kale Crustless Quiche 131
- 228. Quinoa And Oat Breakfast Porridge 131
- 229. Quinoa And Salmon Breakfast Torte 132
- 230. Quinoa And Vegetable Chorizo Salad 132
- 231. Quinoa And Wild Rice Casserole With Kale, Leeks, And Gruyère Biscuit Crust 133
- 232. Quinoa And Cold Sauce 134
- 233. Quinoa Date Pudding 135
- 234. Quinoa Pudding Paletas With Plums 135
- 235. Quinoa Salad With Avocado 136
- 236. Quinoa Salad With Radishes, Avocado, And Citrus Vinaigrette 137
- 237. Quinoa With (Almost) Caramelized Onions And Shiitake Mushrooms Two Ways 137
- 238. Quinoa With Broccoli "Dust", Haloumi Cheese, And Mint 138
- 239. Quinoa With Butternut Squash And Pumpkin Seeds 138
- 240. Quinoa With Butternut Squash, Cinnamon And Mint 139
- 241. Quinoa With Chard, Sausage, And Corn 140
- 242. Quinoa With Curried Cauliflower & Potatoes 140
- 243. Quinoa With Onions 141
- 244. Quinoa With Roasted Beets And Pear ... 141
- 245. Quinoa With Walnuts, Goat Cheese, And Thyme 142
- 246. Quinoa With Apricot And Pine Kernels 142
- 247. Quinoa With Edamame And Sundried Tomatoes 143
- 248. Quinoa, Beet And Chickpea Burgers 143
- 249. Quinoa, Edamame & Cucumber Salad ... 144
- 250. Quinoa, Fava Bean, And Chard Veggie Burgers 145
- 251. Quinoa, Halloumi And Fresh Corn Salad 146
- 252. Quinoa, Molasses And Peanuts For Breakfast 146
- 253. Quinoa, Oat And Chia Porridge 147
- 254. Quinoa, Wheat Berry, And Chickpea Salad With Green Beans 147
- 255. Quinoa, Cherry Tomato, Tuna And Feta Salad 148
- 256. Quinoa Chicken Meatballs With Garlicky Greens 148
- 257. Quinoa Lentil Taco Filling 149
- 258. Quinoa Oat Chocolate Chip Cookies 149
- 259. Quinoa Stuffed Bell Peppers With Basil

Sauce 150
260. Quinoa Stuffed Mushrooms 150
261. Raddichio Wrapped Quinoa Kale Taco Salad W/ Spicy Avocado Dressing 151
262. Rainbow Quinoa Salad 152
263. Red & White Meditterranean Quinoa 152
264. Red Quinoa Peach Porridge 153
265. Red Quinoa Salad With Citrus And Pistachios 153
266. Red Quinoa Salad With Elephant Garlic And Greens 153
267. Red Quinoa Tomato Avocado Summer Salad 154
268. Red Quinoa With Honey Glazed Carrots, Thyme Pistou And Pistachios 154
269. Red Quinoa, Red Lentils: A Salad 155
270. Red Quinoa And Garbanzo Bean Salad With Salmon 155
271. Red Quinoa And Tofu Miso Bowl 156
272. Red Quinoa Salad With Snow Peas, Spinach, Feta And Poached Egg 156
273. Red Quinoa Tabbouleh 157
274. Roast Vegetable Quinoa Salad With Garlic & Parsley Oil 157
275. Roasted Apricot And Quinoa Cakes With Rosemary 158
276. Roasted Beet & Quinoa Salad 158
277. Roasted Butternut Squash Salad With Quinoa 159
278. Roasted Fig And Hazelnut Quinoa Salad 160
279. Roasted Kale, Squash And Quinoa Salad 160
280. Roasted Quinoa With Potatoes And Cheese 161
281. Roasted Sweet Potato, Quinoa And Arugula Salad 161
282. Roasted Vegetables & Quinoa Tartlets ... 162
283. Roasted Vegetables With Bright & Crunchy Herbed Topping 162
284. Roasted Veggie Quinoa Medley 163
285. Roasted Zucchini And Scallion Quinoa Bowl 163
286. Sautéed Kale & Sun Dried Tomatoes With Mixed Red & White Quinoa 164
287. Seared Scallops Over Pesto And Quinoa Paste 164
288. Sesame, Quinoa & All The Greens Power Wrap 165

289. Shaved Fennel & Asparagus Quinoa Salad 167
290. Shrimp Quinoa Salad With Feta And Tomatoes 167
291. Smoky Coconut Broth With Quinoa 167
292. Soupa De Quinoa Con Pollo (Peruvian Quinoa Soup With Chicken) 168
293. Southwest Quinoa Salad With Sweet & Spicy Honey Lime Dressing 168
294. Southwestern Quinoa 169
295. Southwestern Quinoa Salad 169
296. Southwestern Quinoa Salad, By Way Of The Pantry 170
297. Soy Sauce Quinoa Bowl 171
298. Spicy BLAQ (Bean, Leek, Avocado And Quinoa) Salad Tacos 172
299. Spicy Black Bean And Quinoa Salad 172
300. Spicy Delicata Squash Boats With Fruity Quinoa Pilaf 173
301. Spicy Quinoa Pilaf With Warm Beet Greens 173
302. Spicy Quinoa Tabouli 174
303. Spicy Tempeh Quinoa Tacos 174
304. Spicy Quinoa Pilaf With Beet Greens 175
305. Spinach Potato Quinoa Croquettes With A Spinach Sorrel Pesto 176
306. Sprouted Quinoa Salad With Peanut Ginger Dressing 177
307. Steak Quinoa Salad With Avocado Lime Ranch Dressing 177
308. Strawberry And Quinoa Salad With Tarragon, Soft Goat's Cheese And Poached Egg 178
309. Strawberry Basil Skillet Quinoa Cornbread 178
310. Stuffed Tomatoes With Quinoa 179
311. Summer Chili With Quinoa And Black Chick Peas 179
312. Summer Fresh Quinoa And Kale Salad . 180
313. Summer Herb Salad With Fresh Crab, Quinoa Tabouleh, And Harissa Vinaigrette 180
314. Summer Quinoa Salad, Mexican Style 181
315. Sunshine Quinoa Salad 181
316. Sweet Onion & Corn Quinoa Fritters With Fresh Corn & Basil Salad 182
317. Sweet Potato & Mushroom Quinoa Burgers 183

318. Sweet Potato Quinoa Salad 184
319. Sweet Quinoa 184
320. Sweet And Crunchy Quinoa Salad 184
321. Taco Tuna Quinoa Sliders 185
322. Tandoori Quinoa Cakes With Garden Herbs 185
323. Thai Inspired Peanut Quinoa Salad 186
324. The Best Quinoa Salad Ever 187
325. The Family Waffle 187
326. The Leigh Anne (Farro, Sausage And Brussel Sprouts) 188
327. The Red And The Black. Roasted Red Peppers, Black Quinoa And Allioli (with Apologies To Stendhal) 188
328. The Red And The Black: The Sequel. Black Quinoa, Pearl Couscous ,Tomato Coulis 189
329. Toasted Almond And Coconut Quinoa Porridge 190
330. Tomato Peanut Butter Quinoa Soup 190
331. Tomato Quinoa With Zucchini Red Pepper And Corn 190
332. Tomato And Chard Quinoa Bake 191
333. Tomato And Fresh Herbs Quinoa Salad 191
334. Tomatoes Stuffed With Quinoa, Spinach And Feta 192
335. Top Shelf Trek Mix 192
336. Tropical Quinoa And Fruit Pudding 193
337. Turkey Quinoa Burger 193
338. Vegan Quinoa Lentil Curry Burger 193
339. Vegan Rosh Hashanah Recipe: Pomegranate Glazed Tofu & Quinoa 194
340. Vegetable Quinoa Pilaf 194
341. Vegetable Quinoa Salad 195
342. Vegetarian Summer Rolls With Quinoa .. 195
343. Veggie Fried Quinoa 196
344. Veggie Quinoa Stuffed Chiles 196
345. WHEAT BERRIES, RED QUINOA, AND WILD RICE WITH SUN DRIED TOMATOES 197
346. Walnut & Sage Smothered Lentil Quinoa Pilaf 197
347. Walnut And Quinoa Salad With Goat Cheese, Dried Cherries And Arugula 198
348. Warm Red Quinoa & Squash Salad 198
349. Watermelon Pizza Salad With Curried Quinoa 198
350. White Bean And Quinoa Chili 199
351. Wintry Mushroom, Kale, And Quinoa Enchiladas 200
352. Yogurt With Toasted Quinoa, Dates, And Almonds 200
353. Zesty Red Quinoa Salad 201
354. Beet, Quinoa, Tahini Bowl 201
355. Crunchy Quinoa & Veggie Roaster 202
356. Goat Cheese & Quinoa Stuffed Artichoke Heart Bottoms 203
357. Mandarin Quinoa And Kale Bowl 204
358. Quinoa Salad With Vegetables & Poached Egg 204
359. Quinoa With Roasted Vegetables & Wine Glazed Chicken 205
360. Quinoa With Sauteed Vegetables & Soft Cooked Egg 206
361. Quinoa With Wild Mushrooms, Black Eyed Peas And Dandies 207
362. Roasted Cherry Tomatoes + Pomegranate Molasses Over Quinoa 208
363. Tomates Farcies: Vegetarian & Beef Stuffed Tomatoes, Bonus QUINOA Salad 208
364. Warm Quinoa, Collard Greens, And Squash Salad 209
365. {Veg & GF} Quinoa & Pomegranate Tabbouleh Salad 210

INDEX **211**
CONCLUSION **216**

365 Awesome Quinoa Recipes

***

1. Healthy Chocolate Quinoa Cupcakes

Serving: Makes 24 cupcakes | Prep: | Cook: | Ready in:

Ingredients

- quinoa part
- 2/3 cup Quinoa
- 1 1/3 cups water
- cake mix
- 2/3 cup Milk
- 3 Large eggs
- 1 1/2 teaspoons Vanilla (I use pure)
- 3/4 cup Butter
- 1/2 cup Honey
- 2/3 cup Brown sugar
- 3/4 cup Cocoa powder
- 1 pinch salt
- 1/3 cup Oatmeal or Coconut (optional)

Direction

- Quinoa part
- Soak the quinoa in lots of water for 3-5 minutes. Then wash and rinse quinoa few times to get fully rinsed (or it will have a bitter taste).
- Bring quinoa and 1 1/3 cups of water to a boil, then cover and reduce heat to low for 8 minutes.
- Turn off heat and leave covered for extra 8 minutes. Then fluff quinoa with a fork and set aside to allow to cool.
- Cake mix
- Preheat the oven to 350°F. Grease muffin pans (24) or 2 x 8" cake pans.
- Mix the milk, eggs and vanilla. Add 2 cups of the cooked quinoa, honey and butter and blend until really smooth, no chunks (works really good with food processor).
- Mix brown sugar, cocoa, baking powder and salt in bowl. Add to liquid mixture, blend for 1 minute.
- Put batter into muffin tins or cake pans. Bake for 25-30 minutes, or until toothpick inserted in center of muffin comes out clean. Let cool down, then enjoy!!

2. Refried Beans & Quinoa Burger Patties

Serving: Makes 8 | Prep: | Cook: | Ready in:

Ingredients

- 1 cup cooked Quinoa
- 1 cup fat free refried beans
- 2 1/2 cups Panko bread crumbs
- 1 teaspoon Garam Masala
- 1 small Fresh birds eye chilli deseeded & finely minced
- 1/4 cup Finely diced Shallots
- 1/2 cup Finely chopped Cilantro
- Juice of 1 lemon
- Salt to taste
- Oil for Pan frying
- 8 Hamburger rolls
- 8 slices mozzarella cheese
- lettuce, sliced tomatoes & onions as needed

Direction

- To obtain 1 cup of cooked Quinoa, add 1/2 a cup of the seeds to 1. 1/4 cups of hot water. Bring to a boil, reduce heat, cover & cook for ~ 15 min (until the seeds sprout their little tails

out & turn translucent. Drain off any excess water.
- Combine the Quinoa, refried beans and all the other ingredient along with 3/4 cup of Panko bread crumbs. (Reserve the remaining for coating the patties). Bring together into a mass. Taste and adjust for seasonings. Divide into 8 patties. Coat each patty in the Panko bread crumbs prior to pan frying.
- Drizzle the grill pan with oil and cook until the surface turns a deep brown and the aroma emanates from the patties. Place a slice of mozzarella over the patty and allow it to melt. Warm the burger rolls, slather with your choice of condiments, layer the patties and the onions, lettuce and tomatoes as per your preference. Serve warm with any chutney or aioli of your choice.

3. "Baraka Restaurant" Quinoa & Caramelized Squash And Carrots Salad

Serving: Serves 4 | Prep: | Cook: | Ready in:

Ingredients

- 1 pound quinoa grains (well washed, not soaked)
- 2 quarts water
- 1 pinch salt
- 3 bay leaves
- 1 medium squash, peeled and diced medium size
- 2 large carrots, peeld and diced medium size
- 2 tablespoons butter (or extra virgin olive oil if you want it vegan)
- 4 tablespoons honey
- 1 pinch roasted and ground cumin
- 1 bunch small and tender whole spinach leaves (without stems) - a big bunch -
- 1 bunch fresh cilantro leaves, chopped
- 1 bunch fresh mint leaves, chopped
- 200 milliliters lemon/olive oil vinaigrette (1 part lemon juice; 2 parts olive oil)
- 1 pinch sea salt, for dressing
- 1 pinch freshly ground black pepper, for dressing
- 1/2 pound cherry tomatoes

Direction

- Add the bay leaves to the water, and bring to a boil in a large pot, over high heat.
- Add the quinoa grains and a pinch of salt. Let it boil over high heat and then reduce to medium. Cook until tender, but make sure that you can still see a white dot in the center of each quinoa grain, about 12 minutes.
- Meanwhile, place the carrots and the squash on a baking sheet, making sure you don't mix them. Sprinkle with the butter (or olive oil, if you are making the vegan version), then the cumin, then the honey. Bake for 15 minutes, turn them over, and bake for another 10 or 15, until honey is caramelized. Carrots will remain firm while the squash will be very tender. This is the idea. Keep warm for serving.
- Strain the quinoa in a chinoise, and pour plenty of cold tap water over it, so it doesn't overcook
- SERVING: Mix the quinoa with the herbs, and dress it with the vinaigrette, salt and pepper. Set a nice big bunch of fresh spinach on each plate or salad bowl. Serve 3 or 4 spoonfuls of quinoa on the spinach. Lay some caramelized vegetables on top, and arrange a few nice cherry tomatoes all around.

4. A SHRIMP AND QUINOA PAELLA

Serving: Serves 4-6 people | Prep: | Cook: | Ready in:

Ingredients

- SHRIMP AND QUINOA PAELLA

- 1 pound shrimp, peeled and deveined, thawed if frozen
- 1/2 teaspoon paprika, divided
- 1 lemon, halved
- 4 tablespoons olive oil, divided
- 1/2 medium onion
- 1 clove garlic
- 2 anchovies, packed in oil
- 2 tablespoons tomato paste
- 1 cup quinoa, rinsed
- 2 cups chicken stock, or vegetable stock, or water
- 1/2 bunch chard, greens only, chopped
- 1/8 teaspoon ground saffron or a pinch of saffron threads
- 1/2 cup frozen peas, thawed
- 1/2 cup frozen corn, thawed
- salt
- pepper
- 1 handful parsley, chooped for garnish
- Swiss Chard Stalk Salsa
- 1 tablespoon olive oil
- 1/2 a medium onion
- 1 clove garlic
- 1/2 bunch swiss chard stalks, chopped
- 1 tablespoon lemon, zested and halved
- 1 tablespoon yogurt
- 1 handful parsley, chopped
- salt
- pepper

Direction

- SHRIMP AND QUINOA PAELLA
- In a medium sized bowl season shrimp with salt and pepper, 1/4 teaspoon paprika and the juice of half a lemon. Toss to coat well and set aside for 10-30 minutes if you have time otherwise cook right away.
- Heat 2 tablespoons olive oil in a large pan over medium/high heat. Add shrimp and cook for 2-3 minutes on each side. Do in batches if necessary. Transfer shrimp to a plate and set aside.
- Turn the heat down to medium and add remaining 2 tablespoons of olive oil. Add onion and cook until onion softens. About 6 minutes.
- Add garlic and anchovies. Stir and break down the anchovies. Melting them into the onion and garlic. About 1 minute.
- Add the tomato paste and stir into the onion, garlic, anchovy mix. Cook until fragrant. About 2-4 minutes.
- Add quinoa and stir into the sofrito (the tomato paste mixture). Toast the quinoa for 2 minutes.
- Add the chard, stock or water, remaining 1/4 teaspoon paprika, and saffron. Stir to incorporate and the heat up and bring to a quick boil. Cover and lower heat. Simmer for 10 minutes.
- Remove lid. Stir in the green peas and corn and warm through. About 5 minutes. Season with salt and pepper according to taste. Add the shrimp back to the pan and warm through if necessary. Garnish with parsley and squeeze the other lemon half over the whole thing. Serve with Swiss Chard Stalk Salsa if desirable. Enjoy.
- Swiss Chard Stalk Salsa
- Heat the olive oil in a small pan over medium heat. Add onion with a small pinch of salt cook until onion softens. About 6 minutes. Add Swiss chard stalks, garlic and lemon zest. Saute until stalks soften a little and become fragrant. About 6-8 minutes.
- Remove from heat and allow to cool for a few minutes. Transfer to serving bowl and stir in yogurt, parsley and squeeze in juice from half a lemon. Season with salt and pepper to taste. Add more yogurt or lemon juice as desired. Serve alongside Shrimp And Quinoa Paella.

5. Acorn Squash Stuffed With Quinoa, Golden Raisins, Walnuts & Sage

Serving: Serves 6 | Prep: | Cook: |Ready in:

Ingredients

- 3 Acorn Squash
- 3 tablespoons Olive Oil
- 3 cups Cooked Quinoa
- 2/3 cup Golden Raisins
- 1/3 cup Dried Currants
- 1 1/2 cups Diced Red Onion
- 2 Garlic Cloves, minced
- 1 cup Celery, chopped
- 1/4 cup White Wine
- 2/3 cup Walnuts, toasted and coarsely chopped
- 1 tablespoon Fresh Sage, minced
- 1 teaspoon Grated Orange Zest

Direction

- Preheat oven to 375. Cut squash in half and scoop out seeds. Brush lightly with olive oil and place squash halves flesh side down in baking dish. Bake for 20 minutes. Remove the squash from the oven and turn it cavity side up. While the squash is baking, prepare the filling.
- In a small bowl, combine the golden raisins and currants; cover them with 1/2 cup of hot water and set aside. Heat 2 Tbsp. olive oil in a sauté pan, add the onions and 1/2 tsp salt. Sauté over medium heat until the onions are soft, for about 5 minutes, then add garlic and celery and sauté for 1 minute. Add wine and simmer until the pan is nearly dry.
- Combine cooked quinoa, sautéed onions and celery, drained fruit, walnuts, sage, and orange zest and season with salt and pepper to taste. Divide the filling among the squash halves. Cover and bake for 30-40 minutes.

6. Addictive Quinoa Salad

Serving: Serves 4-6 | Prep: | Cook: | Ready in:

Ingredients

- 1 cup uncooked quinoa
- 1 3/4 cups water
- 1/3 large red bell pepper, 1/4" dice
- 1/3 large yellow red pepper, 1/4" dice
- 2 scallions, finely chopped
- 1/3 cup rinsed and drained black beans (Busch's preferred)
- 1/2 lemon
- 2 tablespoons white balsamic vinegar
- 1 tablespoon extra virgin olive oil
- 1/4 teaspoon ground cumin
- 2 tablespoons finely chopped cilantro
- 1/2 teaspoon kosher salt (or to taste)
- 1/4 teaspoon freshly ground black pepper

Direction

- In a saucepan, bring the quinoa and the water to a boil over medium high heat. When it reaches boiling, cover the saucepan and simmer until the water is absorbed and the quinoa is al dente (about 15 minutes). [Note: I find that when making quinoa to use in a salad, the quinoa will be less "gloppy" if cooked in 1 3/4 cups of water for each cup of uncooked quinoa (vs 2 cups of water as is usually recommended]. Set the cooked quinoa aside to cool to room temperature.
- Add the quinoa to a serving bowl and add the red pepper, yellow pepper, scallions, black beans and red beans, and mix lightly to combine.
- Add to the serving bowl the juice of the 1/2 lemon, the white balsamic vinegar, extra virgin olive oil, cumin, salt, pepper and cilantro. Mix lightly to combine and correct the seasoning.
- Chill the salad and enjoy! Salad will keep, refrigerated and covered, for up to 4 days.

7. African Squash And Peanut Stew With Coconut Milk And Quinoa

Serving: Serves 6 | Prep: | Cook: | Ready in:

Ingredients

- 1 Can Garbanzo Beans, Drained and Rinsed
- 1 Can (14oz) Coconut Milk
- 1 Can (14oz) Fire Roasted Diced Tomatoes
- 1 Large Red Bell Pepper, diced
- 1 Small Yellow Onion, finely diced
- 1 Jalapeno, seeded and diced
- 2 cups Butternut Squash, peeled and diced into small cubes
- 1/2 cup Smooth Peanut Butter
- 1 teaspoon turmeric
- 1 bunch Spinach, washed and shredded
- 2-3 Cloves of Garlic, minced
- 2-3 teaspoons Fresh Ginger, minced
- 1/2 teaspoon Coriander (crushed)
- 1/2 teaspoon Cinnamon
- 1 handful Fresh Cilantro, chopped
- 1 cup Quinoa (dry), cooked according to package
- 1/4 cup Peanuts, roughly chopped

Direction

- In a heavy soup pot (my favorite is enameled cast iron), sauté the onion, red bell pepper and squash over medium heat until slightly golden, about 5-10 minutes. Add the fresh ginger, garlic, jalapeno, turmeric, coriander and cinnamon, sauté for about 1 minute.
- Add the coconut milk, canned tomatoes and about 1 Cup of water (or broth). Bring just to a boil and reduce heat to medium-low, and simmer (covered) just until the squash is tender. To test it, simply stab a piece of squash with a fork, if it seems nice and soft, then it's ready, if it's still firm, it needs to cook a little longer. Better yet, taste a small piece of butternut squash to make sure it's at your preferred consistency. For me, it usually takes about 20 minutes, but it can vary depending on how large the squash pieces are.
- Once the squash is ready, add the garbanzo beans and peanut butter and simmer for a couple minutes. Then add the fresh cilantro and spinach and simmer a couple minutes longer (or until the spinach reaches desired consistency).
- Once it's done, potion it into bowls and top with 1/3 Cup cooked quinoa and 1 Tablespoon of crushed peanuts. YUM!!

8. All Week Long Toasted Almond Quinoa And Arugula Salad

Serving: Serves 4-6 | Prep: 0hours30mins | Cook: 0hours20mins | Ready in:

Ingredients

- 1 cup Quinoa (I prefer red because it's nuttier, but any color will do!)
- 5 ounces arugula or baby arugula, chopped
- 1 cup cherry tomatoes, sliced in half
- 2 large garlice cloves, diced
- 1 shallot, thinly sliced
- 1 hot pepper of your choice, diced (optional kick!)
- 4 ounces crumbled reduced fat feta (skip for vegan version)
- 1/4 cup raw sliced almonds
- 1 tablespoon olive oil
- 1 lime

Direction

- Cook the quinoa based on the instructions until al dente. Drain any extra water and set aside in a large salad bowl.
- Pour olive oil into a skillet over medium heat. Add onions and garlic and toss until crispy, making sure not to burn them. Add hot pepper and sauté for 1-2 minutes. Remove from heat. In same pan, toast almonds for 3 minutes or until light-medium brown.

- In the bowl with the quinoa, add sautéed onions, garlic, and pepper to the quinoa, then add arugula while ingredients are still hot. Toss well. Gently mix in feta, tomatoes, and almond slices. Juice lime into the bowl and mix one last time. (I find the arugula and feta are enough salt and pepper for this recipe! But do add more depending on taste!)

9. Almond, Peach And Quinoa Crumble

Serving: Serves 4 | Prep: | Cook: | Ready in:

Ingredients

- 2 yellow peaches
- 1 cup almond flour
- 1/2 cup quinoa flakes
- 4 tablespoons maple syrup
- 4 tablespoons grapeseed oil

Direction

- Preheat oven to 190°C/375°F and lightly brush with oil either 4 individual ramekins/cups or one medium-sized oven dish
- Wash and cut the peaches into half-inch pieces. Place them into your ramekins or oven dish. Drizzle two tablespoons of maple syrup over the peaches and stir with a knife or spoon
- In a medium bowl, use a whisk or fork to combine the almond meal and quinoa flakes
- Add the grapeseed oil and maple syrup to the bowl. Use a knife to stir the ingredients in a circular motion until the mixture is crumbly. Pour the mixture over the peaches
- Place in the oven and bake for around 30-40 minutes (depending on the size of your oven dishes) until the top has browned and the fruit is bubbling nicely

10. Apple Cinnamon Quinoa Porridge

Serving: Serves 1 | Prep: | Cook: | Ready in:

Ingredients

- 1/4 cup uncooked quinoa
- 1 apple, thinly sliced on a mandolin, some reserved for garnish
- 2 tablespoons chia seeds
- 1 cup almond milk, or your milk of choice
- 1 tablespoon cinnamon
- 1/4 teaspoon nutmeg
- Topping like a dopplop of nut butter, toasted pepitas, chia seeds, shaved apples, greek yogurt, agave, honey, or molasses drizzle.

Direction

- Add the sliced apple to a sauce pan over medium-high heat. Allow to cook and draw sugar out, about 2-3 minutes until apples become fairly translucent. Splash with a bit of water to deglaze the pan and further draw sugar out of the fruit. Add cinnamon, nutmeg, quinoa, chia seeds, walnuts and almond milk. Cover and cook quinoa until done while stirring occasionally. About 12-15 minutes.
- Serve with desired toppings and enjoy.

11. Apple And Red Quinoa Salad

Serving: Serves 2 as a main dish | Prep: | Cook: | Ready in:

Ingredients

- 1 tablespoon Red Wine or Champagne vinegar
- 1 tablespoon Flax Oil (grapeseed or olive will sub fine)
- 1 tablespoon Orange Juice
- 2 handfuls Baby Spinach, chopped
- 2 Fuji (or favorite) apples, chopped

- 1/2 cup pickled or roasted beets, chopped
- 2   scallions, sliced thin
- 1 cup toasted pecans, chopped
- 2 tablespoons crumbled stilton cheese with cranberries
- 2/3 cup Cooked Red Quinoa

Direction

- Whisk together the vinegar, oil and orange juice in the bottom of a salad bowl.
- Add chopped spinach, apples, beets, scallions, pecans and cheese and toss well.
- Add warm quinoa and toss together well.
- Serve and eat!

12. Apple Cinnamon Breakfast Quinoa

Serving: Serves 4 | Prep: | Cook: | Ready in:

Ingredients

- 1 cup uncooked quinoa
- 1 1/2 cups apple cider
- 1/4 teaspoon salt
- 1/2 teaspoon cinnamon
- 1/4 teaspoon allpsice
- 1   medium apple (I used Fuji)
- 1/2 cup dried fruit/nut mixture

Direction

- Quinoa should be rinsed before cooking. A mesh wire sieve would be best because quinoa is pretty small. If you don't have a mesh sieve, you can kind of slosh it carefully around in a bowl. You want to run water over the quinoa in the sieve for a good 1-2 minutes.
- Add the washed quinoa, apple cider, salt, cinnamon, and allpsice to a medium pot.
- Bring to a boil. Allow to simmer for 15 minutes.
- Remove from heat, cover, and let stand for 10 minutes.
- While waiting, chop your apple and measure out your nut/dried fruit mixture.
- Fluff the quinoa with a fork and add the chopped apple and nut/dried fruit mixture. Stir to combine and serve.
- Optional: add a touch of vanilla almond milk on top.

13. Asian Style Red Quinoa Salad With Tofu

Serving: Serves 5 | Prep: | Cook: | Ready in:

Ingredients

- 2 tablespoons sesame oil
- 3 tablespoons coconut oil
- 3 tablespoons tamari
- 2 tablespoons raw honey
- 2 tablespoons white wine vinegar
- 2   red chilies, chopped
- 2 teaspoons fresh ginger, grated
- 1   garlic clove, minced
- 1.5 cups red quinoa, cooked according to package
- 1 cup snow peas, trimmed and thinly sliced
- 6 ounces firm tofu, cut into 1 inch dice
- 4   green onions, trimmed and thinly sliced
- 2 tablespoons sesame seeds, toasted

Direction

- Preheat oven to 425oF.
- In a bowl combine coconut oil, sesame oil, tamari, vinegar, honey, chilies, ginger and garlic. Adjust to taste with extra tamari if need be. Divide the sauce in half.
- Toss the tofu with half the sauce, place in a single layer on a baking sheet. Bake, stirring occasionally, until golden, about 15-20 minutes. Allow to cool slightly on baking sheet.
- Meanwhile, cook quinoa, according to direction. And then toss in a large bowl with the remaining sauce; set aside.

- Toss tofu into quinoa, along with snow peas and half the amount of green onions. Divide into bowls and garnish with toasted sesame seeds and the remaining green onions.

14. Asparagus, Avocado, And Caramelized Onion Quinoa

Serving: Serves 3-4 | Prep: | Cook: | Ready in:

Ingredients

- 3 tablespoons extra virgin olive oil or melted organic clarified butter
- 1 large white onion – peeled and cut into ¼ inch slices
- Unrefined sea salt
- 1 teaspoon sherry or raw apple cider vinegar
- 1 cup organic quinoa
- 2 cups filtered or spring water
- 1 bay leaf
- 10 stalks thin asparagus – bottom portion of stalk removed
- Fresh ground black pepper to taste
- 1 medium avocado
- 1 tablespoon fresh lime juice
- 6 baby tomatoes – diced
- 1/2 cup watercress
- 3 red globe radishes – thinly sliced and julienned

Direction

- Heat 1 tablespoon of olive oil or clarified butter over medium heat. Add sliced onions and sprinkle with ½ teaspoon of sea salt and vinegar. Cook onions over medium heat for 20-30 minutes until golden brown in color, stirring occasionally so they don't stick or burn. While the onions are cooking make the quinoa. Once the onions are done cooking, remove from heat, cover and keep warm until the quinoa is done cooking.
- Rinse and drain quinoa. Heat 1 tablespoon of olive oil or clarified butter over medium heat in a medium saucepan with lid until hot but not smoking. Add drained quinoa, sprinkle with 1 teaspoon of sea salt, and cook over medium heat for 2-3 minutes until lightly toasted.
- Add 2 cups of filtered water to the quinoa and the bay leaf. Bring quinoa to a boil over medium-high heat, reduce heat, cover and cook quinoa for around 15 minutes or until liquid is absorbed and quinoa is tender. Remove from heat, stir in caramelized onions, cover, and set aside while you cook the asparagus.
- Toss cleaned asparagus with 1 tablespoon of olive oil or melted clarified butter. Sprinkle asparagus with sea salt and fresh ground black pepper. Place a grill pan over high heat and get the pan hot but not smoking. Add asparagus in a single layer turn down heat to medium-high and cook asparagus on one side for 2-3 minutes until golden brown. Turn asparagus over and continue cooking for an additional 2-3 minutes until brown and tender. Remove cooked asparagus from heat and cool slightly.
- Cut asparagus into bite size pieces and add to quinoa. Remove skin and seed from avocado and cut avocado into small cubes. Toss with lime juice and immediately stir into quinoa. Stir diced tomatoes, watercress leaves, and radishes into quinoa, stir together and taste. Add additional sea salt, black pepper, and lime juice to taste if needed. Serve immediately.

15. Autumn Harvest Quinoa Muffins

Serving: Makes 12 muffins | Prep: | Cook: | Ready in:

Ingredients

- 1 1/2 cups All Purpose Flour
- 1 cup Whole Wheat Flour
- 1 teaspoon Baking Soda

- 1 teaspoon Baking Powder
- 1/2 teaspoon Salt
- 1 teaspoon Cinnamon
- 1/2 cup Dark Brown Sugar
- 1 1/2 cups Buttermilk
- 1 Egg
- 1/4 cup Unsalted Butter, melted and browned
- 1 teaspoon Vanilla Extract
- 1 cup Cooked Quinoa
- 1 cup Grated Apple (1 medium apple)
- 1/2 cup Grated Butternut Squash
- 1/2 cup Golden Raisins
- 1/2 cup Pecans, chopped

Direction

- Preheat oven to 375°. Butter or spray a 12 cup muffin tin.
- Combine flours, baking soda, baking powder, salt, brown sugar, and cinnamon in large bowl. Mix well.
- In medium bowl, whisk together egg, buttermilk, browned butter, and vanilla.
- In another medium bowl, combine quinoa, apple, squash, raisins, and pecans.
- Add wet ingredients to dry and mix until just combined.
- Fold quinoa mixture into muffin batter and scoop into prepared muffin cups.
- Bake until golden and tester comes out clean, about 30 minutes.

16. Autumnal Quinoa Salad

Serving: Makes 4 small servings; 2 main dish servings | Prep: | Cook: |Ready in:

Ingredients

- For the Salad
- 1 cup quinoa (color of your choice!)
- 1 acorn squash, cut into 1 inch slices
- 2 northern spy apples, diced
- 1 cup Arugula
- 1 small bunch of chard, about 5 leaves
- 2 tablespoons Olive Oil
- 1/4 teaspoon Cardamom
- 1/2   teaspoon vietnamese cinnamon
- 1/4 teaspoon cayenne pepper
- salt and pepper to taste
- 1/4 cup Toasted Pecans
- 1/4 cup Toasted Pepitas
- Simple Honey Dijon Vinaigrette
- 1 tablespoon honey
- 1 teaspoon dijon mustard
- juice of one lemon
- 2 tablespoons Olive Oil
- Salt and Pepper to taste

Direction

- First, roast the squash. Preheat the oven to 375. Use 1 tablespoon of olive oil to oil the pan- make sure it is evenly coated or the squash will stick. Sprinkle squash with remaining 1 tablespoon of olive oil. Combine the cinnamon, cardamom, cayenne, salt and pepper. Sprinkle the spice mixture on top of the squash. Use your hands to make sure the squash is even coated with oil and spices. Roast in the oven for 15 minutes. Meanwhile, cook your quinoa according to the package instructions.
- At the fifteen minute mark, add the apple pieces. Roast for another 10 minutes. Using a fork, test the acorn squash for doneness. It should be tender, but not mushy.
- While the roasted squash and apples are cooling, strip the leaves from the stalks of chard. Cut the leaves into ribbons. Save the stalks for another use.
- Assemble the vinaigrette. Combine all ingredients in a mason jar or other container with a tight fitting lid. Shake vigorously until ingredients form an emulsion.
- Remove the skin from the squash. Dice the squash into bite size pieces. Combine the squash, apples, warm quinoa, arugula and chard into a bowl. The warm quinoa will gently wilt the arugula and chard, so that they are tender but not overcooked. Add the

vinaigrette and combine well. Top with the toasted pepitas and pecans before serving.

17. Avocado & Kale Quinoa Salad

Serving: Serves 4 | Prep: | Cook: |Ready in:

Ingredients

- Quinoa
- 1 cup quinoa
- 2 cups vegetable broth
- 2 cups chopped kale
- 1 cup frozen shelled edamame
- Creamy Avocado Dressing
- 1 ripe avocado
- 2 tablespoons fresh lemon juice
- 2 tablespoons mayonnaise
- 1 tablespoon white wine vinegar
- 1 small garlic clove, minced
- 1/4 cup chopped fresh parsley
- 2 tablespoons chopped fresh basil
- 1/2 teaspoon ground cumin
- 1/2 teaspoon kosher salt
- 1/4 teaspoon freshly ground black pepper
- 1/4 cup olive oil
- 1 ripe avocado, slice to garnish

Direction

- Combine quinoa and vegetable broth in a medium saucepan. Bring to a boil over high heat. Reduce heat to low, cover and simmer for 15 minutes, until all liquid is absorbed. Place quinoa in a large bowl and set aside.
- Fill a large pot with about an inch of water. Place a steamer on the bottom of the pot and add the kale and edamame. Cover and steam over high heat for 2-3 minutes, until kale turns bright green and edamame is defrosted. Plunge greens into a bowl of cold water to prevent further cooking. Drain well and set aside.
- For the avocado dressing, using a food processor or blender, combine avocado, lemon juice, mayonnaise, white wine vinegar, garlic, parsley, basil, cumin, salt and pepper. Pulse 2 to 3 times, until well combined. Add olive oil gradually and blend well.
- Add kale and edamame to the quinoa and toss with avocado dressing. Garnish with sliced avocado.

18. BBQ Quinoa Burgers

Serving: Serves 6 | Prep: | Cook: |Ready in:

Ingredients

- 2 cups cooked quinoa
- 1 cup shredded carrots
- 1/4 red onion, finely chopped
- 1/2 cup parsley leaves, chopped
- 1/4 cup spelt flour
- 2 eggs
- 2 tablespoons BBQ Sauce
- salt & pepper

Direction

- Preheat oven to 450 and line a baking sheet with parchment paper
- In a large mixing bowl combine quinoa, carrot, onions, parsley, flour, BBQ sauce, eggs, and good pinch of salt and pepper.
- Form into mixture into balls, and then flatten out into patty shape on the baking sheet (mixture will be quite loose, but will firm up)
- Bake for 6 minutes, flip and continue baking for another 7 minutes.
- Serve with your favorite burger toppings… like avocado and tomato

19. Baked Broccoli And Carrot Quinoa Patties

Serving: Makes 18 patties | Prep: | Cook: |Ready in:

Ingredients

- 1 Head of Broccoli with Florets Torn off the Stem
- 3 Carrots Finely Chopped
- 1 Small Sweet Onion (or two shallots) Diced
- 1 Sweet Onion Finely Chopped
- 1 Clove of Garlic Finely Chopped
- 1 handful Fresh Basil Finely Chopped
- 1 cup Cooked Quinoa
- 2 Eggs
- 1/2 cup Grated Cheese (I used Cheddar, but any will do)
- 1 teaspoon Baking Powder
- 3 tablespoons Panko Crumbs (or any bread crumbs)
- 1 splash Balsamic Vinegar
- 2 tablespoons Chickpea Flour (All purpose flour is also fine) - Optional if you want a drier patty
- Salt and Pepper to Taste
- Cayenne Pepper (I would have added some if I wasn't sharing with with a toddler)

Direction

- Steam broccoli and carrots until tender. I steamed mine for about 15 minutes, but you can do it a little more or less to taste.
- Once the veggies are steaming, pre-heat your oven to 400, chop your onions, garlic and basil, and grate your cheese.
- After your broccoli and carrots are steamed, move them to a large mixing bowl and mash with a potato masher. If you want a chunkier texture, you can chop the vegetables instead.
- Add the rest of your ingredients and stir.
- Scoop out your mixture onto two large baking sheets. I used a standard soup spoon to portion out my patties. You can use a Silpat of parchment paper to line your baking sheets, but if you don't, you'll want to grease your baking sheets.
- Bake for 20 minutes, or until the bottoms of the patties begin to brown. Flip over and bake for an additional 10 minutes.
- They are ready to eat! Now, if you'll excuse me, I'm going to make some tzatziki to dip my patties in!

20. Baked Quinoa Pudding With Persimmon And Pistachios

Serving: Serves a crowd | Prep: | Cook: |Ready in:

Ingredients

- • 1 cup organic quinoa
- • 4 extra-large eggs, separated
- • 1 1/2 cups Thai organic coconut milk +1 cup whole milk
- • 2-3 medium-size ripe Hachiya persimmons
- • 1/3 cup organic Maple syrup or honey
- • 1/4 cup organic cane sugar
- • 1/2 teaspoon cinnamon
- • 1/4 teaspoon cardamom
- • 2 teaspoons freshly grated orange or lemon zest
- • 1/3 cup dry roasted pistachios, finely chopped

Direction

- Rinse and drain quinoa thoroughly in cold water; place quinoa, a large pinch of coarse salt and 2 cups water in a 2 quart saucepan and bring to boil. Reduce to the lowest heat possible, cover and simmer until the grains are very tender and translucent, for 15 to 20 minutes.
- While quinoa is still hot, whisk in milks, maple syrup, cinnamon, cardamom, orange zest and egg yolks. Pour the mixture into a large bowl.
- Make a deep cut in the pointed end of each persimmon. Scoop out pulp into bowl of mini food processor and puree until smooth. You should have about 1 cup of the puree. Stir in into the quinoa mixture until fully incorporated.

- Preheat oven to 325 degrees F. Butter a 13by9by2"glass baking dish and sprinkle bottom and sides with 2/3 of the pistachios.
- Put egg whites in the bowl of an electric mixer fitted with the whisk attachment. Beat on medium-high speed until soft peaks form. Gradually add 1/4 sugar, beating until stiff, glossy peaks form. (Do not overbeat.) Whisk one-third of the egg white mixture into the quinoa mixture. Using a rubber spatula, gently fold in remaining egg white mixture.
- Place baking dish in a large pan; pour hot water into the pan to a depth of 1 1/2". Bake for about 1 hour, or until puffed like a soufflé, lightly browned and set. Serve pudding warm or at room temperature with a dollop of whipped cream and a sprinkle of the remaining pistachios. Can be made 2 days ahead. Cover and chill. Bring to room temperature before serving.

21. Baked Quinoa With Roasted Butternut Squash & Gruyère

Serving: Serves 6 | Prep: | Cook: | Ready in:

Ingredients

- 1 cup quinoa (I like red for visual appeal)
- 3 1/2 teaspoons kosher salt, plus more to taste
- 6 tablespoons extra-virgin olive oil, divided plus more for greasing
- 4 cups 1/2-inch cubes butternut squash (about), 1.25 lbs. post peeling
- 2 cups diced red onion
- 2 tablespoons finely minced herbs, any combination of thyme, sage, and rosemary
- 1 cup milk, any milk fat you like (I use whole)
- 4 ounces grated Gruyère cheese (about 1 1/4 cups)
- 1 1/2 cups fresh breadcrumbs (about 1 1/2 English muffins pulsed in the food processor)

Direction

- Preheat the oven to 400°F. In a medium saucepan, combine the quinoa, 2 cups of water, and 1 teaspoon kosher salt. Bring to a boil over high heat. Reduce heat to low, cover, and let cook for 15 minutes. Remove pan from heat.
- Meanwhile, grease a rimmed sheet pan lightly with olive oil. Place cubed squash and diced onion on pan. Drizzle with 3 tablespoons olive oil, sprinkle with 1 to 2 teaspoons kosher salt (depending on your tolerance — if you are sensitive, use 1 teaspoon), and toss to coat. Spread vegetables out into an even layer. Transfer to the oven and roast for 25 to 30 minutes or until squash and onions are just beginning to brown. Remove pan from oven. Increase oven temp to 425°F.
- Uncover quinoa pan and fluff with a fork. Add 1 tablespoon of the herbs, the milk, and half of the cheese, and mix with a spatula to combine. Transfer to a large bowl. Add the roasted squash and onions and fold gently to combine. Transfer mixture to a lightly greased 9x13-inch baking dish. Cover evenly with the remaining cheese.
- In a small bowl, combine the breadcrumbs, the remaining 3 tablespoons of olive oil, the remaining herbs, and the remaining 1/2 teaspoon salt. Toss with your fingers until the breadcrumbs are fully saturated and seasoned. Spread this evenly atop the cheese. At this point, the pan can be stashed in the fridge for as long as a day (maybe longer) and baked when needed. Bake for 20 to 25 minutes or until evenly golden. Let cool briefly before serving.

22. Baked Quinoa Pork Meatballs

Serving: Makes 26 (2 tablespoon–sized) meatballs | Prep: 0hours30mins | Cook: 0hours30mins | Ready in:

Ingredients

- 1/2 cup quinoa, well-rinsed

- 1 pound ground pork
- 1/2 cup minced or grated yellow onion
- 1/2 cup finely grated pecorino
- 1/3 cup finely chopped parsley
- 2 large eggs
- 2 garlic cloves, minced
- 1 tablespoon fennel seeds, preferably toasted
- 1 teaspoon kosher salt
- 1/2 teaspoon dried oregano
- 1/4 teaspoon red pepper flakes

Direction

- Combine the quinoa and 1 cup water in a small saucepan. Bring to a boil, then immediately reduce to a simmer and cover. Cook for 15 or so minutes until the water has absorbed and the quinoa is tender. When it's done, dump onto a plate and spread out to cool completely. (You can stick it in the fridge or freezer if you're in a rush.)
- When the quinoa is no longer warm, combine that and the rest of the ingredients in a big bowl. You can use your hands or a spoon to combine. Just make sure you don't overwork the mixture, lest you'll end up with tough meatballs.
- Heat the oven to 400° F. Line a sheet pan with parchment or a silicone mat.
- Form the pork mixture into 2-tablespoon sized balls. Line up on the sheet pan. If they seem crowded (which will cause steaming versus browning), divide between two lined sheet pans.
- Bake for about 15 minutes until browned and cooked through.

23. Baked Turkey Quinoa Spinach Meatballs.

Serving: Serves 6 | Prep: | Cook: | Ready in:

Ingredients

- 1 2 lbs of ground turkey (I used lean 93%)
- 1 cup cooked quinoa (any color will do)
- 1 medium yellow onion, diced very small
- 6 6 garlic cloves, minced
- 1 cup fresh chopped spinach leaves (I used baby spinach leaves)
- 2 tablespoons low sodium soy sauce, Sriracha sauce or other hot sauce that you love or Worcheshire sauce
- 1 tablespoon dried Italian Seasoning/spices
- 1 teaspoon dried oregano
- 1 tablespoon ground flaxseed
- Salt and pepper
- 1 1 egg, beaten

Direction

- Preheat your oven to 350 and spray your baking pan with sides with baking spray. Set aside.
- In your stand mixer with the paddle attached, add all of the ingredients and mix until incorporated.
- Then form meatballs, rolling in between your hands and then lay out on your baking sheet.
- Repeat until you use all of the meat mixture.
- Bake for 35 minutes or a little more – until golden brown.
- Rotate them half way through the baking time.
- Bake until fully cooked throughout.

24. Balsamic Mushroom Quinoa

Serving: Serves 2-4 | Prep: | Cook: | Ready in:

Ingredients

- 1/2 cup raw quinoa, well rinsed and drained
- 1 cup water
- 1 tablespoon olive oil
- 3 cups mushrooms, roughly diced
- 3/4 teaspoon salt, divided
- 1 dash pepper
- 2 teaspoons garlic, minced (about 2 cloves)
- 1 shallot, chopped
- 4 tablespoons balsamic vinegar

- 1/2 cup dried figs
- 3 tablespoons pinenuts, toasted

Direction

- Place the water, quinoa and 1/4 tsp of the salt together in a pot and bring to a boil. Reduce heat to a simmer, cover, and cook until all the water is absorbed, about 20 minutes.
- While the quinoa is cooking, add olive oil and mushrooms to a sauté pan on medium high heat. Add 1/4 tsp of the salt and pepper to the mushrooms and sauté until they are brown and caramelized, about 10 minutes. Add shallots and garlic and cook for another 5 minute.
- Turn off the heat on the sauté pan. Add the figs to the sauté pan and then add in the balsamic vinegar. Stir the mushroom fig mixture and let the residual heat from the pan reduce the balsamic vinegar. (Be careful not to inhale the vinegar while it is evaporating) Add the remaining 1/4 tsp salt to the mixture and stir to combine.
- Combine the mushroom mixture and the quinoa. Add toasted pine nuts and stir to combine all the ingredients.

25. Banana Bread Granola With Quinoa And Cocoa Nibs

Serving: Makes 4 cups | Prep: | Cook: | Ready in:

Ingredients

- 3 cups rolled oats
- 1/2 cup quinoa
- 1/4 cup flax seed
- 1 teaspoon cinnamon
- 1/4 teaspoon salt
- 1/2 cup chopped peacans
- 1.5 medium bananas (ripe, but not too ripe)
- 2 tablespoons coconut oil
- 3 tablespoons raw honey
- 1/2 teaspoon coconut extract, optional
- 1/4 cup cocoa nibs, or more if you like

Direction

- Preheat oven to 300°F (150°C). Line a rimmed baking sheet with parchment paper and set aside.
- Combine all dry ingredients (oats through pecans) in a medium bowl.
- Blend, or mash really well, the remaining wet ingredients (banana through coconut extract). Add it to the dry ingredients and mix until coated.
- Spread the mixture evenly over the baking sheet and cook in the oven for 45 minutes, stirring every 10 -15 minutes. At the point the mixture should still have a bit of moisture to it. Turn the oven down to 250°F and bake for another 20-30 minutes, or until the granola is dried out to your liking. Remove from the oven and mix in the cocoa nibs.

26. Beet Salad With Apple, Quinoa, Kale And Walnuts

Serving: Serves 4-6 | Prep: | Cook: | Ready in:

Ingredients

- Roasted Beet and Apple Salad
- 3 large red beets, peeled and diced
- 2 large Granny Smith Apples, peeled and diced
- 2 cups sliced kale (stems removed and discarded)
- 1 tablespoon freshly squeezed lemon juice
- 1 tablespoon extra-virgin olive oil
- 3/4 cup cooked quinoa
- 1/2 cup raw or toasted walnuts
- 1/2 cup goat cheese, crumbled
- Walnut Vinaigrette
- 1/4 cup sherry vinegar
- 1 teaspoon Dijon Mustard
- 1/2 cup extra-virgin olive oil
- 1/4 cup walnut oil

- 1/2 teaspoon clover honey
- Pinch kosher salt and freshly ground black pepper to taste

Direction

- Roasted Beet and Apple Salad
- Preheat the oven to 350. Place the diced beets on a sheet of aluminum foil and drizzle with the olive oil. Fold the foil so the beets are sealed and place on a large cookie sheet. Roast in the oven for 15-20 minutes or until a fork pierces easily into the beets. You want them soft but still a little firm. Remove the beets from the oven and set aside to cool. Add the kale, lemon juice and a drizzle of olive oil. Massage until the kale starts to soften and wilt, 2 to 3 minutes. Add the apple, beets. Drizzle some walnut vinaigrette over ingredients and toss. Add the quinoa and walnuts and gently toss again. Garnish with goat cheese.
- Walnut Vinaigrette
- Combine the vinegar, honey and mustard in a bowl. While whisking, slowly pour a steady stream of the olive oil and walnut oil. Season with salt and pepper.

27. Better Than Central Market's Chipotle Quinoa

Serving: Makes 6 healthy side dishes | Prep: | Cook: | Ready in:

Ingredients

- 1 tablespoon Olive Oil
- 1 Red onion, chopped
- 2-3 Cloves of garlic
- 2 Canned chipotle peppers, diced
- 1 tablespoon Fresh oregano or 1 tsp dried
- 1 cup Red quinoa
- Salt and pepper to taste
- 1 15 oz. can black beans, rinsed and drained or 2 cups prepared black beans
- 2 Ears fresh corn with corn cut from the cob or 1 cup frozen
- 2 cups Vegetable or chicken broth
- 1 cup Scallions, chopped, white and green parts
- 1 cup Cherry tomatoes, halved and seeded
- 2-3 tablespoons Cilantro, chopped
- 1 Avocado, diced
- 1 tablespoon Freshly squeezed lime juice

Direction

- Add olive oil to large skillet and place over medium heat. Add onion and garlic. Cook, stirring until the onions are soft, about 5 minutes. Add chipotles and oregano and continue to stir for another minute.
- Turn up the heat to medium high, add the quinoa and sprinkle with salt and pepper. Continue to cook, stirring frequently for about 3-5 minutes.
- Add broth and bring to a boil. Stir, cover and reduce heat to low. Cook undisturbed for approximately 15 minutes.
- Uncover and test quinoa. If the kernels are still crunchy, add a bit more liquid and cook for another 5 minutes or so. When the grain is fully cooked, it will look like it has sprouted.
- Mix in corn and black beans. Top with cilantro, tomatoes, avocados, and scallions. Squeeze lime juice over all and mix lightly. Great served warm or cold.
- Highly recommend doubling this! Quick lunch or dinner for a few days or just share. My favorite way to eat this is in some garlic naan bread but it's wonderful in tortillas too! Just saying, adding the carbs makes it even yummier but it definitely stands on its own!

28. Black Bean And Quinoa Enchiladas

Serving: Serves 4 | Prep: | Cook: | Ready in:

Ingredients

- Sauce Ingredients
- 2 tablespoons neutral-flavored oil
- 2 tablespoons flour (I used oat flour, but others would work)
- 2 tablespoons chili powder
- 2 cups water
- 1/4 cup tomato paste
- 1/2 teaspoon cumin
- 1/2 teaspoon garlic powder
- 1/2 teaspoon red pepper flakes (or to taste)
- 1 teaspoon salt
- Enchilada Ingredients
- 6-7 small corn tortillas
- 2 cups cooked black beans
- 1 avocado, diced
- 1/4 cup diced red onion
- 2/3 cup cooked quinoa
- 1 medium carrot, finely shredded
- 1/4 cup chopped cilantro
- 2 tablespoons lime juice
- 1/4 cup chopped red onion (optional)
- 2 garlic cloves, crushed or put through a press
- 1/2 teaspoon salt (heaping)

Direction

- (Preheat the oven to 350F.) In a small saucepan over medium heat, combine the flour, oil, and chili powder. Whisk together and let it bubble for a minute or 2.
- Whisk in the water, and add the rest of the sauce ingredients. Let the mixture come to a gentle simmer (it will thicken at this point) and then turn off the heat.
- In a mixing bowl, combine all filling ingredients (except the tortillas) and mix well. Adjust the seasoning to taste.
- Fill each tortilla with filling, fold the tortilla, and place it seam side down in a greased casserole dish. Once all the filling has been used up, pour the sauce over the enchiladas.
- Bake until the sauce is bubbly and browned around the edges, around 30 minutes. Top with any toppings you like.

29. Black Bean And Quinoa Veggie Burgers

Serving: Makes 6-8 burgers | Prep: 12hours15mins | Cook: 0hours50mins | Ready in:

Ingredients

- Patties
- 1/2 cup quinoa
- 1 teaspoon olive oil
- 1 small red onion, chopped
- 3 cloves garlic, minced
- 1 pinch Kosher salt
- 2 cans (15.5 ounces each) black beans, rinsed and drained
- 2 tablespoons tomato paste
- 1 large egg
- 2/3 cup cooked corn (fresh or canned)
- 1/4 cup chopped cilantro
- 1 tablespoon minced chipotles in adobo
- 1 1/2 teaspoons ground cumin
- 1 cup rolled oats, ground into crumbs
- Yogurt Sauce
- 1/2 cup fat-free Greek yogurt
- 1 teaspoon minced chipotles in adobo
- 1/2 teaspoon adobo sauce
- 1 teaspoon honey
- 1/2 teaspoon dijon mustard
- 6 multigrain hamburger rolls
- 1 handful Lettuce, avocado slices, and tomatoes, for topping (optional)

Direction

- Place the quinoa in a small saucepan along with 1 cup of water. Bring the water to a boil then reduce heat to medium low and cover the pan. Cook 10 to 15 minutes until the water is absorbed and quinoa is cooked. Remove from heat.
- Heat the oil in a small sauté pan over medium heat and add the onion and garlic. Season them with a pinch of salt and sauté until

onions are softened, 5 to 6 minutes. Place the mixture into a large bowl. Add approximately 1 1/2 cans of black beans to the bowl and, using a potato masher or fork, mash all of the ingredients together until a pasty mixture forms. Stir in the remaining beans along with the tomato paste, egg, corn, cilantro, chipotles, cumin, and 1/2 teaspoon salt. Stir in the cooked quinoa and ground oats until evenly distributed.

- Form the mixture into 6 equal patties, compacting them well with your hands as you form them. Place the patties on a baking sheet, cover them with plastic wrap, and refrigerate for at least a few hours or overnight.
- To make the yogurt sauce, stir the yogurt, chipotles, adobo sauce, honey, and mustard together in a small bowl.
- When ready to eat, preheat the oven to 400° F. Spray a baking sheet with nonstick cooking spray and place the patties on the sheet. Cook 10 to 12 minutes, until the patties are golden brown and crispy, then carefully flip them over and cook another 10 minutes. You can also fry the patties in a pan with a small amount of oil. Serve patties on the buns with the yogurt sauce and toppings of your choice.

30. Black Bean, Quinoa And Citrus Salad [v] [veg] [gf]

Serving: Makes 7-8 cups of salad | Prep: | Cook: |Ready in:

Ingredients

- 2 cans (15 oz) black beans
- 1/2 red onion, minced
- 2 grapefruits
- 1 red pepper, chopped
- 1 cup cooked corn
- 1 cup quinoa, uncooked
- 1 large avocado
- 1 bunch cilantro
- 3 limes, juiced
- 2 teaspoons cumin
- .25 teaspoons sea salt

Direction

- Cook 1 cup of quinoa, according to directions
- Rinse the beans, corn and chop the veggies and garnishes.
- Mix the cooked quinoa, lime juice, cumin, and salt. Place as a bottom layer in the pan.
- Layer with onions, peppers, grapefruit, black beans, corn, avocado and cilantro. Refrigerate to cool.
- Serve with pita chips, atop greens or alone!

31. Black Quinoa Salad With Grilled Vegetables, Basil, Feta And Pine Nuts

Serving: Serves 6-8 as a side dish | Prep: | Cook: |Ready in:

Ingredients

- Salad
- 1 large zucchini
- 1 large eggplant
- 1 cup raw black quinoa, cooked to equal approximately 4 cups cooked quinoa, and then cooled
- 1 1/2 cups chopped fresh basil
- approximately 1/2 cup crumbled feta cheese (I like French feta made with sheep's milk)
- 1/4 cup pine nuts, toasted for a minute or so in a hot skillet
- Dressing
- 1/4 cup extra virgin olive oil
- 2 tablespoons fresh lemon juice
- 1 tablespoon balsamic vinegar
- 1 teaspoon garlic, peeled and minced
- 1/2 teaspoon dijon mustard
- 1/2 teaspoon organic sugar or honey

Direction

- Preheat your grill. Sliced the eggplant and zucchini and toss with olive oil, salt and pepper. Place in grill basket over high heat and grill until tender. Remove and allow to cool before chopping into bite-sized pieces.
- Combine the chopped grilled vegetables with the cooked quinoa and the basil in a large bowl. Add most of the crumbled feta cheese. Mix well.
- Whisk the dressing ingredients together in a small bowl and then pour over the salad. Mix well and adjust seasonings, if necessary.
- Garnish with the toasted pine nuts and the rest of the feta. You can sprinkle a little more basil on top too, if desired.

32. Black Quinoa Salad With Kidney Beans

Serving: Serves 6 | Prep: | Cook: | Ready in:

Ingredients

- QUINOA SALAD
- 1 cup black Quinoa
- 1 can kidney beans rinsed and drained
- 1 1/2 tablespoons Red Wine Vinegar
- 1 1/2 cups Raw Corn cut off of cob
- 3/4 cup Zucchini
- 3/4 cup Cucumbers
- 3/4 cup Tomato
- 3/4 cup Pea Pods or frozen Pea's
- 3/4 cup Torn Spinach Leaves
- 1 or 2 Avocado
- 1/2 cup Asparagus
- 1/4 cup Chopped Parsley
- 1/2 cup Grated Carrot
- 1/2 teaspoon salt
- Cumin Lime Dressing
- 5 tablespoons Fresh squeezed Lime Juice
- 1 teaspoon Salt
- 2 teaspoons Cumin
- 1/3 cup Olive Oil
- 1 or 2 Shakes of Hot Sauce

Direction

- QUINOA SALAD
- Rinse Quinoa well, add 1 1/2 cup of cold water and 1/2 teaspoon salt cook on medium heat for 15 minutes, covered, set aside to allow all the water to get absorbed and to cool, add red wine vinegar.
- Cut vegetables to bite size pieces and add to Quinoa.
- Drain and rinse kidney beans or use fresh cooked and add to Quinoa.
- Prepare Dressing
- Cumin Lime Dressing
- Mix dressing ingredients and add to Quinoa salad. Mix well serve room temperature or cold.

33. Blueberry White Chocolate Granola With A Quinoa Crunch!

Serving: Makes about 8 cups | Prep: | Cook: | Ready in:

Ingredients

- 1/2 cup honey
- 1/3 cup canola oil
- 1 teaspoon cinnamon
- 1 teaspoon cardamom
- 1 pinch salt
- 4 cups oats
- 1/2 cup slivered almonds
- 1/4 cup flaxseed
- 1/2 cup pepitos
- 1/2 cup quinoa
- 1 cup dried blueberries
- 1 cup white chocolate chips

Direction

- Preheat oven to 325°F.

- In a small bowl whisk honey and canola oil until smooth. You'll need a bit of muscle for this! Add cinnamon, cardamom and salt and blend well.
- In a large bowl, mix oats, almonds, flaxseed, pepitos and quinoa.
- Stir in honey oil mixture until granola is well coated.
- Spread oats on parchment lined cookie sheet and bake for 20 minutes, stirring once halfway through.
- Let granola cool and break apart into a clean large bowl.
- Stir in white chocolate and dried blueberries (make sure your granola is COMPLETELY cooked or the chocolate will melt all over).
- Store in an air tight container.

34. Braised Collard Rolls With Lamb And Quinoa

Serving: Makes 12 large rolls | Prep: | Cook: | Ready in:

Ingredients

- 12 large unbroken collard leaves, washed
- 3/4 cup quinoa, thoroughly rinsed
- 3 tablespoons olive oil, divided
- 1 teaspoon whole cumin seeds
- 1/2 teaspoon whole fennel seeds
- 1/2 teaspoon ground cinnamon
- 1/2 teaspoon ground coriander
- 1/4 teaspoon crushed red chili flakes, or to taste
- 1 large yellow onion, half finely diced, half sliced
- 4 large garlic cloves, minced
- 1 pound ground lamb
- 1/4 cup chopped fresh mint
- 1 large egg
- 1 cup tomato sauce
- 1 quart chicken stock, or as needed
- Salt and freshly ground black pepper to taste

Direction

- Cut the thick center ribs and stems away from the collard leaves. Set the leaves aside.
- In a large heavy skillet, heat 2 tbsp. olive oil over medium heat. Add quinoa and toast, stirring frequently, for 8-10 minutes, or until the grains have turned golden and smell nutty. Add cumin, fennel, cinnamon, coriander, and chili flakes, and cook for another 2-3 minutes, or until spices have toasted and the mixture is incredibly fragrant. Add remaining 1 tbsp. oil, diced onion, and a pinch of salt, and cook, stirring frequently, for 5-6 minutes, or until the onion is translucent. Add garlic and cook for 1 minute, or until fragrant. Remove the mixture from the heat and set aside to cool slightly.
- While the quinoa mixture cooks and cools, bring a large pot of water to a boil. Salt the water generously, then add collard leaves and blanch for 2 minutes. Drain the collard leaves and run them under cold water to stop the cooking. Set aside.
- In a large mixing bowl, combine ground lamb, mint, egg, and the cooked quinoa mixture. Season with salt and pepper, and mix until thoroughly combined. Divide the mixture into 12 portions, and shape each portion into a short, squat log. Set aside.
- Preheat the oven to 350º F. Lay a collard leaf out on a work surface, slightly overlapping the cut sides where you took out the stem. Place one portion of the filling mixture towards the end of the leaf closest to you, and fold that end over the filling. Fold in the sides and roll up the leaf over the filling, as if you were making a burrito. (Don't roll too tightly, or the rolls may swell and burst in the pot.) Repeat with the remaining leaves and filling.
- In a large Dutch oven or other heavy oven-safe pot, lay about half the sliced onion on the bottom in a single layer. Place the collard rolls in the pot on top of the onions, seam side down, in an even layer. (You may have to stack some of the rolls on top of each other; if you do, lay down a few onion slices between the layers.) . Season with salt and pepper. Top

with the remaining sliced onion. Add tomato sauce and enough chicken stock to come most of the way up the sides of the rolls. Cover and bake for 1 hour 15 minutes, or until the rolls are fork-tender and the filling is fully cooked.
- Remove the pot from the oven and let sit, covered, for 30 minutes. Serve the rolls with some of the braising liquid spooned over the top.
- The collard rolls will keep in the fridge, tightly covered, for up to 3 days. For freezer storage, lay cooked and cooled collard rolls on a foil-lined baking sheet and freeze until solid, then transfer to a zip-top bag; save the braising liquid and freeze it separately. The rolls will keep in the freezer for up to 3 months; reheat them with some of the braising liquid.

35. Breakfast Quinoa

Serving: Makes 3-4 servings | Prep: | Cook: |Ready in:

Ingredients

- 1 cup uncooked quinoa
- 1 3/4 cups water
- 1/2 cup unsweetened vanilla almond milk
- 1/2 cup fresh berries (blueberry, raspberry, strawberry, etc.)
- 1/4 cup dried cranberries
- 2 tablespoons honey
- 1/4 cup slivered almonds
- 1/4 teaspoon cinnamon
- sprinkling of ground chia seeds
- 1/2 teaspoon salt
- 2 tablespoons creamy peanut butter (optional)

Direction

- This one is super simple! Start by mixing the quinoa, water and a pinch of salt in a medium sauce pan. Bring to a boil. Reduce to a simmer, cover and let cook until all of the water is absorbed, about 15 minutes.
- Add the rest of the ingredients straight to the pot and mix thoroughly. Add some additional fresh berries to the top for serving. Enjoy!

36. Breakfast Quinoa Bowl

Serving: Serves 1 | Prep: | Cook: |Ready in:

Ingredients

- 1/4 quart quinoa
- 1/2 cup water
- 1 cup unsweetened vanilla almond milk
- 1 banana
- 1 tablespoon almond butter
- cinnamon

Direction

- The night before: In a small saucepan, bring water to a boil and add quinoa. Cover, reduce heat to simmer, and cook for 10 minutes. Turn off heat, but keep pot covered and allow to "cook" for an additional 10 minutes. Transfer to container with lid and place in refrigerator.
- In the morning: In a small saucepan over medium high heat, add almond milk. Once it begins to sizzle (like it's about to boil), add prepared quinoa and reduce heat to low. Stir occasionally until the almond milk is absorbed and becomes similar to the consistency of oatmeal (about 15 minutes). Remove from heat and transfer to bowl. Top with sliced banana and almond butter. Enjoy!

37. Breakfast Quinoa With Oats And Chia Seeds

Serving: Serves 1 | Prep: | Cook: |Ready in:

Ingredients

- 1/4 cup cooked quinoa

- 1/4 cup uncooked rolled oats
- 1/2 cup milk (I used 1%)
- 2/3 cup water
- 1 tablespoon chia seeds
- 1/4 teaspoon ground cinnamon
- 1 packet Truvia or 1 tablespoon brown sugar
- 1/4 teaspoon vanilla extrac
- 1 medium banana, sliced
- 1/4 cup chopped pecans

Direction

- In a small saucepan over medium heat, combine the cooked quinoa, rolled oats, milk, water and chia seeds. Cook for 5 to 6 minutes, until oats and chia seeds have absorbed most of the moisture and the mixture is thickened. Add in the cinnamon, Truvia or brown sugar and vanilla extract. Cook for 30 seconds more. Remove from heat and stir in the banana slices. Spoon into a bowl and top with the chopped pecans.

38. Breakfast Quinoa

Serving: Serves 4-6 | Prep: | Cook: | Ready in:

Ingredients

- 1 cup quinoa
- 1.5 cups milk
- 2 tablespoons maple syrup (more to taste if you like it sweeter)
- 4 ounces blueberries, can use fresh or frozen
- 1/2 cup walnuts
- 1/2 teaspoon cinnamon (optional)

Direction

- In a small saucepan on medium-high heat, combine quinoa and milk.
- When milk heats up and starts to foam/simmer, lower heat to low and allow quinoa to cook through till done, approx. 20 mins.
- Add maple syrup, blueberries, walnuts (and optional cinnamon) and mix. Tastes wonderful warm, or cold.

39. Brown Butter Broccoli Over Quinoa And Feta

Serving: Serves 2 as main dish | Prep: | Cook: | Ready in:

Ingredients

- 3/4 cup red quinoa, dry
- 2 tablespoons olive oil, divided
- 1 large head of broccoli, stalks and florets coarsely chopped
- Kosher salt
- freshly ground black pepper
- 2 tablespoons unsalted butter
- 1/4 cup raw pine nuts
- pinch of red pepper flakes
- 1 tablespoon fresh lemon juice
- 1/5 cup feta cheese, crumbled
- 1/4 cup cilantro, chopped

Direction

- Preheat oven to 450F.
- Rinse quinoa thoroughly in a fine mesh strainer for about two minutes to get rid of some of the bitterness. Drain well.
- Meanwhile, toss broccoli with remaining 2 tablespoons olive oil, salt, and freshly ground black pepper. Roast for 15-20 minutes, until broccoli has browned a bit on the edges and is tender.
- In a small saucepan, melt butter over low heat. Add pine nuts and cook for about 5-7 minutes, stirring occasionally, until butter is browned and pine nuts are toasted. Remove from heat, let cool slightly, and stir in red pepper flakes and lemon juice.
- When quinoa is cooked, fluff slightly with a fork. Toss with broccoli, brown butter sauce and pine nuts, feta, and cilantro.

40. Buffalo Style Quinoa Chili

Serving: Serves 2 to 4 | Prep: | Cook: |Ready in:

Ingredients

- 1 tablespoon olive oil
- 1 white onion, diced
- 3 stalks celery, diced
- one 8-ounce can tomato sauce
- one 14-ounce can diced tomatoes
- 1 cup vegetable broth
- 1 cup cooked black beans
- one 14-ounce can hominy
- 1 cup cooked quinoa
- 1/2 cup Frank's red hot sauce, or to taste
- 1 1/2 teaspoons smoked paprika
- 1 1/2 teaspoons cumin
- 1 teaspoon salt
- Freshly ground black pepper
- Blue cheese, for topping

Direction

- Heat the olive oil over medium in a saucepan and, once hot, add the diced onion and celery to the pan. Cook until soft, about 5 minutes.
- Stir in the diced tomatoes, tomato sauce, and vegetable broth. Bring to a boil then reduce to a simmer cook for 15 minutes. Add in black beans, hominy, quinoa, Frank's, smoked paprika, cumin, salt, and pepper. Continue to cook 15 more minutes, until the flavors have melded.
- To serve, ladle chili into broiler-safe bowls. Top with blue cheese and place under broiler until cheese melts, 3 to 5 minutes.

41. California Pizza Kitchen Style Quinoa & Arugula Salad

Serving: Serves 4 | Prep: 1hours0mins | Cook: 0hours45mins |Ready in:

Ingredients

- For the Dressing
- 1/3 cup extra-virgin olive oil
- 2 tablespoons red wine vinegar
- 1/4 teaspoon kosher salt
- 1/8 teaspoon dried oregano leaves
- a few grinds freshly ground black pepper
- For the Salad
- 1/2 cup cooked quinoa
- 8 Sun dried tomatoes in oil, cut small
- 1 teaspoon oil from sun dried tomato jar
- 3 ounces high-quality feta cheese, cut into small chunks
- 1 1/2 cups baby arugula leaves
- 1 1/2 tablespoons toasted pine nuts
- 1 bunch asparagus, stalks cut off and cut into 1 1/2-inch pieces

Direction

- For the Dressing
- Wash the quinoa and then cook according to package directions. Once quinoa finishes cooking, drain any excess water. Transfer quinoa to a large bowl and set aside to cool to room temperature.
- While quinoa is cooling, prepare the dressing. In a smallish bowl, mix together the olive oil, red wine vinegar, salt, oregano, and pepper. Mix well.
- Once quinoa has cooled, add the sun dried tomatoes, sun dried tomato oil, feta cheese, and dressing to the bowl. Toss well to coat. Cover bowl and put into the fridge for about 30 - 45 minutes.
- About 20 minutes before you are ready to serve salad, steam the asparagus. Put asparagus in a large saucepan and cover just barely with water. Put over medium heat and bring to a simmer, then lower the heat and simmer for 3 - 5 minutes. Asparagus is done when you can prick it through with a fork, but still tender. Don't let it get too soft!
- Once asparagus finishes cooking, drain and transfer to a plate to cool.

- When ready to serve the salad, mix in the 1 1/2 cups of baby arugula to the quinoa and toss. Divide the salad between 3 - 4 serving plates. Top each plate with asparagus and toasted pine nuts. Sprinkle with freshly ground pepper, if desired.
- Enjoy!

42. Cauliflower Cheddar Quinoa Fritters

Serving: Makes 12 | Prep: | Cook: | Ready in:

Ingredients

- 1 generous cup of cooked and cooled cauliflower, diced into small pieces
- 2 cups of cooked and cooled quinoa
- 2 cups vegetable broth or one Rapunzel No Salt Vegetable Bouillon Cube and 2 cups of water.
- 1 lemon, a few squeezes of lemon juice
- 4 generous tablespoons finely chopped chives or dill
- 1/2 cup of shredded cheddar. I use sharp cheddar, but extra sharp is wonderful too.
- 2 large eggs
- 1/3-1/2 cups of self rising flour or Pamela's Gluten Free mix
- Salt and pepper to taste
- Olive oil for cooking
- Serving Suggestions: lemon wedges, sour cream, salsa, Greek yogurt, ketchup, hot sauce
- 2 Tablespoons of milk

Direction

- Steam or boil the cauliflower until tender. Don't cook too long or it will get mushy. Chop it into small pieces. Add a generous cup full to a large bowl and set aside.
- Rinse one cup of quinoa. Put it in a pot with some olive oil and toast it on low heat until you can smell the nutty aroma. Then cook the toasted quinoa in two cups of water with one Rapunzel vegetable bouillon cube and some salt. Alternately, you can use two cups of your favorite vegetable broth or stock. Bring the quinoa and broth to a boil. Turn down the heat to low, cover and simmer gently for about 15 minutes. Remove the covered pot from the heat and let it stand for another 5 minutes. Portion out 2 cups of quinoa and put it in the same bowl with the cauliflower.
- Add the diced chives, eggs, lemon, milk, cheddar, salt and pepper to the bowl with the cauliflower and quinoa. Stir in about 1/3 cup of self-rising flour or Pamela's gluten free mix. If the mixture seems too wet, add more self-rising flour or Pamela's mix.
- Heat a large nonstick fry pan over medium high heat with some olive oil. Drop the batter onto the pan by two tablespoons each. Cook each fritter until golden brown on both sides. Serve with suggestions. Enjoy!

43. Chard And Quinoa Crustless Tart

Serving: Serves 1 10 inch tart | Prep: | Cook: | Ready in:

Ingredients

- 1 medium bunch chard, stemmed and chopped into small pieces (Reserve the stems and pickle them to serve on the side.)
- 1 cup chicken stock or broth (You can use water if you want this to be vegetarian.)
- 1/2 cup quinoa
- 1 cup water
- 4 large eggs
- 1/4 cup Greek yogurt
- 4 ounces pecorino romano cheese, finely grated (I used a microplane)
- 1/4 cup golden raisins
- 1 generous pinch red pepper flakes
- 2 tablespoons pine nuts
- 1/4 teaspoon flaky sea salt

Direction

- Bring chicken broth to a boil, and add chard, a little at a time, till submerged. Reduce heat to medium-low, and let chard cook until it is soft and somewhat reduced in volume. Drain chard well.
- In a medium saucepan, bring water to a boil. Rinse the quinoa in a fine mesh strainer, and add to the water. Reduce heat to medium-low, and let simmer till quinoa puffs up and all the water has been absorbed, about 20 minutes. Turn off the heat, and let quinoa cool till nearly room temperature.
- Heat oven to 400. Butter a 10 inch pie pan. Break eggs into a large bowl. Add yogurt, cheese, raisins and red pepper flakes and stir well. Finely chop cooked chard and stir it into the egg mixture. Add cooled quinoa, and stir till thoroughly combined.
- Place mixture into prepared pan and smooth top. Sprinkle pine nuts and a little flaky sea salt over the top of the mixture. Place into the oven, and bake for about 45 minutes. The edges of the pie will be golden brown, and the pine nuts will be toasted.
- Serve hot, warm, or at room temperature. This can be made ahead--let it cool completely and wrap it well. Let it come to room temperature, and then warm it in a 200 degree oven before serving.

44. Chayote, Avocado And Macadamia Quinoa With Coconut Lime Vinaigrette

Serving: Serves 4-5 | Prep: | Cook: | Ready in:

Ingredients

- Quinoa
- 1 cup quinoa
- 1 chayote squash
- 1/2 or small cucumber
- 1 slightly firm avocado,
- 1 small handful cilantro
- 1 small handful of mint
- 1/2 cup macadamia nuts
- Coconut Lime Vinaigrette
- 1/3 cup coconut milk (lite can be substituted)
- 3 tablespoons champagne vinegar
- 1/2 jalepeno pepper (optional)
- 1 small piece of fresh ginger
- 1 lime zested
- 1 lime juiced
- 1 bunch cilantro (to taste)
- 1/3 cup canola or veggie oil

Direction

- Prepare the quinoa as you normally would - rinse well, boil with water or broth, reduce heat and simmer for 15 minutes. For this recipe, I do prefer to let mine cool in the fridge before combining all ingredients.
- While the quinoa is cooking, prepare the dressing. Mince the jalapeno and ginger and add to a bowl or food processor along with the lime zest, lime juice, coconut milk and vinegar. Add as much or as little cilantro as you like. Slowly whisk or blend in the oil. Add salt to taste.
- For the salad: While the quinoa cools, julienne or shred the chayote. You could try doing a small chop as well. Peel and seed the cucumber and chop into 1/2 inch pieces. Note: A little green onion might be a nice addition. Roughly chop the mint and cilantro. Put the macadamias into a baggie and break them up a bit, perhaps give them a light toasting if time permits.
- Combine the chayote, avocado and any other veggies in a large bowl. Add the quinoa once it has been fluffed and cooled, at least to room temperature. Add the dressing a little at a time until you have the texture you like, being careful to toss lightly without mashing the avocado. Add the macadamias at the last minute, they can get a little soggy.... Serve immediately.

45. Cheesy Greek Style Baked Quinoa

Serving: Serves 8 | Prep: | Cook: | Ready in:

Ingredients

- 2 1/2 cups Cooked Quinoa
- 1 1/4 cups Fat Free Feta Cheese
- 1/2 cup Reduced Fat Shredded Mozzarella or Cheddar
- 1 cup Marinated Artichoke Hearts (in Oil)
- 1 cup Chopped Spinach
- 1 cup Diced Cherry Tomatoes
- 1/2 cup Skim Milk
- 1 teaspoon Crushed or Minced Garlic
- 1 teaspoon Lemon Juice
- 1 teaspoon Parsley
- 1 teaspoon Onion Powder
- 1/4 teaspoon Sea Salt & Coarse Black Peppercorn - approx.

Direction

- Prepare the quinoa as directed (preferably with chicken broth instead of water - this gives it more flavor). While quinoa cooks, dice cherry tomatoes and chop spinach leaves, then set aside. Next, in food processor combine 1 cup feta, skim milk, garlic, lemon juice, and parsley, blending until smooth.
- When ready, stir artichoke hearts, cherry tomatoes, and spinach into quinoa, plus 1 tbsp. oil from artichokes, stirring well. Pour over with feta sauce, then season with onion powder and salt & pepper, combining thoroughly.
- Transfer mixture to oven safe casserole dish, spreading evenly. Top with remaining feta and mozzarella (or cheddar), then bake at 400F for 15 minutes until top has melted. Immediately plate and serve.

46. Cherry Tomato Quinoa Caprese

Serving: Serves 6 - 8 | Prep: | Cook: | Ready in:

Ingredients

- 1 cup red quinoa
- 2 cups vegetable broth
- 2 garlic cloves, minced
- 2 tablespoons balsamic vinegar
- 3 tablespoons extra virgin olive oil
- 8 ounces fresh mozzarella balls (Bocconcini), drained
- 1 cup fresh basil leaves, torn
- 4 cups heirloom cherry tomatoes in a variety of colors (examples – Sungold, Sweet Million,
- salt and pepper, to taste

Direction

- - In a medium saucepan, combine red quinoa, broth and garlic. Bring to a boil, reduce heat to a simmer, cover & cook 10 – 15 minutes until all broth is absorbed. Cool and set aside.
- - In a small bowl, combine balsamic vinegar and olive oil.
- - In a large mixing bowl, combine the cooked quinoa, dressing, mozzarella cheese balls, basil and heirloom cherry tomatoes. Salt and pepper, to taste.

47. Chicken & Quinoa Stuffed Peppers

Serving: Serves 5 | Prep: | Cook: | Ready in:

Ingredients

- 5 Red Bell Peppers
- .5 tablespoons Coconut Oil
- 1 Onion
- 2 tablespoons Minced Garlic
- 1 pound Diced Chicken Breast
- 1 teaspoon Italian Seasoning
- .25 teaspoons Black Pepper

- .25 teaspoons Red Chili Flakes
- .25 cups Shredded Carrots
- 3 Campari Tomatoes
- 2 handfuls Chopped Baby Spinach
- .33 cups LowFat Cottage Cheese
- 1 cup Cooked Quinoa

Direction

- Pre-Heat Oven at 400 degrees
- Heat 1/2 TB Coconut Oil in a Sauté Pan on a medium flame. Add 1 small Onion, Diced and 2 TB Minced Garlic. Cook for 2-3 minutes.
- Then add 1 lb. Diced Chicken Breast, Italian Seasoning, Black Pepper & Red Pepper Flakes (optional).
- Stir occasionally and when Chicken is nearly cooked through, add 1/4 Cup Shredded Carrots, 3 Chopped Campari (or 2 Plum) Tomatoes. Sauté for about 4-5 more minutes.
- Turn heat off and Stir in 2 Handfuls of Chopped Baby Spinach, 1/3 Cup Low-fat Cottage Cheese & 1 Cup Cooked Quinoa.
- Cut off the tops of peppers, remove seeds and place in a deep pan. Fill Peppers with Chicken Mix and cover with foil. Bake for 20 minutes. Remove Foil and turn oven up to broil for about 5 minutes (to crisp up the top of the filling)

48. Chicken Quinoa

Serving: Serves 2 | Prep: | Cook: | Ready in:

Ingredients

- 1.5 cups quinoa
- 3 cups broth or water
- 4 chicken thighs
- 1 onion or leek
- olive oil

Direction

- Heat olive oil in pan with onions or leeks
- Add chicken... cook on both sides for a few minutes
- Add 3 cups broth or water
- Add 1.5 cups quinoa
- Cover and cook on lower temperature
- Serve warm!

49. Chipotle Peach Quinoa Salad

Serving: Serves 4 | Prep: | Cook: | Ready in:

Ingredients

- Quinoa salad
- 1 cup uncooked quinoa
- 1 zucchini, diced
- 1 cup corn (fresh, frozen, or canned)
- 1 tablespoon olive oil
- 1 peach, pitted and diced
- 3 ounces cotija cheese, crumbled
- 3 tablespoons chopped green onions
- Chipotle-peach vinaigrette
- 1 peach, pitted and diced (no need to peel)
- 1-2 chipotle peppers in adobo, diced
- 2 tablespoons olive oil
- 1 tablespoon apple cider vinegar
- 1 tablespoon honey or agave nectar

Direction

- Cook the quinoa according to the directions on the package.
- Place all the ingredients for the vinaigrette in a blender and blend until smooth.
- Heat 1 tablespoon olive oil in a skillet over medium heat for 1-2 minutes. Test the oil with a piece of zucchini – once it sizzles upon contact, add the rest of the zucchini and sauté until softened (but not squishy), about 2 minutes. Transfer the zucchini to a plate or bowl. Add the corn to the skillet and sauté until tender (about 8-10 minutes for fresh corn, 1-2 minutes for frozen or canned). If you are using frozen corn, heat it in the microwave

and drain any excess liquid before adding it to the skillet.
- In a large bowl, combine the quinoa, zucchini, corn, diced peach, and vinaigrette. Stir in half of the Cotija, and sprinkle the remaining half on top, along with the chopped green onions.

50. Chocolate Quinoa Crackers

Serving: Makes one batch | Prep: | Cook: |Ready in:

Ingredients

- 3 tablespoons vegetable oil
- 1/2 cup water, room temperature
- 1 cup quinoa flour
- 1/4 cup white rice flour
- 1/2 cup unsweetened cocoa powder
- 1 teaspoon baking powder
- Pinch salt (generous)
- 1/2 cup coconut sugar

Direction

- Preheat the oven to 400 degrees.
- Mix the flours, sugar, cocoa powder, baking powder and salt together in a medium bowl. Drizzle the oil in and mix with your fingers until it resembles sand.
- Add the water slowly until the dough comes together in a ball. If it's too sticky, add some more flour (quinoa or white rice flour).
- Roll out the dough on a lightly floured surface as thin as you can (unless you like slightly thicker and less snappy crackers). Score the dough into squares and pierce them slightly with the tines of a fork.
- Bake them on a parchment lined baking sheet for 10-11 minutes (they will crisp as they cool).

51. Chopped Parsley Salad With Quinoa, Comte + Pumpkin Seeds

Serving: Serves 4 | Prep: | Cook: |Ready in:

Ingredients

- 1 cup quinoa (I used "rainbow")
- 2 cups chopped parsley (leaves and stems from 2 bunches)
- 1/2 cup toasted pumpkin seeds
- 1 1/2 cups grated Comte or sharp cheddar cheese
- 1 small shallot, finely chopped
- 2 tablespoons olive oil
- 2 teaspoons red-wine vinegar
- Kosher salt and freshly ground black pepper

Direction

- Place quinoa and 1 cup water in a medium saucepan. Cover and soak quinoa for 6 to 8 hours. When ready to prepare salad, add 1/4 cup water to saucepan and place over high heat to bring to a boil, then simmer 5 minutes. Pour cooked quinoa onto a rimmed baking sheet and spread to a thin layer to cool (about 10 minutes).
- While quinoa cooks and cools, heat a medium, heavy skillet over medium heat. Add pumpkin seeds and cook, tossing occasionally, until they are toasted, about 5 minutes. Transfer to baking sheet with quinoa to cool.
- Chop parsley and transfer to a large bowl with shallot and cheese. Add quinoa and pumpkin seeds and toss to combine. Stir in oil and vinegar and season with salt and pepper.

52. Cilantro And Lime Quinoa

Serving: Serves 4 to 6 people | Prep: | Cook: |Ready in:

Ingredients

- 1 small onion diced
- 1 lime, zest of half juice of whole lime
- 1/4 cup choped cilintro
- 1 tablespoon butter
- 1 tablespoon olive oil
- 1.5 cups quinoa
- 3 cups chicken stock
- 1 to 2 bay leaves
- 1 teaspoon Adobo
- Salt and pepper to taste

Direction

- Melt the butter with the olive oil in a Dutch oven. Add the onions and sweat until translucent about 5 mins. Add the bay leaves and Adobo. Season with salt and pepper. Add the quinoa and mix to coat, and toast for 3 to 5 mins. Add the lime zest, lime juice and the chicken stock. Adjust for seasoning if needed. Bring to boil, reduce to simmer and cover. Cook the quinoa on low simmer for about 20 mins or until cooked though. At the end add the cilantro and fluff with a fork. Serve!!

53. Cinnamon French Toast Breakfast Quinoa

Serving: Serves 1 | Prep: | Cook: | Ready in:

Ingredients

- 1/4 cup white quinoa
- 1/2 cup coconut milk
- 1 teaspoon honey
- 2 teaspoons ground cinnamon
- 1/2 teaspoon vanilla extract
- 1/4 cup pecans, chopped
- 1 teaspoon maple syrup
- 1/2 cup blueberries
- 1 teaspoon chia seeds (optional)

Direction

- In a small pot combine quinoa, milk, honey, 1 1/2 tsp cinnamon and vanilla. Stir and bring to a boil.
- When quinoa reaches a boil, turn down the heat and let simmer for 15 minutes.
- When quinoa is done cooking, scoop into a bowl and top with pecans, blueberries, chia seeds, maple syrup and additional cinnamon.

54. Cinnamon Maple Quinoa With Roasted Apples, Dried Fruit And Toasted Almonds

Serving: Serves 3 | Prep: | Cook: | Ready in:

Ingredients

- 2 apples (I like Fujis or Pink Ladies; a granny smith would work here, too)
- 2 1/2 tablespoons olive oil
- 1/4-3/8 teaspoons kosher salt
- 2-3 tablespoons sliced almonds, toasted
- 1 cup quinoa, rinsed and drained
- 1 1/2 cups water
- 1 cinnamon stick
- 2-3 teaspoons Maple syrup; Grade B is best
- 1/4 cup dried cranberries
- 1/4 cup dried apricots, chopped into 1/4-inch pieces

Direction

- Preheat oven to 350 degrees.
- Peel, core and chop the apples into 1/4-inch pieces and place on a cookie sheet. Drizzle with 1/2 Tablespoon olive oil and sprinkle a pinch of salt over the apples. Mix them with your hands until the apples are coated with oil.
- Roast them in the oven for 20-25 minutes. They're done when they're barely tender and the edges have begun to brown.
- Remove from oven and add to a large bowl with the dried cranberries and apricots.

- Toast the almonds in small saucepan over low-medium heat until fragrant and very light brown. Spread on a paper towel on the counter to cool.
- Make the quinoa: rinse and drain the quinoa. Toast the quinoa in a dry, medium saucepan, over medium heat for 3-5 minutes, until you begin to hear popping sounds and the nutty aroma is release. Add the water, cinnamon stick, 1/4 teaspoon salt, 2 teaspoons of maple syrup and 1 Tablespoon of olive oil to the pan. Bring to a boil and then turn the heat down, simmering until the water has been absorbed; about 20 minutes.
- When the quinoa has finished cooking, remove the cinnamon stick and add the quinoa to the bowl with the fruit, stirring with a rubber spatula.
- Add the remaining 1 Tablespoon of olive oil and taste for seasoning (you may opt to add 1 more teaspoon of maple syrup). Serve in a bowl and top the quinoa mixture with the toasted almonds.

55. Coconut Quinoa Crunch Yogurt Parfait With Gingered Maple Syrup

Serving: Serves 2 | Prep: | Cook: |Ready in:

Ingredients

- 3/4 cup uncooked quinoa, rinsed in a fine mesh strainer, drained
- 1/2 cup sliced almonds
- 4 tablespoons unsweetened shredded coconut
- 1/4 teaspoon kosher salt
- 1/2 cup pure maple syrup
- 1/2 teaspoon peeled, grated ginger root (from a 1-inch piece)
- 1 1/2 cups mixed berries or your favorite fruits, washed and cut into bite-sized pieces
- 2 cups plain yogurt (your favorite)

Direction

- Make the syrup: In a small saucepan bring maple syrup and ginger to a boil. Remove from heat and stir. Set aside to cool.
- Make the topping: Heat a large skillet over medium heat. Add quinoa (don't worry if it's damp. The water will evaporate) and cook, stirring and tossing with a spatula, for a minute or so. Add nuts and coconut. Cook, stirring frequently, for 7-8 minutes more until quinoa is a making frequent popping sounds and becomes toasted and golden brown. Sprinkle with salt and mix. Spread toasted quinoa mixture out on a plate to cool.
- Assemble the Parfaits: When the syrup & toasted quinoa have cooled, about 15 minutes, assemble the parfaits: Using two bowls or parfait glasses, make alternate layers of quinoa, yogurt, fruit, syrup. Repeat. Top with a light sprinkling of quinoa. Enjoy!

56. Coconut Quinoa Porridge With Berry Compote

Serving: Makes 4 servings | Prep: | Cook: |Ready in:

Ingredients

- Porridge
- 1 cup oats
- 1/2 cup quinoa
- 6 cups coconut water
- 1 pinch salt
- Compote
- 3 cups mixed berries, such as strawberries, raspberries, blueberries and blackberries
- 1 teaspoon sweetener, such as coconut sugar
- 1 teaspoon vanilla

Direction

- Porridge
- Measure the oats and quinoa and place into a medium sized saucepan.

- Add the coconut water.
- Bring the porridge to a simmer over a low heat.
- Allow to simmer for 10-15 minutes, stirring frequently. It's ready when the porridge is smooth and you can see the quinoa grains starting to open up.
- Compote
- If using strawberries, cut them in half so they're about the same size as the other berries.
- Combine the berries, sweetener, and vanilla in a medium sized saucepan.
- Heat the berries slowly over a low flame.
- Allow to simmer for 10-15 minutes, stirring frequently. It's ready when the compote has created a sauce, but you can still see some whole berries.
- Top the porridge with compote, then drizzle with maple syrup or your favorite sweetener. Leftover porridge and compote can be stored in the fridge for a few days. To reheat the porridge, just add a little bit of extra water and reheat on the stove.

57. Coconut Quinoa Pudding

Serving: Makes about 6 servings | Prep: | Cook: | Ready in:

Ingredients

- For the quinoa and topping
- 1 cup rinsed and drained quinoa
- 2 cups coconut milk (I used Silk original from the dairy case)
- 1/2 cup grated sweetened coconut
- 1/2 teaspoon cinnamon
- Putting it all together
- 2 cups coconut milk
- 1/3 cup semolina
- 1 tablespoon cornstarch
- A pinch of salt
- 2/3 cup sugar, divided
- 2 large eggs
- 1 cup grated sweetened coconut
- 1 tablespoon grated fresh orange zest
- Juice of one orange
- 2 teaspoons vanilla extract
- Cooked quinoa
- Coconut-cinnamon topping

Direction

- For the quinoa and topping
- In a medium saucepan combine the quinoa and coconut milk. Bring to a boil and then cover and lower the heat to a simmer for about 15 minutes until the liquid is absorbed into the grain. Set aside.
- Spread the coconut on a baking sheet and place in a 350° F oven for 5 to 8 minutes, stirring occasionally, until the coconut starts to slightly brown. Place in a small bowl and stir in the cinnamon. Set that bowl aside.
- Putting it all together
- Whisk the semolina, cornstarch, 1/3 cup sugar and the pinch of salt in a small mixing bowl and set aside.
- In a medium saucepan, begin slowly heating the coconut milk to boiling. While watching the milk, beat the eggs with an electric mixer, add the remaining 1/3 cup sugar and continue beating until thick and a little fluffy.
- Once the milk comes up to a boil, whisk in the semolina mixture and continue stirring until the mixture thickens and just starts to boil again. Take off the heat and let rest for about 2 minutes.
- Stir in the egg mixture, cooked quinoa, orange zest, orange juice, coconut, and vanilla. Pour into a greased 8 x 11-inch baking pan. Bake at 350° F for 35 to 40 minutes.
- Serve warm in small dessert dishes topped with a teaspoon or two of the cinnamon-coconut topping.

58. Coconut Quinoa And Warm Broccoli Bowl With Ginger Lemongrass Dressing

Serving: Serves 2 to 4 | Prep: | Cook: | Ready in:

Ingredients

- For the quinoa and broccoli bowl:
- 3/4 cup quinoa
- 1 1/2 cups coconut milk
- 1 pinch sea salt
- 1/2 head broccoli florets
- 1/2 cup snow peas, thinly sliced
- 1 spring onion, thinly sliced
- 1/4 cup large coconut flakes, toasted
- 1 tablespoon black sesame seeds
- For the dressing:
- 1 stalk lemongrass
- one 2-inch knob fresh ginger, peeled and sliced
- 1 teaspoon brown rice syrup
- 1 lime, juiced
- 1/4 cup grapeseed or olive oil

Direction

- In a metal sieve, rinse the quinoa under cold water for about 30 seconds. In a medium pot, add the rinsed quinoa, coconut milk, and sea salt. Bring to a boil, then cover and simmer for 15 minutes, until quinoa has increased in sized and absorbed most of the water. Remove from heat and let sit with the lid on for another 5 minutes before fluffing with a fork.
- Lightly steam the broccoli in a double boiler until just tender and vibrant green, no more than 5 minutes once the water boils, then rinse under cold water so it retains its color and texture.
- Divide the coconut quinoa evenly between 2 to 4 bowls. Add the warm broccoli on top and top with snow peas, spring onion, toasted coconut flakes, and sesame seeds.
- To make the dressing, remove the woody outer layer of the lemongrass and trim off the tough ends. Bash the stalk to release some flavor, then give it a rough chop. Place lemongrass, fresh ginger, brown rice syrup, lime juice, and oil in a small blender and combine until smooth. Add a teaspoon or two of water to help the process along, as needed.
- Serve the dressing over the quinoa bowl.

59. Coconut Ginger Quinoa With Carrots And Shrimp

Serving: Serves 2 | Prep: | Cook: | Ready in:

Ingredients

- Olive oil
- 1 cup Quinoa
- 2 cups Chicken stock
- 3 tablespoons Unsweetened coconut flakes
- 1/2 cup Grated carrots
- 1/4 cup Diced onion
- 1 teaspoon Grated fresh ginger
- 1/2 teaspoon Minced garlic
- 10 Peeled and deveined shrimp
- Splash Fresh lime juice
- Cilantro for garnish

Direction

- Cook quinoa and stock according to package's directions. Meanwhile, toast coconut flakes in a pan, and set aside.
- Coat the pan in olive oil and sauté carrots and onions until tender. Add the ginger and garlic and cook for just about a minute. Set aside with the toasted coconut flakes.
- In the same pan, sauté the shrimp until browned.
- Once the quinoa is cooked, toss with coconut flakes, carrots, onions, ginger, and garlic. Add minced cilantro and a splash of fresh lime juice. Top with the shrimp and enjoy!

60. Colca Cañon Quinoa Soup

Serving: Serves 8 | Prep: | Cook: | Ready in:

Ingredients

- Quinoa
- 1.5 cups white quinoa, rinsed in a mesh strainer under cold water for 1-2 minutes
- 3 cups cold water
- 1 bay leaf
- 1 teaspoon vegetarian beef or vegetable broth powder
- Soup
- 3 medium carrots, diced
- 1 medium onion, diced
- 3 cloves of garlic, minced
- 2 tablespoons olive oil
- 1 pound bag of frozen chopped kale (or one 10 oz box, defrosted)
- 6 cups vegetable stock or boxed broth
- 8 ounces cotija cheese (OR queso duro blanco), diced and set aside
- 1 small lime, cut in wedges

Direction

- Use your favorite method to cook the quinoa. I dump everything into my programmable rice cooker and use the "quick cooking" setting, fluffing it when the timer goes off. If you are cooking it stovetop: after rinsing the quinoa put it in a large sauce pan and add the water and bay leaf. Bring to a boil and then add the broth powder. Stir and turn down the heat to a simmer. Cover and cooker for another 15 minutes. Remove from heat and turn off the stove. After 5-7 minutes uncover and fluff the quinoa as you would rice. Set aside and keep covered until ready to add to the soup.
- In your soup pot (4 qtr. or larger), heat the olive oil over medium heat. Cook the carrots and onion until soft, then add the garlic. Stir often. Cook until the onion is translucent and just starting to brown (about 15 minutes).
- Add the stock/broth to the onion mixture in the soup pot and bring up to a simmer.
- Once the broth is simmering, add the bag of frozen kale and let the soup heat up until it's just starting to bubble around the edges again.
- Add the quinoa.
- Turn off the heat and add the diced Cotija cheese and serve immediately. OR you can just top what you want to eat immediately with cheese and let it cool before adding the cheese to pint jars of soup (this soup travels well for lunches and freezes well -minus the cheese- too).

61. Colorful Rice Cooker Blueberry Morning Quinoa

Serving: Serves 4 | Prep: | Cook: | Ready in:

Ingredients

- 1 cup Rainbow Quinoa
- 2 cups Unsweetened Almond Milk
- 1 cup Blueberries
- 1 teaspoon Vanilla Extract
- 2 tablespoons Sugar
- 1 teaspoon Nutmeg
- .5 teaspoons Cloves
- 1 teaspoon Cinnamon

Direction

- Rinse Quinoa
- Mash Blueberries (Optional)
- Add all ingredients to rice cooker
- Set rice cooker to White Rice setting
- Take out of Rice Cooker and serve with additional non-dairy milk and/or sugar if desired.

62. Corn Salad With Tomatoes, Avocado, Quinoa And Feta

Serving: Serves 4 as a side, 2 as a main course | Prep: | Cook: | Ready in:

Ingredients

- 1 ear of corn
- 2 medium-sized tomatoes, diced
- 2 avocado, diced
- 100 grams feta, crumbled
- 1/2 teaspoon paprika
- 1 teaspoon dried thyme
- 1 pinch of espelette pepper (or other mild pepper)
- 2 tablespoons lemon juice

Direction

- Bring a large pot of water to boil. Remove and discard the green outer husk and silky threads from the corn. Cook the ear of corn for 5 minutes then cool in a cold water bath. Remove the corn kernels and reserve in a bowl
- Rinse the quinoa under cold water. Put the quinoa and twice its volume in water in a pot and bring to boil. Reduce the heat and cook for 10 minutes with a lid. Let it stand for 5 minutes
- Make the dressing: mix the olive oil, lemon juice, pepper, cumin, paprika, thyme, salt and pepper
- Add the tomatoes, avocado, quinoa and corn. Stir well
- Top with the crumbled feta and serve

63. Cranberry Almond Quinoa Pilaf

Serving: Serves 4-6 | Prep: | Cook: | Ready in:

Ingredients

- 1/2 cup slivered almonds
- 1 cinnamon stick, about 3 inches long
- 1 bay leaf
- 1 cup uncooked quinoa
- 1/2 cup dried cranberries
- 1 3/4 cups chicken broth

Direction

- Heat a medium sauce pan over medium high heat. Add almonds and toss a few times, until they are toasted and smell fragrant. Remove from pan and set aside (if a few remain in the pan, that is ok)
- Return pan to heat and add cinnamon stick and bay leaf, allow to toast for about 1 minute. Add quinoa and toast as well, about 4-5 minutes. There will be popping sounds and a lovely, toasty fragrance will fill the air.
- Add cranberries and chicken broth, carefully! Chicken broth will sputter and hiss as it hits the hot pan. Stir well and bring mixture to a boil. Cover, reduce to simmer, 20 minutes.
- Turn off heat and keep covered. Let sit for about 5 minutes. Fluff with fork and add salt, as necessary (depending on broth used, you may not need much, if any, salt).Top with toasted almonds and enjoy!

64. Cranberry Smoothie Quinoa Pudding

Serving: Makes 2 | Prep: | Cook: | Ready in:

Ingredients

- 1/2 cup frozen cranberries
- 1/2 cup frozen blackberries
- 1/2 cup unsweetened almond milk
- 1-2 packets sweetener of choice
- handful of ice
- 3/4 cup cooked quinoa
- 1 cup unsweetened almond milk
- 1/2 teaspoon cinnamon

Direction

- Prepare the pudding by mixing the milk, vanilla extract, cinnamon & cooked quinoa together in a jar or bowl the night before
- Refrigerate overnight for the pudding to thicken
- The next day, blend all ingredients for the smoothie together
- In a glass, layer the smoothie on top of the quinoa pudding, top with more fruit & enjoy!

65. Creamy Quinoa Custard Pie Layered With Bananas And Date Toffee

Serving: Serves 8 | Prep: | Cook: | Ready in:

Ingredients

- Quinoa Custard & Coconut Cream Topping
- 1 c quinoa flakes
- 3 1/2 c milk (regular or soy)
- 1/2 c maple syrup
- 3 tsp vanilla extract
- 1 tsp espresso powder
- 1/4 tsp salt
- 1 c coconut milk
- 1 tbsp cornstarch
- Date Toffee & Bottom Layer
- 1 pie crust (use your favorite recipe)
- 1/4 c dates, finely chopped
- 3/4 c milk (soy or regular)
- 2 tbsp coconut oil
- 2 tbsp brown sugar
- 1 tsp blackstrap molasses
- 2 bananas, sliced

Direction

- Preheat the oven to 350 degrees and grease an 8" pie pan. To prepare the toffee, soak the chopped dates in 3/4 C milk.
- Place the quinoa flakes and 1 1/2 C of milk in a saucepan, bring to a boil, and then simmer for 15 minutes. Add another 1 1/2 C soy milk and beat well with an electric mixer or handheld blender. Simmer for another 5 minutes.
- Add the maple syrup and divide the mixture between 2 bowls.
- To one, add the espresso powder, 2 tsp vanilla, and salt, mix thoroughly and set aside. To the second bowl, add coconut milk, 1 tsp vanilla, and 1 heaping tbsp. cornstarch, then beat until smooth.
- To make the toffee, blend the dates soaking in milk (and extra milk), coconut oil, brown sugar, and molasses in a food processor until smooth. Then, spread date toffee into the pie crust and top with a layer of sliced bananas.
- Smother bananas with quinoa custard, smooth with a rubber spatula, and chill pie in the refrigerator. Serve cold, topped with coconut cream and cocoa powder.

66. Creamy Quinoa Onion Soup

Serving: Makes about 2 quarts | Prep: | Cook: | Ready in:

Ingredients

- 1 cup sprouted quinoa
- 2 cups water
- 2 tablespoons butter
- 2 tablespoons olive oil
- 2 medium sweet onions
- 2 medium leeks (white and pale green part only)
- 1 large clove garlic
- 1 teaspoon granulated sugar
- 1/2 teaspoon aleppo pepper (optional)
- 1/2 cup dry white wine
- 4 cups chicken broth(plus more if you want a thinner soup..see note*)
- 2 cups beef broth
- Salt and pepper for seasoning
- Thinly sliced green onion and crumbled bacon for garnish

Direction

- Cook the quinoa per package instructions. Normally you rinse the grain and combine it with the 2 cups water, bring to a boil and then gently simmer, covered, for 12 to 15 minutes until the liquid is absorbed. Set aside.
- Slice the onions and leeks thinly and mince the garlic clove. In a 4 quart soup pot melt the butter and oil and add the onions, leek, garlic, sugar and Aleppo pepper(if using). Gently saute until everything softens but doesn't brown. This might take about 20 minutes.
- Add the wine, chicken broth and beef broth and bring the soup to a boil. Add the cooked quinoa and then simmer the soup for about ten minutes.
- After 10 minutes cool the soup a bit and then in batches, puree the soup until very creamy. Return the soup to a clean pot and then re warm and taste for seasoning.
- To serve, ladle soup into bowls and garnish with green onion and crumbled bacon.
- Note: If you feel the soup is thicker than you like, thin it a bit by whisking in a little more chicken broth after pureeing.

67. Crispy Quinoa Chocolate Bars

Serving: Makes 4 bars | Prep: | Cook: |Ready in:

Ingredients

- 1/4 cup Quinoa
- 1/2 cup Water
- 2 tablespoons Coconut Cream
- 1 1/2 tablespoons Unsweetened Cocoa Powder
- 1 dash Salt
- 1/2 tablespoon Coconut Oiil
- 1/2 tablespoon Coconut Sugar

Direction

- Cook 1/4 cup of Quinoa with 1TB Coconut Cream, 1/2 cup of water & a dash of Salt on low heat (covered) until water is evaporated - about 25 minutes.
- In a small bowl, mix: 1 1/2TB Unsweetened Cocoa Powder; 1TB Coconut Cream; 1/2TB Coconut Oil; Sweetener of Choice (I used 1/2TB Coconut Sugar). Add cooked Quinoa
- Spoon into square Tupperware, lined with parchment paper
- Optional: Top with nuts or Unsweetened Coconut Flakes (Chocolate Chips if you dare!)
- Let set in refrigerator until hardened
- Cut into 4 pieces & Enjoy!

68. Crispy Quinoa And Mustard Green Cakes

Serving: Makes 10 to 12 patties | Prep: | Cook: |Ready in:

Ingredients

- 3/4 cup dried quinoa
- kosher salt
- 1/2 pound mustard greens, rough ends trimmed and discarded
- 2 teaspoons cumin seed or ground cumin
- 1 cup diced red onion
- freshly cracked pepper to taste
- 1 cup fresh bread crumbs
- 1/2 cup grated Parmigiano Reggiano, see notes above
- 4 eggs
- grapeseed or other neutral oil, for frying
- lemons, cilantro, naan, tahini-yogurt sauce for serving, optional, see notes above

Direction

- Fill a large pot with water and place over high heat. Bring to a boil. Add the quinoa and 1 tablespoon kosher salt and simmer for 9 minutes, just until the quinoa begins to unfurl. Drain through a fine-meshed strainer.

- Meanwhile, pulse the greens in a food processor. It's best to do this in two batches: fill the processor with greens. Pulse until the greens fall to the bottom. The pieces should be small but not puréed or mushy. Transfer them to a large bowl. Repeat with the remaining greens.
- In a small skillet over medium heat, toast the cumin seeds or powder until fragrant and slightly darker in color. If using seeds, crush them gently with a mortar and pestle or in a spice grinder. Transfer to the bowl with the greens. Add the drained quinoa, onion, 1 teaspoon of salt, pepper to taste, bread crumbs, cheese and eggs. Mix with your hands or a spatula until everything is well blended.
- Test the mixture for seasoning and structure: Place a small skillet over high heat. Add a small amount of oil — just enough to cover the bottom of the pan in a thin layer. Cup a small amount (less than ¼ cup) of the mixture with your hands. Mixture will feel wet and will loosely hold together. Form into a ball, packing and cupping with your hands. When the oil shimmers, immediately lower the heat to medium and gently place the ball into the pan. Flatten with your hand or spatula to form a patty. Season with a pinch of salt. Let cook undisturbed for 2 to 3 minutes, or until evenly golden. Flip, and brown the other side for another 2 minutes or until evenly golden. Remove patty from pan and let cool briefly. Taste. If necessary, adjust mixture with more salt and pepper to taste. If the patty fell apart in the pan, crack in another egg to the bowl of quinoa/greens and mix to combine. When the mixture is tasting and holding together to your liking, use a 1/4-cup measure to portion out the remaining mixture into balls — you should get 10 to 12.
- Place a large skillet over high heat. When it simmers. Add balls to pan — they should sizzle when they hit the oil — then turn the heat down to medium or medium-low. Flatten balls gently with a spatula. Season with a pinch of salt. Cook undisturbed for 2 to 3 minutes or until golden. Use a spatula to flip the patties and cook for another 2 minutes or until golden. Pile onto a platter and serve with lemon, cilantro, naan, and sauce, if you wish.

69. Crispy Shrimp & Red Quinoa Patties

Serving: Makes nine 3-inch patties | Prep: | Cook: | Ready in:

Ingredients

- 1 1/2 cups red quinoa, cooked** and cooled to room temperature
- 9 to 12 shrimp, peeled, deveined, chopped into 1/2-inch pieces, and cooked
- 2 to 3 tablespoons coarse bread crumbs
- 3 tablespoons flax meal
- 1 small red onion, minced
- 2 cloves garlic, chopped
- 1/2 jalapeño, minced
- 3 eggs (free-range if possible)
- 1 pinch red pepper flakes
- Sea salt and freshly cracked black pepper to taste
- 2 tablespoons Greek yogurt, plus 1/2 cup for topping
- 2 teaspoons harissa paste, for topping

Direction

- **If you can spare the time to make stock from the shrimp shells and use that as the cooking liquid for the quinoa, you will have extra-shrimpy, even more flavorful patties.
- In a good size bowl, fold together the quinoa, shrimp, eggs, onion, garlic, jalapeño, flax meal, bread crumbs, red pepper flakes, 2 tablespoons of Greek yogurt, and salt and pepper until well combined.
- If the mixture is too wet, add more flax meal or bread crumbs. If it is too dry, add a little water or a bit more yogurt. This is not an exact science -- It is important that the mixture binds together, but you don't want it cakey.

- Mix together the remaining 1/2 cup Greek yogurt and harissa paste; I like to partially mix, so that some of the experience is creamier yogurt, and some is more fiery/ savory harissa. Do as you like in combining them. Place back in the refrigerator until ready to top the patties.
- Over medium heat in a heavy bottomed skillet, sear the patties in a glug of good olive oil for 5 to 7 minutes on the first side. Cook spaced judiciously but without crowding the pan.
- You're looking for a nicely crisped surface without any blackening. Use a spatula and flip, browning the second side for 3 to 5 minutes. Adjust heat as needed so that you get golden brown, crispy-edged patties, and of course, add more olive oil as needed as you cook subsequent rounds.
- Serve patties dolloped with the harissa yogurt and serve with a zingy cucumber salad or other crunchy, juicy vegetable.

70. Crockpot Chicken Quinoa Soup

Serving: Serves 6 | Prep: | Cook: |Ready in:

Ingredients

- Yellow Onion, garlic, celery, carrots, chicken, chicken broth, smoked paprika, cayenne pepper, bay leaves, tomato, salt, pepper,
- 1/2 Yellow onion, diced
- 1   Clove garlic, diced
- 4   stalks celery, diced
- 2 cups carrots, diced
- 2   chicken breasts, cooked and diced (can use rotisserie as well)
- 1 1/2 teaspoons Smoked paprika
- 3   Fresh bay leaves
- 1   medium tomato, diced
- 1 teaspoon cayenne pepper (or to taste)
- 1/2 cup quinoa, rinsed
- 6 cups low-sodium chicken broth
- fresh ground pepper and kosher salt, to taste
- N/A

Direction

- Yellow Onion, garlic, celery, carrots, chicken, chicken broth, smoked paprika, cayenne pepper, bay leaves, tomato, salt, pepper,
- Add the above ingredients to crockpot and stir.
- Set to low for about 8 hours.
- Enjoy!

71. Curried Quinoa With Cherries And Roasted Chickpeas

Serving: Serves 4 | Prep: | Cook: |Ready in:

Ingredients

- 1 cup Quinoa
- 1 1/2 cups Vegetable broth
- 15 ounces Can garbanzo beans/chickpeas
- 1   Roma tomato (diced)
- 1/4 cup Dried cherries
- 1 tablespoon Olive oil
- 1 teaspoon Salt
- 1 teaspoon Curry powder
- 1/4 teaspoon Cumin
- 1/4 teaspoon Garlic Powder
- 1/8 teaspoon Cinnamon
- 1/8 teaspoon Cloves

Direction

- Soak the quinoa in cool water for ten minutes. Strain, rinse and let drain for 20 minutes. Lightly toast the quinoa in a saucepan to remove excess liquid. Remove from the pan and set aside.
- While the quinoa is draining, prepare the garbanzo beans. Preheat the oven to 400 degrees F. Drain and dry the beans with a paper towel. Toss them with the olive oil and 1/2 tsp of salt and place them on a cookie

sheet. Let them roast in the oven for 15 minutes. When it's finished roasting remove them from the oven and set them aside in a separate dish, keeping them as warm as possible.
- Mix the curry, cumin, cinnamon, cloves, garlic powder and 1/2 tsp salt together and whisk it in the vegetable broth in a saucepan. Add the dried cherries to the broth and bring to a rapid boil.
- Add the quinoa to the broth and turn down the heat to a simmer. Cover the saucepan, leaving a little bit open for ventilation, and let it simmer until the liquid is no longer visible and the seeds show a white center spot with a ring around them (like Saturn's rings) This should take about 20 minutes.
- Fluff quinoa with a fork and place into serving bowl. Toss in the roasted chickpeas and diced tomato. Enjoy!

72. Curried Quinoa With Spinach And Avocado

Serving: Serves 4 | Prep: | Cook: | Ready in:

Ingredients

- 2 cups Cooked quinoa
- 1 tablespoon Oil (vegetable)
- 1 Small onion, finely chopped
- 2 Tomatoes (I usually use Roma)
- 1 Green jalapeño, chopped (or to taste)
- 2 teaspoons Cumin seeds
- 1/4 teaspoon Turmeric
- 1/2 teaspoon Salt (or to taste)
- 2 cups Baby spinach, roughly chopped
- 1/2 cup Cilantro leaves, roughly chopped
- 1 Large avocado, cubed
- 1 Lemon, to juice over the avocado cubes

Direction

- Heat oil in a 12" skillet. Add onions and sauté until soft and translucent.
- While the onions cook, toss the cumin seeds onto a cast iron pan (or any other kind of pan that is not non-stick will work) and heat over medium high heat until you can smell the fragrance of the seeds. Keep an eye on it and stir often so that the seeds don't burn. **Don't add oil. The point is to dry roast the cumin.
- Toss the dry roasted cumin seeds into a blender with the tomatoes and the green chili. Puree and set aside.
- When the onions are soft and translucent, add in the tomato puree. Stir and cook until the puree begins to look more like a paste. About 5 minutes.
- Add in the turmeric and salt. Stir.
- Add in the cooked quinoa. Stir until the quinoa is evenly coated in the spicy tomato mixture and cook for about 2 minutes.
- At this point, you can let the quinoa cool and refrigerate until you're ready to eat.
- Add in the chopped spinach, cilantro and lemon juice coated avocado when ready to serve.
- If you're like me and want to eat this for lunch in small portions, this is what I do: I portion out 1/2 cup of quinoa. Toss a big handful of chopped baby spinach leaves (you don't really have to chop them, I like to because I prefer to eat quinoa with a spoon and not a fork).Liberally sprinkle lemon juice over half a small avocado (I also add salt) and toss into the salad. Top with cilantro leaves.

73. Curried Red Quinoa, Peas And Paneer Salad

Serving: Serves 3 | Prep: | Cook: | Ready in:

Ingredients

- 1/2 cup red quinoa, cooked
- 2 tablespoons olive oil
- 1 teaspoon cumin seeds
- 1/2 teaspoon red chilly powder

- 3/4 cup peas
- 1/2 cup paneer
- 1 teaspoon garam masala
- 1 pinch kasturi methi (optional)
- 1 teaspoon lemon juice
- Salt and peper to taste

Direction

- Heat oil in a wok and add the cumin seeds. Once they crackle, add the ginger paste and spices.
- Tip in the peas and paneer and stir well to coat the spices on paneer and peas. Cook till the peas have softened. Add the garam masala and crushed kasturi methi.
- Add the cooked quinoa and toss well. Add lemon juice and season with salt and pepper.
- Serve warm or room temperature with yogurt. We serve it with a tablespoon of green chutney stirred in a cup of yogurt.

74. Curried Eggplant & Sweet Onion With Quinoa

Serving: Serves two. | Prep: | Cook: | Ready in:

Ingredients

- 1 small/medium eggplant
- 1 yellow onion
- 3 tablespoons coconut oil
- 1 teaspoon curry powder
- salt & pepper
- 1 cup cooked quinoa
- 2 tablespoons pinenuts

Direction

- Heat 3 tablespoons coconut oil over high heat.
- In the meanwhile, thinly slice onion into rings (about 1/4 inch; very thin!). Set aside.
- Half your eggplant, if using a whole eggplant. Then half it again, so that it's in quartered spears. Now thinly slice the eggplant, also 1/4 inch thick (it's not really important how you cut it; just make sure it's sliced thin- otherwise it will take forever to cook).
- When oil is hot (it will slide around the pan easily), add sliced eggplant and onion to the pan and lower the heat to medium-low. Sprinkle on the curry powder, and season generously with salt and pepper. Turn everything around gently with a spatula to make sure everything is evenly coated with oil and spices.
- Add a couple tablespoons of water to the pan, as it has probably already absorbed the oil. Turn the heat to very low and cover the pan (if you don't have a lid, use foil as I did).
- Cook over low heat for 25-30 minutes. Check every 5-10 minutes, turning the veggies so everything cooks evenly. If it seems very dry, add additional water.
- You can tell when the veggies are cooked when the eggplant is no longer opaque- it should look clear-ish and break easily with a spoon. Remove from heat. Taste and add additional salt if necessary.
- Remove eggplant and onions from pan and add pinenuts. Put the pan over high heat and shake around frequently for a couple minutes, until the pinenuts are toasty.
- Serve the eggplant and onions alongside your cooked quinoa. Garnish with toasted pinenuts and a little mint, as I did.

75. Curry Quinoa Pilaf With Roasted Butternut Squash And Raisin Mix

Serving: Serves 2 as a dish/ 4 as a side | Prep: | Cook: | Ready in:

Ingredients

- 1/2 butternut squash
- 1 tablespoon ground sea-salt
- 1 onion, finely chopped

- 2 garlic cloves, finely chopped
- 2 tablespoons extra virgin olive oil
- 1 tablespoon honey
- 1/2 tablespoon hot madras curry
- 1 cup quinoa grain
- 2 1/2 cups vegetable broth
- 2 tablespoons ghee
- 1/2 cup blonde raisins
- 1/2 cup dark raisins
- 1/4 cup pine-nuts

Direction

- 1. Cut the butternut squash into ½" inch dices and add the ground sea-salt
- 2. Preheat oven to 220 C and place the diced butternut squash on an oven tray lined with parchment paper for 20 minutes or until crisp and golden
- 3. In a pan, on medium fire, pour the 2 tbsp. extra virgin olive oil and sauté the chopped onion with the chopped garlic cloves
- 4. Add the honey and the curry and stir. Allow to cook for a minute
- 5. Wash the quinoa thoroughly, add to the pan and stir
- 6. Pour 2 cups of vegetable broth and allow to boil
- 7. Lower the fire and allow the liquid to evaporate, if necessary add ½ a cup more of the broth until the quinoa is tender
- 9. Add the raisins and the pine nuts and stir a few seconds until they are lightly toasted
- 10. In a serving bowl combine the curry quinoa pilaf with the roasted butternut squash
- 11. Add the raisin mix as a topping
- *For this presentation I molded the Curry Quinoa Pilaf with Roasted Butternut Squash and garnished it with the raisin mix as a topping

76. Dark Chocolate Cherry Quinoa Bark

Serving: Makes 1 tray | Prep: | Cook: | Ready in:

Ingredients

- 1/4 cup quinoa
- 6 ounces dark chocolate, roughly chopped
- 1/3 cup dried tart cherries, roughly chopped

Direction

- Heat a medium sized, high sided pot over medium-high heat until it's really hot (I actually found it most efficient to set the pan heating, then chop up the chocolate and cherries while I waited for it to come to temperature).
- Once pot is screaming hot, add the quinoa, making sure the seeds are spread evenly across the bottom of the pot. Reduce heat to medium, put a lid on the pot, and shake it to agitate the quinoa. If your pot is hot enough, you should start hearing the quinoa popping almost immediately (if not, keep heating and shaking the pot periodically until you hear popping). Continue shaking until you no longer hear popping. If it smells like the quinoa is getting too toasty, just remove pot from heat and continue shaking. Once popping has stopped, dump popped quinoa out onto a baking sheet to cool off.
- Place the chocolate in a microwave safe bowl and microwave for 30 second intervals, stirring after each, until chocolate is smoothly melted. Stir in the dried cherries and all but 1-2 tsps. of the popped quinoa.
- Place baking sheet in refrigerator to cool until chocolate has solidified (about 1 hour). Peel bark off of parchment paper and break into pieces. Store in an airtight container.

77. Double Chocolate Quinoa Brownies

Serving: Serves 16 | Prep: | Cook: | Ready in:

Ingredients

- 1 1/2 cups cooked quinoa (1/4 cup dry)
- 1/2 cup cocoa powder
- 2 flax eggs - 2 tbsp golden flaxseed meal + 6 tbsp water
- 1/4 cup coconut oil
- 3/4 cup almond butter
- 1/3 cup unsweetened applesauce
- 1/2 cup maple syrup
- 2 teaspoons almond extract
- 1/2 teaspoon sea salt
- 1/2 cup dark chocolate chips

Direction

- Prepare flax egg by combining flaxseed meal with water & sitting in the refrigerator for 30 minutes
- Preheat oven to 350 degrees
- Prepare an 8x8 baking dish with cooking spray if not non-stick
- In a large bowl or standing mixer, combine all ingredients and mix well
- Add batter to baking dish
- Bake 35-45 minutes until a toothpick can be removed cleanly
- Allow to cool in the pan 30 minutes before cutting
- Cut with a plastic knife for a clean cut

78. Double Corn, Quinoa & Cheddar Muffins

Serving: Makes 12 muffins | Prep: | Cook: | Ready in:

Ingredients

- 1 1/2 cups stone-ground cornmeal
- 1/2 cup quinoa flour
- 2 teaspoons sea or kosher salt
- 1/2 teaspoon black pepper
- 1 teaspoon baking powder
- 1/2 teaspoon baking soda
- 1 cup buttermilk
- 2 large eggs
- 4 ounces butter, melted
- 1 cup corn kernels, roasted
- 1 cup shredded sharp cheddar cheese
- 1/2 cup scallions, 1/4-inch dice, greens only

Direction

- Preheat the oven to 375 degrees. Fill a 12-cup muffin tin with liners. Spray the top with pan spray so that the muffins don't stick to it as they rise.
- Line a sheet pan with parchment. Spread a cup of thawed frozen corn kernels on it. Roast in oven until nicely browned, about 15 minutes. Remove from oven and allow to cool while mixing batter. Alternatively, husk a fresh ear of corn and roast it on the grill, then strip the kernels and toss them into your batter.
- Sift the dry ingredients together into a mixing bowl. Add the eggs, buttermilk, and melted butter. With a wooden spoon or a spatula, stir only until the dry ingredients are moistened. Add the corn, cheese, and scallions and stir to blend.
- Use an ice cream scoop to fill each muffin cup to the top. Bake until perfectly risen and golden brown, about 12-15 minutes. Remove from oven and allow cool for a few minutes. If you find that they are still a bit crumbly, don't worry -- they'll firm up as they cool.

79. Earthy Quinoa "Tabbouleh"

Serving: Serves 4 | Prep: | Cook: | Ready in:

Ingredients

- Qunioa, Sunburst Squash, Water, Kosher Salt

- 1/2 cup Quinoa
- 1 Sunburst Squash
- 1/2 teaspoon Kosher Salt
- 1 cup Water
- Kohlrabi, Anaheim Pepper, Pickling Cucumber, Radish, Fresh Shallot, Italian Flat Leaf Parsley, Extra Virgin Olive Oil, Lemon, Kosher Salt, Black Pepper, Red Pepper
- 1 Medium Kohlrabi
- 1 Pickling Cucumber (or Persian Cucumber)
- 1 Large Radish
- 1 Anaheim Pepper (very thin and very green)
- 1 Fresh Shallot or Scallion
- 1/3 cup Shelled Walnuts
- 2 tablespoons Fresh Lemon Juice
- 1 tablespoon Fresh Lemon Zest
- 3 tablespoons Very Good Extra Virgin Olive Oil
- Salt, Black Pepper, and Red Pepper (optional) to taste
- 1/3 cup Italian Flat Leaf Parsley, chopped coarsely

Direction

- Quinoa, Sunburst Squash, Water, Kosher Salt
- Rinse quinoa in cold water and strain well.
- Slice sunburst squash into about 10 wedges.
- Bring water to a boil, add salt, quinoa, and squash pieces, stir, cover, and simmer for 15 minutes. Once the quinoa has absorbed all the water, allow it to rest until it reaches room temperature (about 1/2 hour).
- Kohlrabi, Anaheim Pepper, Pickling Cucumber, Radish, Fresh Shallot, Italian Flat Leaf Parsley, Extra Virgin Olive Oil, Lemon, Kosher Salt, Black Pepper, Red Pepper
- Peel the kohlrabi and using a sharp knife cut into match-like "julienne" sticks.
- Cut cucumber in half, lengthwise, and slice into thin semi-circles.
- Cut radish into quarters, and similarly slice into thin quarter-circles.
- Remove seeds from Anaheim pepper at the stem, and slice the pepper into very thin rings.
- Slice and dice the fresh shallot (or scallion), including most of the green portion.
- Sprinkle a bit of salt on the sliced vegetables.
- Toast the walnuts for about 5 minutes in a dry frying pan, allow them to cool, and chop them very coarsely
- In a large bowl, combine the cooked quinoa and squash with all the chopped vegetables and walnuts. Toss gently and add olive oil, fresh lemon juice, fresh lemon zest, half the chopped parsley, salt, pepper, and optional red pepper. Taste and adjust seasonings, transfer to a serving dish, and garnish with remaining parsley.

80. Easy Greek Quinoa Salad With Shrimp

Serving: Serves 8 | Prep: | Cook: |Ready in:

Ingredients

- Greek Quinoa Salad with Shrimp
- 1 tablespoon olive oil
- 1 red pepper, chopped
- 1/2 cup chopped red onion
- 3/4 pound peeled and deveined shrimp (raw or cooked), chopped
- 1/2 cup chopped kalamata olives
- 4 teaspoons drained capers, lightly chopped
- 3/4 cup crumbled feta cheese
- 10 basil leaves, julienned
- 2 cups cooked quinoa
- 3/4 cup balsamic vinaigrette (recipe below)
- salt and freshly ground pepper to taste
- Balsamic Vinaigrette
- 2 tablespoons balsamic vinegar
- 1 tablespoon fresh squeezed lemon juice
- 1 tablespoon dijon mustard
- 1 clove of garlic, minced
- 1/3 cup olive oil
- salt and freshly ground pepper to taste

Direction

- Greek Quinoa Salad with Shrimp

- Sauté the red pepper and onion in olive oil until soft. Put in large bowl.
- Sauté the shrimp in the same pan (if raw, until cooked or if already cooked, just a few minutes for flavor). Add the shrimp to the bowl with the red pepper and onion. Let cool slightly.
- Add the remaining ingredients and then put in the fridge for at least 20 minutes so that it can chill and the flavors can marinate.
- Enjoy!
- Balsamic Vinaigrette
- Blend all ingredients in a blender to emulsify, or just add to a glass jar and shake until well incorporated.

81. Easy Quinoa Sweet Porridge

Serving: Serves 2 | Prep: | Cook: | Ready in:

Ingredients

- 1 cup water
- 1/2 cup quinoa, washed and ready
- 1/4 teaspoon sea salt
- 1/4 teaspoon ground nutmeg
- 1/4 teaspoon ground cloves
- 1/4 teaspoon ground cinnamon
- 1/4 cup raisins
- 1/2 tablespoon honey
- 1 handful chopped blanched almonds

Direction

- Bring water, quinoa, and salt to a boil in a small saucepan. Stir, cooking approximately 15 minutes, with spices and raisins. Cook until water is sufficiently absorbed and quinoa is fluffable.
- Stir in honey. Serve topped with chopped blanched almonds.

82. Easy Scallion, Green Pea And Lemon Quinoa Pilaf With Sesame Seeds

Serving: Serves 6-8 | Prep: | Cook: | Ready in:

Ingredients

- 1 cup organic Quinoa
- 2 cups vegetablebroth, chicken broth or water
- 1 1/2 cups defrosted frozen green peas
- juice of 2 lemons
- zest of one lemon
- 1/8-1/4 cups toasted sesame seeds
- 2 tablespoons walnut oil
- 3-4 scallions diced
- Pinch salt
- Pinch black pepper

Direction

- 1. Rinse Quinoa2. Cook Quinoa in broth or water3. Place cooked Quinoa in large bowl and add in sliced scallions, defrosted peas, lemon zest, lemon juice, walnut oil, toasted sesame seeds, salt and pepper.4. Good served chilled or warm.
- Great served with roasted vegetables or grilled fish etc.

83. Eat Your Peas & Carrots Quinoa Pasta (with Bacon!)

Serving: Serves 2 - 3 | Prep: | Cook: | Ready in:

Ingredients

- 3 slices bacon, cut crosswise into 1/2-inch pieces
- 2 medium carrots, peeled and finely chopped
- 1 leek (white and light green part only), halved lengthwise then cut crosswise into thin slices
- 1/4 teaspoon kosher salt
- 1/4 teaspoon freshly ground black pepper

- 1/2 cup half-and-half
- 1 teaspoon finely chopped fresh rosemar
- 8 ounces quinoa spaghetti or regular spaghetti
- 1/2 cup grated Parmesan cheese
- 1/3 cup frozen or fresh green peas

Direction

- In medium saucepot, cook bacon over medium heat 5 to 7 minutes or until crisp, stirring occasionally. Add carrots, leek, salt and pepper and cook 6 to 8 minutes or until carrots are softened, stirring occasionally. Add half-and-half and rosemary; heat to boiling. Reduce heat to medium-low and simmer 5 to 7 minutes or until sauce has thickened (should coat the back of a spoon); stirring occasionally. Remove from heat but keep in a warm place on the stove.
- Meanwhile, cook the pasta in salted water as the box instructs for al dente. Drain the pasta, but save about 2 cups of the cooking water.
- Add Parmesan, peas, pasta and 1 cup of pasta cooking water to sauce. Heat over medium heat, stirring constantly, until sauce completely coats pasta and peas are warmed through. Add more pasta cooking water as needed.

84. Edamame And Quinoa Salad

Serving: Serves 6 | Prep: | Cook: | Ready in:

Ingredients

- for the salad:
- 1 cup quinoa
- 2 cups water
- 1 cup edamame
- 1/2 cup thinly sliced radishes
- 4 scallions, thinly sliced
- 1/3 cup chopped parsley
- 2 tablespoons chopped mint
- 1/4 cup red onion, thinly sliced
- for the vinaigrette:
- zest and juice of 1 lemon
- 1 large clove garlic, minced
- 1 tablespoon red or white wine vinegar
- 1/4 cup olive oil
- 2 tablespoons chopped mint
- 1/2 teaspoon kosher salt
- 1/4 teaspoon black pepper

Direction

- Place the quinoa in a fine mesh strainer and rinse under running tap water. Transfer quinoa to a saucepan and add 2 cups water. Bring to a boil, cover and reduce heat to a simmer. Cook for 15 minutes or until quinoa is tender and spirals are visual on the surface. Remove from heat and let sit uncovered, until quinoa is at room temperature.
- Meanwhile, prepare the vegetables, slicing the onions, scallions, radish, parsley and mint and transferring them to a large bowl.
- In a small bowl, add all the ingredients for the vinaigrette and stir to combine.
- When quinoa is cool, fluff the quinoa with a fork and add it to the vegetables. Add the vinaigrette and toss to combine. Can be made ahead and served chilled or at room temperature.

85. Epic Quinoa Kale Salad With Orange Miso Dressing & Teriyaki Cashews

Serving: Serves 2-4 (main-starter) | Prep: | Cook: | Ready in:

Ingredients

- For the cashews
- 1 1/2 cups cashews
- 1/4 cup tamari (gluten free soy sauce)
- 2 tablespoons date paste (or maple syrup, honey...)
- 1/4 teaspoon chili powder
- 1/4 teaspoon sea salt

- For the salad & dressing
- 1/2 cup dried quinoa, white or red
- 1 cup water
- 1 bunch kale, thoroughly washed and dried
- 2 tablespoons sweet 'Shiro' miso (white mellow miso)
- 1/2 medium avocado, pitted and mashed
- 2 teaspoons date paste (or maple syrup, honey...)
- 1/8 teaspoon sea salt
- 2 pinches chili powder (or more if you like it hot)
- 2 handfuls sprouts, of your choice
- 1/4 cup orange juice, freshly squeezed
- 1 tablespoon Dijon mustard
- 2 tablespoons mellow white miso (I like sweet 'Shiro' miso)
- 1/2 tablespoon sesame oil, extra virgin
- 2 teaspoons date paste (or maple syrup, honey...)
- 1/4 teaspoon orange zest
- 1/8 teaspoon sea salt
- 2 pinches chili powder (or more if you like it hot)

Direction

- For the teriyaki cashews, combine tamari, date paste, chili powder and sea salt in a small mixing bowl, and stir well. Add the cashews and mix well until every cashew is covered with the marinade. Set aside for 15-30 minutes to allow the cashews to soak up the flavors. Place the marinated cashews on top of a Teflex covered dehydrator tray. Dehydrate at 115°F for 12 hours or longer. You can also just roast your cashews in a pan or a regular oven until they are crunchy. This recipe makes more teriyaki cashews than you need for one salad - they make a great snack & delicious pasta topping too!
- Using a fine mesh strainer, rinse your quinoa until the water is clear. Drain well. Combine rinsed quinoa, water and a pinch of sea salt in a pot. Turn on to medium heat and bring to a rolling boil. When the quinoa is simmering, cover it and reduce to low heat. Let it cook for another 15-20 minutes until all the water is absorbed. Turn off the heat and remove the pot from the burner. Let stand for 5 minutes, covered. After 5 minutes, remove the lid, fluff the quinoa gently with a fork, and let it cool down.
- Remove the stems from the kale, arrange the leaves in a flat pile and roll them up tightly. Slice into very thin strips and put into a large mixing bowl. By finally slicing your kale, it will be easier to digest, and you'll be able to absorb the nutrients more effectively too.
- Trim off the ends of the Brussels sprouts and remove the outer leaves. Cut the Brussels sprouts in half and mince. Finely chop the green onion. Add both to the mixing bowl, together with the mashed avocado, lemon juice and sea salt.
- Use your hands to mix everything together and 'massage' the kale salad by gently squeezing it between your fingers.
- Add pomegranate seeds, chilled quinoa, teriyaki cashews and sprouts of your choice.
- Make your dressing by combining orange juice, Dijon mustard, miso, sesame oil, date paste, orange zest, sea salt and chili powder in a small blender or food processor. Blend until smooth. Serve on top of the salad and enjoy immediately. Bon appétit!

86. Everything Bagel Quinoa Cakes With Smoked Salmon And Crème Fraîche

Serving: Serves 2 | Prep: | Cook: | Ready in:

Ingredients

- Everything Bagel Seasoning
- 2 teaspoons dried minced garlic
- 2 teaspoons poppy seeds
- 2 teaspoons sesame seeds
- 1 teaspoon caraway seeds
- 1 teaspoon kosher salt

- Quinoa Cakes
- 2 eggs
- 1 1/4 cups cooked quinoa, cooled
- 1/2 cup panko breadcrumbs
- 2 tablespoons shredded Parmesan cheese
- 1 tablespoon Everything Bagel Seasoning
- Nonstick cooking spray
- 3 ounces smoked salmon
- 1/3 cup crème fraîche or sour cream
- 1 tablespoon chopped fresh chives

Direction

- Make the Everything Bagel Seasoning: In small bowl, stir together all the ingredients. Store in an airtight container at room temperature until ready to use. You will have a little bit left over to sprinkle on other things.
- Make the Quinoa Cakes: In a medium bowl, lightly beat the eggs. Add the quinoa, breadcrumbs, and cheese; then stir until well combined. Form the mixture into four 1/2-inch thick cakes. Sprinkle both sides of the cakes with Everything Seasoning, then lightly pat to adhere.
- Heat a large nonstick skillet over medium-high heat. Spray skillet with cooking spray, then carefully add the cakes. Cook 4 to 6 minutes per side, or until cakes are golden brown.
- Serve quinoa cakes topped with smoked salmon, crème fraîche, and chives.

87. Everything I Want To Eat Quinoa And Lentil Salad

Serving: Serves 6 to 8 | Prep: | Cook: |Ready in:

Ingredients

- 1/4 cup tart dried cherries
- 2 tablespoons apple cider vinegar
- 3/4 cup dried brown lentils, rinsed
- 3 garlic cloves, divided
- 3/4 cup quinoa, rinsed
- 1 small/reasonably-sized sweet potato, peeled and cut into 1/4-inch cubes
- 1 small/reasonably-sized butternut squash, peeled and cut into 1/4-inch cubes
- 1 teaspoon ground coriander
- 1 teaspoon smoked paprika
- 1/2 teaspoon cayenne
- Olive oil, for roasting and seasoning
- Salt and pepper, for roasting and seasoning
- one 8-ounce package tempeh, cut in half widthwise, then cut into very thin (1/8-inch) strips
- 1 slice stale wheat bread, crumbled into small bits
- 1 handful sesame seeds
- 1/2 cup toasted sunflower seeds
- 1/3 cup chopped toasted pistachios
- 2 scallions, green parts only, finely chopped
- 1/2 cup crumbled ricotta salata
- Freshly squeezed lemon juice, for seasoning (you'll want at least 1 tablespoon)
- 1 avocado, cubed

Direction

- Preheat the oven to 425° F. In a small bowl, add the tart dried cherries, apple cider vinegar, and 2 tablespoons of hot water. Let the cherries plump up while you plow onwards.
- In a small saucepan, add the lentils, 1 1/2 cups water or vegetable broth, 1 crushed garlic clove, and a generous pinch of salt. Bring to a rapid simmer over medium-high heat, then reduce the heat and cook, uncovered, for 20 to 30 minutes, until the lentils are cooked but not soft or mushy. Add water as needed to keep the lentils barely covered.
- In another small saucepan (I know, I'm pushing it here!), add the quinoa and 1 1/2 cups water. Bring to a boil, then reduce the heat to low, cover the pot, and let it simmer for 15 minutes, or until the quinoa is finished (you'll see that the seed is translucent and the germ is a thin white circle around it).
- While the grainy and beany stuff cooks, it's time to roast the vegetables. Toss the squash

and the sweet potatoes with the coriander, paprika, cayenne, the 2 remaining garlic cloves, minced, and 1 to 2 tablespoons olive oil (you want the pieces to be well-coated but not swimming). Spread onto a parchment-lined baking sheet (or two) and bake for about 30 minutes, flipping vegetables once or twice during baking, until crisp and browned in areas.
- Tempeh time! Cut the block in half widthwise, then cut it into very thin (1/8-inch) strips. Coat the bottom of a pan in a thin layer of olive oil and, when hot, fry the tempeh until brown and crispy on each side (you might have to work in batches). Drain it on a plate lined with paper towels.
- When the tempeh is done, fry the bread pieces in the leftover tempeh oil until crisp and crunchy.
- HALLELUJAH: You're ready to assemble. In a big bowl, mix together the roasted vegetables, quinoa, and lentils. Drain the cherries and add those, along with the fried tempeh, bread pieces, sesame seeds, scallions, sunflower seeds, pistachios, and cheese. Season with lemon juice, olive oil, salt and pepper. Gingerly place avocado cubes on top, and season with a bit more salt.
- Reward yourself for you hard work!!!!

88. Flax And Quinoa Seed Bread (LC, GF)

Serving: Makes 2 small loaves | Prep: 0hours30mins | Cook: 0hours40mins | Ready in:

Ingredients

- 4 eggs
- 0.5 cups sour cream
- 2 tablespoons sweetener (Swerve granular)
- 1 tablespoon Italian Seasoning
- 1 teaspoon rosemary leaves
- 0.75 cups parmesan cheese (shredded)
- 1.25 cups flaxseed meal
- 1 cup quinoa flour
- 2.5 tablespoons baking powder
- some sesame seeds
- some caraway seeds
- some low salt sunflower seeds

Direction

- Combine well the wet ingredients and herbs
- Add the dry ingredients (baking powder last)
- Ladle out into 2 EVOO-sprayed small loaf pans
- Bake for 35-40 minutes at 325F
- Turn out and cool on a rack

89. Flourless Quinoa Chocolate Cake

Serving: Serves 8 | Prep: | Cook: | Ready in:

Ingredients

- For the Cake
- 1/2 cup plain almond yogurt (or plain yogurt of choice)
- 4 large eggs
- 1 teaspoon pure vanilla extract
- 2 cups Alter Eco Royal Pearl Quinoa
- 3/4 cup melted coconut oil
- 3/4 cup raw honey
- 2 bars of Alter Eco Blackout
- 1 1/2 teaspoons baking powder
- 1/2 teaspoon baking soda
- For the Vegan Frosting
- 3/4 cup mashed sweet potato
- 1/4 cup maple syrup
- 3 tablespoons melted coconut oil
- 2 tablespoons unsweetened applesauce
- 2 tablespoons cocoa powder
- 1 tablespoon tapioca starch
- 2 teaspoons vanilla
- 1/4 teaspoon fine sea salt

Direction

- Preheat oven to 350°F. Grease a 9-inch springform pan with non-stick cooking spray and line the bottom with parchment paper.
- Combine yogurt, eggs and vanilla in a food processor fit with the steel blade, and process until smooth. Add quinoa, oil and honey, and process until fully combined and as smooth as possible, 2 – 3 minutes.
- Whisk together dry ingredients in a separate mixing bowl. Melt chocolate and add wet ingredients to the dry mix until combined.
- Transfer batter to the prepared pan and bake for 40 – 45 minutes, until a cake tester inserted into the center comes out clean.
- While the cake is cooking, prepare frosting by adding all ingredients to a food processor and blending until smooth. Let frosting cool before covering the cake.
- Remove cake from the oven and let it cool completely in the pan, then transfer to a wire rack.
- When completely cooled, carefully slice the cake in half, making two layers. Frost the top of the bottom layer, then add the top layer and frost the rest of the cake.

90. Fresh Stuffed Red Pepper Shells With Pearl Couscous, Forbidden Rice, Kamut Or Red Quinoa

Serving: Serves 4 or even 8 (with half portions) | Prep: | Cook: | Ready in:

Ingredients

- 4 sweet select red peppers
- 2-3 cups whole grains, soaked and then cooked accordingly, such as forbidden rice, pearl couscous, kamut, or red quinoa
- 2 teaspoons cumin, optional
- 1/4 teaspoon tumeric, optional
- 1 cup feta or similar cheese
- 1 ounce toasted pinion pine nuts, almonds, or pecans
- 4 tablespoons fresh chopped mixed herbs, such as mint, basil, parsley and cilantro
- 1 teaspoon pink or kosher salt
- 1-2 tablespoons chopped scallions
- 1-2 tablespoons dried currants, yellow raisins or cranberries, optional
- 2 tablespoons grated carrot and fresh ginger
- 4 tablespoons EVOO
- juice of a fresh lemon or lime
- 1 tablespoon champagne vinegar
- 1 teaspoon dijon mustard
- 1 tablespoon sweet or hot pepper jelly, or honey
- salt, paprika and pepper to taste
- paprika for garnish
- fresh herbs for garnish

Direction

- Cut the tops of the peppers and take out all the seeds as well as the white fleshy interior bits. Cut triangles out of the top of the pepper saving the cuts for use in the filling. (You can bisect or even trisect the remaining triangle border of the pepper shell for effect if desired. This can also make eating easier with these pre-cuts).
- Mix your cooked grains of choice with feta and whatever other fillings and seasonings you want to include in a bowl. Be sure to add the leftover red pepper triangles diced further into the filling. I have used turmeric and cumin with the pearl couscous in one version, but not in the forbidden rice version.
- Mix the oil, juice, mustard, jelly or honey, vinegar with salt, paprika, and pepper to taste for the dressing. Pour this over the grain salad filling and lightly toss. Adjust the seasoning if needed.
- Fill each cut pepper with the grain filling. Garnish with fresh herbs and paprika. You can serve whole or even consider slicing these in half.

91. Fried Quinoa, Apples, Beets & Herbs

Serving: Serves 4 | Prep: 0hours45mins | Cook: 0hours10mins | Ready in:

Ingredients

- 1 cup black or red quinoa, rinsed
- 1 cup beets, peeled, julienned (about 2 medium)
- 1 cup carrots, peeled, julienned (about 3 large)
- 2 apples, julienned
- 1/2 lemon
- 1/4 cup brown or turbinado sugar (white would be fine as well)
- 1/4 cup sherry vinegar
- 1/2 cup water
- 1 orange
- 1/2 teaspoon salt
- pepper
- 1 tablespoon chives or green onions
- 2 tablespoons walnut oil
- 1/4 teaspoon coriander, toasted, ground
- 1/4 teaspoon aleppo or red chile
- 1/4 teaspoon dijon mustard

Direction

- Heat oven to 400. Bring quinoa to a boil in 3-4 cups salted water and cook 10 minutes. Drain and then let sit, covered for about 10 minutes. Drizzle with oil, toss to coat, spread out on a baking sheet and bake 10-15 minutes until crunchy. Can be made ahead and kept in an airtight container in the fridge.
- Toss carrots and apples together, cover with water. Squeeze lemon into bowl, add peel and chill in fridge (up to a day).
- Simmer vinegar, sugar, water, salt and 4 thick strips of zest from orange until sugar is dissolved then let cool. Pour over beets and chill at least an hour and up to two days.
- Heat about 1/2" vegetable oil in a small pot and working in batches, fry quinoa. Drain on paper towel and salt lightly.
- Mix 2 T juice from orange with mustard, chives, coriander, chili and salt to taste. Whisk in walnut oil until emulsified.
- Drain carrots and apples pressing gently. Drain beets. Toss together with dressing and parsley. Stir in quinoa just before serving.

92. Garden Herbed Quinoa

Serving: Serves 4 | Prep: | Cook: | Ready in:

Ingredients

- 1 cup quinoa
- 1/3 cup cilantro
- 1/3 cup parsley
- 1/3 cup basil
- 4 tablespoons extra virgin olive oil
- 1 lemon (juice)

Direction

- Add 1 cup Quinoa to 2 cups boiling water until water evaporates- med to low heat for 10+ min.
- Wash and remove stems from herbs.
- Add juice from lemon, olive oil, and herbs in a food processor and grind together. Once your quinoa has absorbed all the water, stir in herb mixture until it is well combined.

93. Garden Tomato, Ceci And Black Pepper Feta Quinoa

Serving: Serves 6 | Prep: | Cook: | Ready in:

Ingredients

- 1 cup organic quinoa
- 1/8 teaspoon salt

- 1 3/4 cups water
- 1 cup canned ceci beans (garbanzo), drained
- 2 large garden tomatoes, chopped
- 1 clove garlic, minced
- 4 tablespoons lime juice
- 4 teaspoons lemon juice
- 5 tablespoons extra virgin olive oil
- 1/2 teaspoon ground cumin
- Pinch of sea salt and fresh black pepper to taste
- 1/2 teaspoon of dried oregano
- 1/2 cup of crumbled black pepper feta
- 1 stalk of celery chopped
- 2 tablespoons of red wine vinegar

Direction

- Place the quinoa in a fine mesh strainer and rinse under cold water until the water no longer foams. Bring the quinoa, salt and water to a boil in a saucepan. Reduce heat to medium-low cover and simmer until the quinoa is tender about 20-25 minutes.
- Once done, stir in the ceci beans and garden tomatoes (marinated in olive oil, salt, oregano and red wine vinegar), garlic, lemon and lime juice, and olive oil. Add in crumbled black pepper feta cheese (I discovered this at Whole Foods). Then season with cumin, salt, and pepper. Add tortilla chips for presentation and to serve.

94. Garlic Roasted Vegetables And Quinoa

Serving: Serves 10 | Prep: | Cook: |Ready in:

Ingredients

- Garlic Roasted Vegetables
- 2-3 Yellow Squash
- 2-3 Green zucchini
- 1-2 handfuls Fresh Green Beans
- 1 Large Red Bell Pepper
- 2-3 tablespoons Fresh Chopped Garlic
- Splash Olive Oil
- Pinch Sea Salt
- Pinch Black Pepper
- Garlic Quinoa
- 1 cup Rinsed Quinoa
- 2 cups Organic Chicken Broth
- 1 tablespoon Fresh Chopped Garlic
- Splash Olive Oil
- Dash Black Pepper

Direction

- Garlic Roasted Vegetables
- Preheat oven at 400 degrees
- Rinse Vegetables and remove stems.
- Chop Squash, Zucchini, Red Bell Pepper, Green Beans (I leave my green beans long & un-cut) & garlic
- In large bowl add Chopped squash, zucchini, red bell pepper, green beans, & garlic. Coat vegetables in Olive oil generously, Add salt & pepper.
- Pour coated vegetables on a cooking sheet, spread vegetables out evenly (it's okay if some are layered) on the sheet.
- Put in pre-heated 400 degree oven & cook for 45 mins until edges are golden brown or depending on how you like you vegetables.
- Garlic Quinoa
- Rinse 1 cup of Quinoa for at least 2 mins.
- Add Two Cups of Chicken broth to Pot * bring to a simmer
- Add Quinoa, Garlic, Olive Oil, Black pepper to Simmering Chicken Broth.
- Simmer & Cover, Cook for 10 mins (or whatever the quinoa cooking directions say.)
- When done Cooking add In the Garlic Roasted Vegetables toss & serve Hot or Cold!

95. Georgian Quinoa Salad With Eggplant & Sour Cherries

Serving: Serves 4 | Prep: | Cook: |Ready in:

Ingredients

- Salad
- 1/2 cup dried tart or sour cherries
- 2 teaspoons pomegranate molasses
- 1/2 cup water
- 1 pound small eggplants
- 3 cloves garlic
- 1/2 teaspoon salt
- 1 tablespoon sweet paprika
- 1 pinch cayenne (to taste)
- 2-3 tablespoons olive oil
- 4 scallions, slivered, greens and all
- 1/2 cup toasted walnuts, chopped
- 1/2 cup parsley, chopped (I permit you to use curly leaves)
- Salad greens of choice
- 1 cup quinoa
- 2 cups water
- Dressing
- 1 tablespoon freshly squeezed lime juice
- 1/2 teaspoon pomegranate molasses
- 1 teaspoon Pedro Ximenez or Spanish sherry vinegar
- 1/4 cup preferred salad oil (see below)
- 1 pinch sugar
- salt and pepper to taste

Direction

- Dissolve pomegranate molasses in half a cup of hot water before adding sour cherries. Leave them to plump and assume a tarter, intriguing flavor as they grow increasingly unattractive.
- Dump spices, salt and garlic in bowl large enough to accommodate eggplant before dicing the latter into half-inch cubes and, let's face it, polygons, given rounded sides. I favor white eggplants from the farmers market, but thin Asian or Graffiti work well, too. The object is to use a variety with thin skins that becomes tender rather quickly. Once you've done with the knife, throw eggplant into bowl and coat with seasonings. Or hand a wooden spoon to a child and let him do it; it's fun.
- Meanwhile, place the enameled Dutch oven you bought for No-Knead bread on the stove to heat a few minutes, then raise heat to medium high and add enough olive oil to coat the bottom of pan. When you think the fat is hot enough, toss in a piece of eggplant just to make sure it sizzles. Okay? Then start adding the rest of eggplant bit by bit. Stir with your wooden spoon from time to time. The eggplant should turn golden and soft in 10 minutes or so.
- Then, read this carefully: reserve soaking water from tart cherries as you drain them. Add a little more water if necessary to measure half a cup and add this to eggplant. Turn down heat to medium low and cover, letting eggplant stew until tender. Check in 5 minutes, then again in 10. Uncover and let any excess water evaporate before turning off burner and draining eggplant on paper towel.
- As eggplant cools, prepare the quinoa. I recommend running it under cold water and straining the grains just like everyone else does. I also belong to the toasting school and think a minute of stirring the strained quinoa in a pot with a thick bottom until the tiny seeds that didn't remain stuck to your strainer, fingers and stove top become dry. No need to coat them with oil first, though, you could. Add 2 cups boiling water and simmer, covered, 15 minutes. When water is fully absorbed and you see your cute little spirals, remove lid briefly to place clean dishtowel in between top of the pot and the lid. Let this contraption sit a spell off the burner as steam rises to become one with fabric and as you move on to final things.
- Mix dressing. Here's where I am going to leave matters up to you and ask you to just keep stirring vigorously as you emulsify and combine ingredients to your liking. Start with only a wee bit of pomegranate molasses as recommended and the same, trifling amount of Spanish vinegar. A strong, bitter olive oil is going to make this taste ghastly, but do not despair. Pinch of sugar and a glug of neutral oil (Bittman dislikes canola, but not me) evens

out disparate elements and as you adjust, there will be a joyful "ah!" moment. Go with that. The point is to retain that original citrus accent and don't let the molasses play more than a very minor role.

- Assemble salad by dressing a bed of greens first. Pour the remain dressing over the cooled eggplant and combine your nightshade family-member with fork-fluffed grains. Coarsely chop cherries and mix with the remaining ingredients before serving all on the bed of greens.

96. Golden Quinoa Cakes With Salsa Fresca

Serving: Makes twelve 3- to 4-inch cakes, or many bite-sized ones | Prep: 0hours20mins | Cook: 0hours40mins | Ready in:

Ingredients

- For golden quinoa cakes
- 1 Hatch chile
- 1/2 teaspoon whole coriander seed
- 1/2 teaspoon whole cumin seed
- 1 1/2 tablespoons unsalted butter
- 1 cup quinoa
- 2 cups water
- 1 pinch kosher salt
- 2 large eggs
- 3 tablespoons buttermilk
- 1/2 cup green onion, sliced
- 1 large garlic clove, minced
- 1/2 cup cheddar, grated
- 1/2 teaspoon kosher salt
- 1/4 cup sweet rice flour (also labeled "Mochiko")
- 1 splash canola oil for frying the cakes
- For the salsa fresca
- 2 French breakfast radishes, diced (or 4 round radishes, diced)
- 8 to 10 sweet cherry or pear tomatoes, diced
- 1/2 avocado, diced
- 1/4 cup lemon juice
- 1 pinch kosher salt, to taste
- 1/4 cup cilantro, chopped
- 1 tablespoon sour cream

Direction

- Preheat your broiler and roast the chile (might as well roast a few and then freeze for use in another recipe, like Huevos Rancheros) until wrinkled and blackened, turning once. Place roasted chile in a heat-proof bowl and cover with plastic wrap to make it easier to remove the skin. When cool, carefully remove skin (the tip of a sharp knife is helpful), stem, and as much of the membrane and seeds as you'd like -- keeping more will yield a spicier result. Dice chile, using gloves if desired.
- While chile is roasting, toast whole coriander and cumin over medium heat, until fragrant, in a Dutch oven or similar pot. Transfer whole spices to a bowl and crush with the back of a spoon or pestle.
- Place Dutch oven back onto the burner and melt butter, stirring, until it begins to brown and smells nutty. Add quinoa and stir, constantly, until it begins to get golden and toasty. At this point I always think it smells a little bit like deliciously roasted cheese.
- Add two cups of water, crushed whole spices, and a good pinch of salt. Bring mixture to a boil, cover, and lower heat to a simmer. Cook until quinoa is tender and water is absorbed, about 15 to 17 minutes. Spread hot quinoa out on a large rimmed baking sheet to cool.
- In a large bowl, combine the cooled quinoa, the diced Hatch chile, and the remaining ingredients (from egg through sweet rice flour). Stir to thoroughly combine and then let mixture sit for a few minutes to hydrate the flour.
- Meanwhile, combine radishes, tomatoes, avocado, and lemon in a bowl. Add salt to taste and let mixture sit until ready to eat.
- Heat a large skillet over medium heat with 1 tablespoon of canola oil. Set out a large rimmed baking sheet lined with wax paper. If

you want to make larger (3- to 4-inch) cakes, scoop quinoa mixture with a quarter cup measure, tap against your open palm to release, and then flatten the cake with the back of the cup measure before placing on the waxed paper. Repeat with remaining cake mixture. For bite-sized cakes, use a tablespoon to scoop and flatten the mixture.
- Cook the cakes in the skillet for about 3 minutes per side, until crisp and golden. Transfer to a serving platter. Continue cooking the remaining cakes, using additional oil if necessary.
- Right before serving, stir cilantro and sour cream in to salsa fresca. Top cakes with salsa fresca and enjoy.

97. Gourmet Vegetarian Pâté With Walnuts And Quinoa

Serving: Serves a crowd | Prep: | Cook: |Ready in:

Ingredients

- • 2 cups homemade or store-bought low-sodium organic vegetable stock
- • A large pinch of saffron threads
- • 3/4 cups organic white quinoa, well rinsed in cold water and thoroughly drained
- • 3/4 cups organic Green French lentils
- • 1/4 cups pure olive oil
- • 2 large Vidalia or other sweet onion, diced
- • A generous splash or two of good quality dry white wine
- • 1 heaping cup walnuts, toasted
- • Kosher or Sea coarse salt + freshly ground black or white pepper
- • 3 large hard boiled eggs, coarsely chopped + 1more hard boiled egg
- • 2 teaspoons Dijon or Spicy Brown mustard
- • 1/4 cups freshly chopped parsley

Direction

- In a medium saucepan combine the vegetable stock and saffron threads. Add and mix in the quinoa and lentils. Bring to simmer over medium heat, reduce to low, cover and cook until each grain of quinoa is translucent, white germ is clearly visible, lentils are tender and the stock is completely absorbed, about 20 to 22 minutes. Let stand until ready to use.
- Heat oil in a large sauté pan over medium-low heat. Add onions, season with salt and pepper and slowly sauté them, adding the wine halfway through and then continue cooking until deeply caramelized, but not burned, about 40 to 50 minutes. Let cool in the pan.
- While the onions are cooling slightly, grind the walnuts in food processor to a fine paste and transfer to a large mixing bowl.
- Working in batches, start adding the quinoa and lentil mixture, the 3 chopped cooked eggs and the caramelized onions to the food processor. Pulse and then process until smooth.
- Add this pureed mixture into the bowl with walnut paste, add mustard and mix everything together until homogeneous mixture forms. Taste and add salt, pepper or mustard if needed.
- Line an 8-by-4-inches loaf pan with plastic wrap, allowing about 3 inches to hang over each long side. Spoon the pate into the loaf pan, smooth the top and fold plastic over top. Top with something heavy and refrigerate for at least 4 to 5 hours or overnight. Can be made a few days in advance and kept refrigerated.
- When ready to serve, unwrap the top, and invert Pate onto a rectangular platter. Bring to room temperature. Shred the remaining cooked egg on a large hole side of a box grater and mix it with parsley, add a little salt and freshly ground pepper (garnish should be tasty also) and sprinkle on the top.
- Serve with toasts or crackers or use only yolks in the filling, stuff the whites and you'll have delicious vegetarian Deviled Eggs.

98. Greek Quinoa Salad

Serving: Serves 8 | Prep: | Cook: | Ready in:

Ingredients

- Dressing
- 1/4 cup olive oil
- 1 small spring fresh oregano
- 1 clove garlic, grated
- 2 lemons, juiced
- Salt to taste
- Salad
- 1 cup cherry tomatoes cut in half
- 2 small Persian cucumbers, cubed
- 6 ounces Feta cheese, crumbled
- 1 red bell pepper, diced
- 1/4 cup red onion, diced
- 1 cup pitted kalamata black olives
- 1/2 cup Italian parsley, chopped
- 1 cup quinoa, cooked according to package

Direction

- In a small bowl or Mason jar, add dressing ingredients and whisk or shake – set a side.
- In a large bowl, toss the chopped salad ingredients together, add the quinoa, pour dressing on top, and mix. Salad is best if it sits out at room temperature for 30 minutes prior to serving.

99. Greek Salad And Parsley Tabbouleh With Quinoa

Serving: Serves 2-3 | Prep: | Cook: | Ready in:

Ingredients

- Parsley quinoa
- 1/2 cup uncooked quinoa
- 2 cups water
- 1 bunch fresh parsley
- 1/2 lemon
- olive oil
- salt and pepper
- Greek salad
- 1 bowl of parsley quinoa
- 2 peppers
- 1 avocado
- 1/2 cucumber
- 2 handfuls arugula
- feta
- cider vinegar or lemon juice
- olive oil
- salt and pepper

Direction

- Parsley quinoa
- Cook your quinoa in 2 cups of water approximately 15 minutes over medium heat. Once cooked, let it cool.
- Cut your parsley in more or less big pieces. It depends of your tastes if you prefer big pieces or not.
- In a bowl, mix the quinoa and the parsley with a fork, season with 2 tbsps. of olive oil, add the juice of 1/2 lemon, and salt pepper.
- Greek salad
- Bake your peppers, cut there in two pieces, remove membranes and pips and put them on a cooktop. Put in the oven in 350°F (180°C) during 30 minutes. When you perceive that the skin forms blisters, take out them of the oven and put them in a plastic bag which you will close. Leave 10 minutes. You can then remove the skin in all simplicity. Peppers will be also tender and delicious!
- Take your bowls or plates and set your plates with 1/2 bowl of quinoa for each, peppers cut in small strips, cucumber in slices, avocado, the arugula and feta cheese.
- Season with 1 tbsp. cider vinegar (or lemon juice), 2 tbsps. olive oil, salt and pepper.
- Note that you can also marinate the peppers slices overnight in balsamic vinegar and olive oil. It will be delicious!

100. Green Quinoa Patties

Serving: Makes approximately 25 patties | Prep: | Cook: | Ready in:

Ingredients

- 2 cups Organic Quinoa
- 1 packet Organic Spinach (large clamshell, about 11 oz), chopped finely
- 2 Large Zucchinis, grated
- 2 Large Leeks, chopped finely
- 2 Organic Eggs
- 1 teaspoon Cayenne Pepper, or more if you like spice!
- 1 dash Chili Flakes
- 1 cup Goat Cheese (or 1 10 oz package)
- 1 teaspoon Olive Oil
- 1 dash Salt
- 1 dash Pepper

Direction

- Rinse quinoa. Bring 4 cups of salter water to a boil and add quinoa. Cook covered for 15 minutes. Let stand for 5 minutes, covered, and transfer to a bowl to cool.
- Heat olive oil in a large sauté pan. Add chopped leeks and sauté with salt and pepper until soft but not brown. Add zucchini and sauté for about 2 minutes. Add spinach and let wilt. Allow vegetable mixture to cool.
- Combine quinoa and vegetable mixture together in a large mixing bowl. Add eggs, goat cheese, cayenne, and chili flakes. Combine thoroughly. Season with salt and pepper to taste.
- Fill a quarter cup measurement with quinoa mixture. Place upside down on a lined baking sheet to form patty shape (the same way you may build a sand castle!). If the quinoa is not sliding out easily, rinse the measuring cup with water between each patty. Continue until all patties are formed.
- Bake for about 40 minutes at 400 degrees, or until brown and crispy.

101. Grilled Avocado Halves With Cumin Spiced Quinoa And Black Bean Salad

Serving: Serves 4 to 6 | Prep: | Cook: | Ready in:

Ingredients

- For the grilled avocados:
- 3 avocados
- 1 to 2 tablespoons olive oil
- 2 lemons, juiced
- Salt and pepper, to taste
- For the cumin-spiced quinoa and black bean salad:
- 1 cup dry quinoa
- 3 tablespoons extra-virgin olive oil
- 2 tablespoons apple cider vinegar
- 2 teaspoons maple syrup
- 2 teaspoons Dijon mustard
- 1 teaspoon ground cumin
- 1/2 teaspoon salt
- black pepper, to taste
- 1 cup diced cucumber
- 1 cup diced red bell pepper (or substitute cherry tomatoes)
- 1/2 cup raw corn kernels (from about 1 ear)
- 1 1/2 cups cooked black beans (or 1 can beans, rinsed)
- 10 to 15 basil leaves, cut in a chiffonade
- 1/4 cup chopped fresh cilantro, plus extra for garnish

Direction

- Lightly oil your grill or grill pan and set over medium heat.
- Rinse the quinoa through a fine sieve for about a minute. Place quinoa in a medium sized pot with 2 cups of water and a pinch of salt. Bring the water to boil, then reduce it to a simmer. Cover the quinoa and simmer for 15 minutes, or until all of the liquid has been absorbed. Fluff the quinoa with a fork and allow it to rest, covered, for 10 minutes.

- While the quinoa cooks, cut the avocados in half and remove the pits. Brush the avocados lightly with olive oil and drizzle with lemon juice. Sprinkle them with salt and pepper. Place the avocados, cut side down, on the grill. Allow them to cook for 5 minutes, or until they have nice grill marks. Remove them from heat and set aside.
- In a small bowl, whisk together the olive oil, vinegar, maple syrup, mustard, cumin, salt, and pepper to taste.
- To a large mixing bowl, add the cooked quinoa, cucumber, pepper, corn, black beans, basil, and cilantro. Dress the salad and toss gently. Season to taste.
- Fill each avocado half till it's brimming over with a cup of quinoa salad. Serve, garnished with extra cilantro if desired.

102. Grilled Pineapple And Red Curry Quinoa

Serving: Serves 4 | Prep: | Cook: | Ready in:

Ingredients

- 210 grams quinoa
- 500 milliliters water
- 1 piece stalk lemongrass
- 1,5 teaspoons salt
- 150 grams pineapple slices
- 14 grams fresh basil leaves, chopped
- 14 grams fresh mint leaves, chopped
- 2 teaspoons red curry paste
- 2 tablespoons coconut oil
- 62,5 milliliters olive oil
- 2 teaspoons lime juice
- 2 pieces kaffir lime leaves

Direction

- Combine water, lemongrass, kaffir lime leaves, 1 teaspoon salt and 1 tbsp. coconut oil in a pot and bring to a boil.
- Add quinoa, reduce heat to low, cover, and simmer for 15 minutes.
- Leave lid on for another 5 minutes.
- Fluff cooked quinoa with a fork. Discard lemongrass and kaffir.
- Set pineapple slices on a grill set to 220C/430F. Char for 3 minutes on each side. Chop into bit-size chunks.
- Whisk red curry paste, lime juice, 1 tbsp. coconut oil, olive oil, and 1/2 teaspoon salt in a bowl.
- Toss cooked quinoa, pineapples, dressing, basil, and cilantro in a bowl.

103. Guacamole Quinoa

Serving: Serves 4 | Prep: | Cook: | Ready in:

Ingredients

- 1 ripe avocado, pitted, peeled, and diced
- Juice of 1 1/2 limes
- 1/4 teaspoon kosher salt
- 3 cups cooked quinoa
- 1 garlic clove, crushed with a press or minced and ground into a paste
- 1 Roma tomato, diced
- 1/2 jalapeño pepper, seeded and minced (I only add SOME of the seeds to the dish. Do as you please).
- 1/4 cup chopped fresh cilantro
- 1/4 cup diced red onion
- 1/4 teaspoon ground cumin
- 1/2 teaspoon cayenne

Direction

- In a medium bowl, mash together avocado, lime juice, and salt. Add remaining ingredients, then toss to combine well. Serve warm or cold.

104. Harissa Steak & Eggs With Quinoa Tabbouleh Hash

Serving: Serves 2 | Prep: | Cook: | Ready in:

Ingredients

- For Hash:
- russet or Yukon gold potatoes
- 1 small yellow onion, diced
- 1 green bell pepper, diced
- 2 cloves garlic
- 2 tablespoons olive oil
- 1/2 stick butter
- salt and pepper to taste
- 1/2 cup quinoa tabbouleh
- 1/2 tablespoon za'atar seasoning
- For Steak:
- 2 strip steaks
- 1/2 cup Harissa
- olive oil
- butter
- salt and pepper to taste

Direction

- Place the whole potatoes in a large pot, cover with water, and bring to a boil. Lower the heat and simmer until half-cooked and almost tender, about 15 minutes. Drain and let sit until cool enough to handle. Cut into a 1/2-inch dice.
- Heat the oil and melt the butter in a skillet over high heat. Add the onions and peppers and cook, stirring, for 2 minutes. Add the garlic, and cook, stirring, for another minute or two. Add the potatoes, salt, and pepper, and cook without stirring, but shaking the pan occasionally to keep from burning, until the potatoes begin to color and crisp on the underside, about 4 minutes. Turn the potatoes with a spatula being careful not to mash, and continue cooking until uniformly golden. Stir in quinoa tabbouleh and top with za'atar seasoning.
- Heat cast iron skillet over high heat.
- Lightly brush the steaks on both sides with oil and season evenly with salt, pepper, and harissa. Allow the steaks to stand at room temperature for 15 to 30 minutes.
- Bring cast iron skillet to medium-high heat and sear steak on both sides, 4-5 minutes per side for medium-rare (or to your preference).
- Prepare quick-scrambled eggs and serve steak with eggs and hash browns. Enjoy!

105. Harvest Quinoa And Mixed Veggie Salad

Serving: Serves 6-8 | Prep: | Cook: | Ready in:

Ingredients

- 1 cup quinoa
- 1 1/2 cups cherry or grape tomatoes, quartered
- 1 kirby or small cucumber peeled (if not organic), seeded, and cut into small dice
- 1/3 cup crumbled feta
- 2 ears of corn, blanched and cut off cob...or cut the kernels off the cob and microwave for 30 seconds or so
- 1/4 cup olive oil, enough to moisten and flavor
- juice and finely grated zest of half a lemon or more zest
- 1/4 cup finely minced red onion
- 5 sliced peppadew peppers with 2 tablespoon of their juice
- 1/2 cup or more chopped Italian parsley
- 1/2 cup or more chopped cilantro
- sea salt and freshly ground pepper to taste

Direction

- COOK THE QUINOA: Toast the quinoa over medium heat in a medium saucepan for five minutes, stirring. This is step is optional but does bring out the nutty flavor of the grain. Add 2 cups of water and bring to a boil. Cover and reduce to a simmer. Cook until the grains

have become translucent and begun to split apart, about 10 minutes. Cool completely and set aside.
- In a large salad bowl mix the lemon juice and zest and olive oil with all the ingredients except the quinoa and the cheese.
- Toss in the cooled quinoa and then the cheese.
- Taste and adjust seasonings….you may need pepper, salt, oil, and/or lemon juice.
- This salad keeps for several days covered and refrigerated and is best if let to sit at least an hour before serving.

106. Heirloom Tomato, Basil And Goat Cheese "Pie" (With A Rice, Millet, And Quinoa Crust)

Serving: Serves 6-8 | Prep: | Cook: | Ready in:

Ingredients

- Brown Rice, Millet, and Quinoa Crust
- 1/3 cup short grain brown rice
- 1/3 cup millet
- 1/3 cup quinoa
- 2 1/2 cups water
- 2 tablespoons olive oil
- 1/2 tablespoon honey
- 1 teaspoon sea salt
- Tomato Pie
- 1 prebaked rice, millet, and quinoa crust (see above)
- 3-4 large tomatoes (or 2-3 large tomatoes and several smaller tomatoes)
- about 20 fresh basil leaves
- 1/2 cup crumbled goat cheese (you could also use feta or sliced mozzarella), or more to taste
- olive oil

Direction

- Brown Rice, Millet, and Quinoa Crust
- Combine brown rice, millet, and quinoa with water. Bring to a boil, cover and reduce heat to a simmer, and cook until water is absorbed and the grains and quinoa are tender (or prepare in a rice cooker, like I did).
- Allow to cool and add olive oil, honey, and salt. Mix well and press evenly into a deep-dish pie plate.
- Bake in a 300-degree oven for 40 minutes. Remove from oven and allow to cool.
- Tomato Pie
- Slice tomatoes and layer them in the pie, alternating layers with basil leaves, crumbled goat cheese, and a drizzle of olive oil. If your tomatoes are different colors, you can make 1 layer for each color. I sliced my tomatoes fairly thick, so I had three total tomato layers (if you slice them thinner, you might end up with more).
- Bake in a 300-degree oven for 30-40 minutes, until crust is brown and tomatoes and cheese are cooked and bubbly.

107. Heirloom Tomato Avocado Quinoa Lettuce Wraps

Serving: Serves 4 | Prep: | Cook: | Ready in:

Ingredients

- 3 Heirloom tomatoes - chopped
- 1 avocado - chopped
- 1 cup uncooked quinoa - makes ~2 cups cooked quinoa (I used black and red quinoa)
- juice of 1 lime
- 2 tablespoons chopped cilantro
- salt and pepper, to taste
- 1 head of butter lettuce

Direction

- In a mixing bowl, toss the chopped tomatoes, avocado, cilantro, salt, pepper and lime juice. Once everything is mixed and coated well with the condiments, refrigerate the mixture while you cook the quinoa. You want all the flavors to seep into the veggies.

- Cook the quinoa as directed on the box/bag it came in. I usually cook it in water (1 cup uncooked quinoa to 1 1/4 cup water) and add some salt and a slice of lemon or lime to flavor it.
- Wash and dry the lettuce and set the individual leaves on a platter. Scoop 3 tbsps. of cooked quinoa onto each leaf of lettuce and then spoon the tomato-avocado mixture.
- Serve cold as an appetizer, side dish or even a healthy lunch.

108. Herb, Feta, And Quinoa Filled Frittata

Serving: Serves 2 with leftovers for 1 | Prep: | Cook: | Ready in:

Ingredients

- 4 eggs or 3 whole eggs and 2 whites
- 1/2 cup cooked quinoa
- Small pinch of freshly grated nutmeg
- 3 tablespoons fresh bread crumbs
- 2 teaspoons butter, melted
- Olive oil for the pan
- 1 medium shallot, thickly sliced lengthwise
- 1 tablespoon chopped fresh herbs, like marjoram and thyme, or oregano and basil, or rosemary and sage, etc.
- 2 tablespoons coarsely chopped or torn Italian parsley leaves
- 1 to 2 tablespoons crumbled feta cheese, to taste (or any other similar cheese)
- 1 tablespoon finely grated Parmigiano Reggiano, Pecorino Romano, or Asiago
- Salt
- Freshly ground pepper

Direction

- Crumble bread crumbs into a small bowl and drizzle the melted butter over them with a tiny pinch of salt and some freshly ground pepper. Toss gently to coat. (If your bread crumbs are a bit moist, toast them first briefly in a skillet over medium heat.)
- Turn on broiler.
- Beat the eggs with the quinoa. Add the nutmeg, a pinch of salt, and freshly ground pepper to taste.
- On the stove, drizzle a teaspoon or two of oil into a medium-sized oven-proof skillet, and sauté the shallots over medium heat to soften, about one minute.
- Still using medium heat, pour the eggs and quinoa into the skillet. Sprinkle on the herbs. Use a spatula to lift the edges, tilting the pan to allow the uncooked egg to flow into the exposed areas under the lifted edges. As soon as the eggs begin to set on the stove, remove the pan from the heat.
- Sprinkle the cheeses on top. Put under the broiler for 30 seconds, remove, sprinkle on the buttered crumbs, and put back under the broiler for another 30 seconds, or until the crumbs and cheese are nicely browned.
- Enjoy!! ;o) This also tastes great at room temperature.

109. Herbed Quinoa Salad With Roasted Shrimp

Serving: Serves 2 | Prep: | Cook: | Ready in:

Ingredients

- 2 cups vegetable stock
- 1 cup quinoa
- 3/4 pound extra-large shrimp, peeled and deveined (about 12 shrimp)
- 4 tablespoons olive oil, divided
- Kosher salt and ground black pepper
- 2 tablespoons Meyer lemon juice, or juice of any organic lemons
- 2 teaspoons champagne vinegar
- 1 teaspoon Meyer lemon zest, or zest of any organic lemon
- 3 tablespoons pine nuts

- 2 tablespoons flat-leaf parsley, chopped
- 1 tablespoon fresh chives, chopped
- 1 tablespoon fresh dill, chopped
- 1 teaspoon fresh lemon thyme leaves

Direction

- Preheat oven to 400 degrees.
- Using a medium-sized saucepan, heat the stock until it boils. Add the quinoa, stir, cover, and reduce heat to low. Cook 15 to 20 minutes, until stock has been absorbed. Remove pan from heat and allow quinoa to "rest", covered, for 15 minutes.
- Spread the shrimp on a sheet pan. Drizzle with 1 tablespoon of the olive oil, then add salt and pepper. Roast in the oven for 3 minutes, then turn the shrimp and cook for 2 more minutes. Remove from oven and set aside.
- To make the vinaigrette, whisk together the remaining 3 tablespoons of olive oil, lemon juice, vinegar, and lemon zest. Set aside.
- Heat a small frying pan and toast the pine nuts, stirring, until they turn golden brown. Remove from heat.
- Fluff the cooked quinoa with a fork and turn into a salad bowl. Add the shrimp, vinaigrette, toasted nuts, and fresh herbs. Toss and allow salad to sit for 15 minutes before serving. If you wish to serve the salad chilled, refrigerate for 2 hours before serving.

110. Herbed Yellow Cherry Tomato, White Lima Bean And Black Quinoa Medley

Serving: Serves 4 | Prep: | Cook: | Ready in:

Ingredients

- Preliminaries
- 1 cup dried lima beans
- 1 teaspoon sea salt
- 1/4 cup black quinoa
- water
- The tagine or casserole
- cooked lima beans (@2 cups)
- cooked black quinoa (about 1/2 cup)
- 1/3 cup pitted olives, nicoise, gaeta or kalamata, cut in halves
- 1 pint yellow cherry tomatoes, cut in halves
- @1.5 ounces extra virgin olive oil
- zest and juice from half a lime
- 1 teaspoon fresh oregano or 1/2 tsp. Mexican dried oregano
- pinch of kosher salt or Maldon sea flakes
- fresh milled pepper to taste
- 1 anchovy cut into small pieces (or roasted garlic or pancetta as substitutions)
- 2 tablespoons chopped flat leaf parsley, divided
- splash of white wine

Direction

- Preliminaries
- Soak the lima beans in 3-4 cups of water overnight. The drain and cook in 3 cups of water with 1 tsp. of salt for about 45 minutes until tender. Drain (and reserve the broth for another soup).
- Rinse the quinoa well under cool water. Then add 2/3 cup of water to a pan with the quinoa. Bring to a boil. Simmer for 15 minutes until the water is absorbed. Fluff up and set aside.
- The tagine or casserole
- Toss the beans, quinoa, olives, and cherry tomatoes together. Drizzle with olive oil. Add salt, pepper, dried herb, half of the fresh parsley, and lime zest.
- Place in a heated tagine or casserole dish. Mix in the anchovy. Splash with lime juice and wine.
- Bake covered in a 350 degrees oven for 40-45 minutes or until the tomatoes are tender when poked. Adjust seasoning if needed. Let the flavors develop as the dish rests and the sauce thickens on its own. Garnish with fresh parsley. Serve warm with crusty bread, couscous or rice.

111. Holiday Pomegranate Quinoa Salad

Serving: Serves 6 | Prep: | Cook: |Ready in:

Ingredients

- 1 cucumber, peeled seeded and diced
- 1 green or red pepper, finely diced
- 1 cup uncooked quinoa
- 1/2 cup pomegranate arils
- 1/2 cup feta, optional can use tofu feta or omit for vegan option
- 1/2 cup toasted slivered almonds or pine nuts
- 2 tablespoons chopped mint
- 1 lemon, zested and juiced
- 1/4 cup extra virgin olive oil
- 1 clove garlic, minced

Direction

- Cook quinoa according to directions.
- Let cool completely. I like to cook my quinoa on the stove, keep covered and remove from heat. Let sit for an hour until completely cooled, fork to fluff the quinoa kernels.
- In a large bowl, combine cucumber, pepper, pomegranate arils, feta (if using), toasted nuts, and mint.
- Whisk together the minced garlic clove, lemon, olive oil and pinch salt/pepper.
- Toss to combine and serve!

112. Holy Shitake Quinoa Sushi

Serving: Serves a crowd | Prep: | Cook: |Ready in:

Ingredients

- 1 cup quinoa
- 2 cups water
- 1 pinch sea salt
- 2 tablespoons tahini
- 2 tablespoons rice wine vinegar
- 3 sheets nori seaweed
- 1/2 cup shitake mushrooms
- 1 tablespoon low-sodium tamari
- 1 tablespoon sesame oil
- 2 tablespoons daikon sprouts
- 2 tablespoons baked shallots

Direction

- Preheat oven to 300 degrees Celsius. Rinse quinoa well, place in a pot with water and sea salt, cover and bring to a boil
- Reduce heat and simmer until all the liquid is absorbed.
- In the meantime, thinly slice shitake mushrooms. Mix tamari, sesame oil, and mushrooms in a bowl.
- Spread mushroom mixture on a baking pan and bake for 7 minutes or until mushrooms are browned but not burnt (this will depend on how thinly you have sliced your mushrooms).
- Once quinoa is ready, remove from heat and stir in rice wine vinegar. Cool, add tahini to help the grain stick together.
- Proceed with regular sushi making. Place nori sheet, shiny side down on a bamboo mat. Spread quinoa evenly over the first 2/3 of the sheet. Place mushrooms, daikon sprouts and shallots down the center. Roll and squeeze tight. Slice rolls into bite size sushi pieces.

113. How To Cook Quinoa

Serving: Serves 3 | Prep: 0hours5mins | Cook: 0hours20mins |Ready in:

Ingredients

- 1 cup quinoa grains
- 2 cups water

Direction

- Rinse the quinoa in water in 5 minutes and drain it well.
- Bring rinsed quinoa to a saucepan and start cooking in high heat until the quinoa has absorbed all of the water.
- After 5 minutes counting from the boiling point, reduce the heat to medium level. Start stirring the quinoa up, then get a lid to cover and let it sit in 15 minutes.
- Open the lid and fluff it over one last time. Shut down your stove and remove the saucepan from heat. Cover it up and let the quinoa steam for 5 more minutes.
- Serve your quinoa versatility. Sprinkle some pepper flakes, sliced olives or fresh chopped herbs will also help brighten the whole thing up. If you still find it a bit flat in taste, then some additional drops of soy sauce going in can always stimulate your appetite big time.

114. Hungarian Stuffed Reds With Red Quinoa

Serving: Serves 4-6 | Prep: | Cook: | Ready in:

Ingredients

- 1/2 cup whole red quinoa, uncooked, soaked in water
- 1/2 pound farm quality ground beef
- 1/2 pound farm fresh quality ground pork
- 1/4 cup finely chopped red cabbage
- 1/4 cup finely chopped red onion
- 1/4 cup grated carrot
- 1/2 teaspoon fresh chopped thyme leaves
- 1/2 teaspoon fresh chopped marjoram leaves
- 1/2 tablespoon premium quality Hungarian smoked (or sweet) paprika
- dash of kosher salt
- pinch of pepper
- 4-6 plump red sweet bell peppers
- 2-4 cups fresh vegetable broth, made from fire roasted as well as uncooked red pepper, tomatoes, carrots, onions and herbs (see photo) with canned stewed tomatoes as alternative
- 1/2 tablespoon sweet red Hungarian paprika
- 1 bay leaf
- 1 bouquet garni of fresh herbs (thyme, marjoram, parsley, even some basil)
- sweet paprika for garnish
- dollop of sour cream, creme fraiche, or fage for serving
- fresh chopped parsley for serving
- 4 cups red pepper semolina soup as a richer alternative to the vegetable broth

Direction

- Soak the quinoa in water for an hour and then drain off the water. Mix gently the next ten ingredients on the recipe list together with the quinoa for the filling.
- Cut a border of triangles out of the top edge of the peppers, about an inch in height. Clean out their seeds and interior membranes. Take the cut out triangles and dice smaller. Add these into the filling mixture.
- Stuff the peppers up to the beginning of the triangular border. The quinoa will expand when cooking.
- Arrange these in a large Dutch oven and add the broth. Make sure to add sweet paprika to the broth. Bring to a boil, then simmer for 40 minutes. While cooking ladle some broth over the peppers. Make sure the quinoa is fully cooked. Remove the peppers carefully to a bowl and peel off their skins, if desired. Replace back into the broth to keep warm until serving. If you do not mind the skins, you can simply skip this step.
- Serve with a generous ladle-ful of broth in a bowl, or alternatively for a richer meal with my red pepper semolina soup. Fold the triangles inwards. Garnish with sour cream, crème fraiche or fage, chopped flat leaf parsley and sweet paprika.

115. Italian Tuna, Quinoa And White Bean Salad

Serving: Makes 5 cups | Prep: | Cook: | Ready in:

Ingredients

- 1/2 cup tricolor dry quinoa, or 1 cup cooked leftover quinoa
- 10 ounces Italian canned tuna, I like Genova
- 1/2 cup fresh parsley, minced
- 2 juicy lemons
- Kosher salt
- Ground black pepper
- Extra virgin olive oil
- 1/2 cup scallions, sliced thin, about 3
- 15 ounces can of cannellini beans, rinsed well in cool water
- Avocado, optional

Direction

- In a small pot bring 1 cup of water boil and add 1/2 teaspoon of salt. Add the quinoa cover and cook at low rolling boil for 10 minutes. Turn off the heat, leave the lid on and steam for another 5 minutes. While the quinoa is cooking prepare the rest of the salad.
- Dump the tuna from the can(s) in a fine mesh strainer in the sink. Break up the tuna with your fingers. Place the tuna in a large bowl. Resist the urge to rinse it. Italian tuna packed in oil has a lot of flavor!
- Add the parsley, zest and juice of one lemon, 2 tablespoons of olive oil and 1/2 teaspoon each of salt and pepper. Mix well to combine in the tuna. Taste for seasoning.
- Add the scallions and cannellini beans. Toss to combine, taking care to not have the beans break apart.
- When the quinoa is done drain in the same colander you used for the tuna. Toss and fluff it up a bit. Let it cool down for 5 minutes and then toss it into the tuna salad. If needed squeeze a little more lemon over the salad and add a good drizzle of olive oil. Toss gently to combine and taste for seasoning. It may not be necessary if your lemons are on the large size.
- You have two options with the avocado if desired: you can half it and scoop the tuna into it, or you can cut it up and toss it into the salad. Either way squeeze a little lemon juice over the avocado and a pinch of salt and pepper. The lemon juice will help keep it from turning brown.
- Serve cold or at room temperature.

116. KOSHERMOMS RECIPE: BABY QUINOA SALAD WITH ROASTED VEGETABLES

Serving: Serves 4 | Prep: | Cook: | Ready in:

Ingredients

- 1 cup Baby quinoa
- 1 sweet potato
- 1 red onion

Direction

- Prepare Baby Quinoa according to package directions
- Dice the onion, sweet potato and pepper into small pieces
- Put on a sheet pan, coat with olive oil, salt and pepper. Roast veggies till golden brown and soft (about 25 minutes)
- Mix honey, ¼ cup of olive oil and balsamic vinegar in a container, until completely mixed. Once the Baby Quinoa has cooked and rested, mix with the roasted veggies and dressing.

117. Kale & Quinoa Salad

Serving: Makes approx 4 cups | Prep: | Cook: | Ready in:

Ingredients

- 2 handfuls baby Kale (or 1/2 of 7 oz package)
- 1 cup dry Quinoa, cooked (approx 2 cups cooked)
- 2 tablespoons extra virgin Olive Oil
- 1/2 Cucumber, peeled, seeded and chopped (approx 1/2 cup)
- juice and zest of one Lemon (wash and rinse lemon well), approx 4 tablespoons of juice and 1 teaspoons of zest
- 1/2 cup dried currants
- 1/2 cup shelled pistachios
- sea salt & freshly ground pepper to taste

Direction

- After cooking, allow quinoa to cool in cooking pot, with lid on, for 20-30 minutes and then fluff with a fork.
- Stack kale leaves together and roll up like a cigar, then slice thinly with a sharp knife ("chiffonade").
- Peel cucumber and remove seeds. Dice into 1/8 inch cubes.
- Combine kale, quinoa, and cucumber in a large non-reactive mixing bowl. Add currants and mix well.
- Add olive oil, zest the lemon over the bowl (to capture the essential oils), and add lemon juice. Add a large pinch of salt and grind pepper into the bowl.
- Mix well to combine all ingredients. The slightly warm quinoa will absorb the seasonings, and the warmth and lemon juice will slightly "cook" the kale. To serve a larger crowd, simply double or triple the recipe.
- PLEASE NOTE: When making this, I didn't measure. These measurements are approximations; however, you can add more or less of anything to suit your taste.
- Just before serving, sprinkle pistachios on top. Bon Appetit!

118. Kale And Quinoa Salad

Serving: Serves 4 | Prep: | Cook: |Ready in:

Ingredients

- 1 cup Quinoa
- 1 bunch Curly kale
- 1/2 Red capsicum
- 1 Small lebanese cucumber
- 1 Small fennel bulb
- 1 Lemon, juiced
- 6 tablespoons Extra virgin olive oil
- 1 teaspoon Nutritional yeast (optional)
- Salt & pepper
- 1/4 cup Slivered almonds, toasted

Direction

- Rinse and rub the quinoa grains with your fingers under running water. Drain and place in a medium saucepan. Add 1 plus 3/4 cup water and bring to the boil. Once boiling add 1/2 tsp salt, reduce heat to a gentle simmer and cover the pot. Cook for about 15 minutes or until all liquid is absorbed and you can see the tiny spirals curling around the seed. Remove from the heat, and place a clean dishcloth over the pot and pop the lid back in place. Rest for 10 minutes before turning out into a deep serving bowl.
- Wash the kale and trim off the stems, tear into bite size pieces and set aside. Remove the capsicum seeds and membranes and slice into thin strips, cut in half if they are too long. Slice the cucumbers in quarter's length-ways and cut out seeds and membranes. Slice these on an angle into thin strips too. Trim the fennel and slice at an angle into equivalent strips.
- Squeeze the juice from the lemon and place in a glass jar with a lid. Add the extra virgin olive oil, nutritional yeast, and some salt and pepper. Shake for a uniform consistency, taste, you're looking for a slight tang. Adjust accordingly.
- Add the vegetables to the cooled quinoa and add 4 tbsp. of the vinaigrette, mix thoroughly

before topping with the toasted almonds. Serve with the remaining dressing on the side.

119. Kale And Tomato Quinoa Bowl With Lemon Mint Vinaigrette

Serving: Serves 4 | Prep: | Cook: |Ready in:

Ingredients

- Quinoa Bowl
- 2 cups Quinoa, cooked
- 3 cups Kale, shredded (choose any salad greens)
- 2 cups Cherry Tomatoes, halved or quartered
- 1 cup Feta Cheese, crumbled (choose any cheese)
- 1 cup Avocado, diced
- *Any fresh diced vegetable would go well in this.
- Lemon Mint Vinaigrette
- 1/4 cup Olive Oil
- 1/4 cup Lemon Juice, freshly squeezed
- 1/4 cup Mint, chopped
- 1-2 teaspoons Sugar

Direction

- Toss salad ingredients together.
- Whisk olive oil, lemon juice, mint and 1 tsp sugar together until blended.
- Taste and add more sugar if needed.
- Pour over salad and toss right before serving
- Tip: For a stronger mint essence make this dressing ahead and leave extra mint sprigs in until ready to serve.

120. Lemon Cranberry Quinoa Salad

Serving: Serves 4 people | Prep: | Cook: |Ready in:

Ingredients

- 1 cup raw quinoa (yellow or tri-color)
- Water
- 2 tablespoons fresh lemon juice
- 1/2 tablespoon ground coriander
- 1/2 tablespoon ground cumin
- 1 teaspoon paprika
- Table Salt
- Freshly ground black pepper
- Half a red bell pepper, deseeded and finely chopped
- 1/3 cup sweetened dried cranberries
- 1/3 - 1/2 cups of any 1-2 of the following ingredients: halved grape tomatoes, chopped walnuts, chopped cucumbers, OR crumbled goat cheese
- 3 green onions, white and green parts, thinly sliced
- 1/4 cup chopped fresh cilantro leaves

Direction

- Pour quinoa into a mesh strainer and rinse with tap water. Rinse the quinoa a few times, rubbing the quinoa between your fingers to remove bitter taste on outside of quinoa grains.
- Pour quinoa into a small pot with water (about 2 inches of water above quinoa) and cover saucepan to bring to a boil. Once pot comes to a boil, reduce the heat to low and allow to simmer for 6-10 minutes, or just until quinoa is tender and slightly firm still. Do not overcook quinoa; drain any excess water in the saucepan and transfer the cooked quinoa to a large bowl.
- Add lemon juice, ground coriander, ground cumin, paprika, ½ teaspoon salt, and ¼ teaspoon ground black pepper, and toss quinoa until evenly mixed. Add chopped bell pepper, sliced green onions, cranberries, cilantro, and your preferred optional ingredients, and mix with quinoa until combined. If necessary, adjust for seasoning by adding additional spices, lemon juice, ¼

teaspoon salt, and pepper. Serve quinoa salad at room temperature or chilled.

121. Lemon Herb Quinoa With Hemp Seeds, Spring Peas, And Basil

Serving: Serves 4 | Prep: | Cook: | Ready in:

Ingredients

- 1 cup Quinoa, dry
- 2 cups Water, cold
- 1 cup Green peas, fresh or frozen
- 1/4 cup Fresh basil, finely chopped
- 1/4 cup Shelled hemp seeds
- 2 tablespoons Olive oil
- 2 tablespoons lemon juice
- 2 teaspoons Dijon mustard
- 1 teaspoon Maple syrup
- 1/4 teaspoon Sea salt (plus a little extra)
- 1 dash Black pepper

Direction

- Rinse quinoa in a mesh strainer with cold water. Transfer to a pot and add the 2 cups cold water and a nice pinch of salt. Bring to a boil.
- Reduce heat to a simmer, and leave the lid of the pot slightly ajar while cooking. Simmer for about 15 minutes, or until quinoa is plump, the water is absorbed, and you see the tiny little outer "shells" of the quinoa grain coming loose in the pot.
- Remove quinoa from heat and let sit, covered, for 5 minutes or so. Fluff with a fork and set aside.
- While quinoa is cooking, boil fresh or frozen peas till warm and tender. Drain and set aside.
- Mix quinoa, peas, basil, and hemp seeds in a large bowl. Whisk together the oil, lemon juice, maple syrup, Dijon mustard, 1/4 tsp sea salt, and black pepper. Pour over the quinoa salad mixture, and serve warm or cold. Dish

will keep excellently (though the basil might turn a little dark) in the fridge for 2-3 days.

122. Lemon Tri Color Quinoa Tabbouleh

Serving: Serves 6-8 | Prep: | Cook: | Ready in:

Ingredients

- 1 cup tri-color quinoa
- 1 1/2 cups water
- 1/2 bunch watercress or other green (like parsley or cilantro)
- 1/2 bunch mint
- 6-8 mini red, yellow orange peppers, diced (or use 1/2 each of red, yellow, orange bell peppers)
- 1/2 cup heirloom cherry tomatoes, diced
- 1 cucumber, seeded and diced
- 1/4 cup flavored olive oil (I used a harissa flavored one)
- 1/4 cup neutral oil
- 1/4 cup orange champagne vinegar (I used the one from trader joes)
- 1 lemon, juiced
- kosher salt and fresh cracked pepper, to taste.

Direction

- Boil quinoa in 1 1/2 c. of salted water...turn down immediately to a low simmer, cover and cook 10 minutes. Take off heat, let stand 5 minutes. You can then chill grains overnight. If prepping for the next day, wait to add dressing before using, or bring an additional amount to add.
- Add diced veggies and herbs. Original tabbouleh calls for flat leafed parsley but I like the peppery flavor of watercress and the zing of mint.
- Mix together oils and vinegar with lemon juice and salt and pepper with a whisk. If you want a bit of sweetness, but don't have an orange Muscat champagne vinegar, add 1 T. orange

marmalade or honey and 1 T. OJ to 1/4 c. vinegar.
- Serve with baked pita chips or torn pieces of warm pita bread.
- This salad is great for vegans, vegetarians and those with gluten sensitivities...if you want to make it more of a main dish salad, add some roasted chicken or fish (or for those vegan/vegetarian friends, grilled tempeh)

123. Lemon Quinoa With Fresh Pesto

Serving: Serves 2 | Prep: | Cook: |Ready in:

Ingredients

- 2/3 cup dry quinoa
- 1 1/3 cups water
- 1/4 cup slivered almonds, toasted
- 1 bunch fresh basil, about 3 cups
- 1/4 cup parmesan, freshly grated
- 1/2 cup walnuts, toasted
- 3 cloves garlic
- 3 tablespoons high quality olive oil, plus more to taste
- juice of 1 lemon
- 1 cup chickpeas, drained and rinsed
- handful sun-dried tomatoes, for garnish
- salt and pepper, to taste

Direction

- Place the basil through the olive oil in the bowl of a food processor. Pulse until smooth. Set aside.
- Place quinoa and water in a small saucepan over medium heat. Bring to a boil, then reduce heat to a simmer, cover and let cook about 15 minutes, until the water is absorbed
- When quinoa is finished, remove from heat, fluff with a fork and toss with almonds, chickpeas, pesto, and lemon juice. Garnish with sun-dried tomatoes

124. Lemony Quinoa Broccoli Salad

Serving: Serves 2, very generously | Prep: | Cook: |Ready in:

Ingredients

- 1/3 cup quinoa
- 2 lemons, zest and juice
- 80 milliliters olive oil
- 2 cups broccoli florets, cut into bite sized pieces
- 2 ounces feta, cubed
- 1/4 cup pepitas, dry toasted
- plenty of salt and pepper, to taste
- 1/2 avocado, cubed

Direction

- Rinse your quinoa in a fine mesh sieve under running water for about 30 seconds. It is best cooked by absorption method, 1 part quinoa to 1 and 1/2 parts cold water. Place water and quinoa in a saucepan over high heat until it comes to the boil, then turn the heat to low and pop a lid on. When the quinoa is ready it will swell, and a curly little tail will pop out. Quinoa should be al-dente and not mushy – this generally takes about 10-12 mins. Once it is cooked, rinse it again in a fine mesh strainer under cold running water. Make sure it gets drained very well, water logged quinoa is not at all nice.
- While the quinoa is cooking you can also blanch the broccoli florets in salted boiling water for 1 minute. Resist the urge to cook them for any longer. Drain under cold running water until cool. Pat dry with a tea towel.
- Place your lemon juice, zest, olive oil and a big pinch of salt and freshly ground pepper into a jar and shake vigorously to combine. Set aside.
- Place the cooked and drained quinoa into a large serving bowl with the broccoli and chopped herbs. Pour on half the lemon

dressing and toss to combine. I use my hands for this.
- Add the feta and avocado, very gently toss again and taste for seasoning – adjust if necessary (I almost always will add more salt). Sprinkle on toasted pepitas and drizzle a little more dressing on if you wish. It is now ready to serve!

125. Lemony Quinoa Salad With Summer Vegetables

Serving: Serves 6 | Prep: | Cook: | Ready in:

Ingredients

- Dressing
- Finely grated zest and juice of 1 large lemon
- 3 tablespoons olive or vegetable oil
- 1/2 teaspoon ground coriander
- 1/2 teaspoon ground cumin
- 1/2 teaspoon paprika
- salt and pepper to taste
- Quinoa Salad
- 1 cup Red or White quinoa, rinsed well
- 1/2 teaspoon salt
- 2 cups cold water
- 1 cup dried cranberries
- 2 ripe avocadoes, diced
- 1 red or yellow bell pepper, diced
- 2 scallions or red onions, sliced
- 1/4 cup toasted sunflower seeds

Direction

- Dressing
- Whisk or shake together dressing ingredients and set aside.
- Quinoa Salad
- In a saucepan, combine quinoa, salt and cold water; bring to a boil over medium-high heat. Stir, reduce heat to low, cover and simmer for about 15 minutes or until water is absorbed and quinoa is tender. Drain if necessary. Fluff with a fork and allow to cool.
- Add remaining salad ingredients to quinoa and toss with dressing to coat. Can be served room temperature or cold. Can be refrigerated in an airtight container for up to 1 day.

126. Lemony Shrimp And Quinoa

Serving: Serves 2 | Prep: | Cook: | Ready in:

Ingredients

- Lemony Quinoa
- 1 cup Quinoa
- 2 juice of 2 lemons
- 2 zest of 2 lemons
- 1 cup frozen mixed vegetables
- Lemony Shrimp
- 10-12 Shrimp (31-40 size)
- 2 Asparagus stalks
- 2 cloves minces or grated garlic
- 1 pinch pepper (if you have lemon pepper use it)
- 1 teaspoon Olive oil to sauté

Direction

- Cook quinoa according to package directions - I substituted 1/4 cup of lemon juice to the liquid to give it more of a lemon hit
- While quinoa is cooking add the frozen vegetables (since the vegetables have moisture because they are frozen I tend to add a touch less liquid to the quinoa)
- In a separate pan, heat oil and garlic and then throw in the chopped asparagus.
- Let it sauté for a couple of minutes to get the asparagus slightly cooked. Add the shrimp, whatever is left from the lemon juice and some pepper. Stir and cook until shrimp is light pink and turn off heat.

127. Light Chicken Quinoa Divan

Serving: Serves 6 | Prep: | Cook: | Ready in:

Ingredients

- 1 cup quinoa
- 2 cups water
- 6 cups broccoli florets
- 1 1/2 pounds chicken breasts
- 1 tablespoon plus 1 tsp olive oil
- 1 cup extra sharp cheddar cheese
- 1 cup freshly grated parmesan cheese
- 2 tablespoons flour (or 2 Tbsp of arrowroot flour if avoiding gluten)
- 2/3 cup white wine
- 1/2 cup chicken broth
- 1 cup milk
- 1 1/2 cups light sour cream
- 1/4 cup lemon juice
- 2 tablespoons plus 2 tsp yellow curry
- 1/4 teaspoon sea salt
- olive oil cooking spray

Direction

- Like many casseroles, this one involves prepping a bunch of ingredients, mixing them together, and then baking the dish with delicious results. To begin, rinse the quinoa, place it in a sauce pan with 2 C of water, and bring to a boil over medium-high heat. Once boiling, cover, reduce heat to medium-low, simmer, and allow it to cook until all of the water is absorbed. This will take about 12 minutes. Note that it's important to rinse your quinoa before cooking, otherwise it may have a slightly bitter flavor.
- While your quinoa is cooking, cut your broccoli, place it in a pot so that it's submerged in water, bring to a boil, and boil for 2 minutes. You will then drain off the hot water and submerge the broccoli in cold water until you are ready to use it. This will make it so the broccoli is not under-cooked or mushy in your casserole, but just right.
- After you have the quinoa simmering and have begun bringing the broccoli up to a boil, cube your chicken breast into bite-sized pieces and brown over medium-high heat with 1 tsp of olive oil. You're just browning, so your chicken shouldn't cook through (no nibbling!).
- At this point, your quinoa is just about ready to remove from the heat. Fluff with a fork and set aside. Your broccoli is also ready to place into a cold water bath. Set both aside until you're ready to assemble your casserole.
- Shred 1 cup each of extra sharp cheddar cheese and fresh parmesan.
- All of your filling is now prepped, so it's time to prepare the sauce that makes this recipe so delicious. First, Place 1 Tbsp. of olive oil in a saucepan and heat over medium heat for 1 minute. Next, add 2 Tbsp. of flour (or arrowroot flour), mix together, and cook for 1 minute. Now add 2/3 C of white wine and 1/2 C of chicken broth and whisk in with the flour and oil mixture. Bring the sauce to a simmer, continuously whisking, and simmer until the sauce has thickened. Add 1 cup of milk and continue whisking until the sauce begins to simmer again, and then immediately remove from the heat. Finally, mix in the sour cream, lemon juice, yellow curry and salt.
- In a large mixing bowl, fold together all of your ingredients: quinoa, broccoli, chicken, shredded cheese, and your sauce.
- Once combined, place your casserole mixture into a baking dish that has been sprayed with olive oil cooking spray.
- Bake uncovered at 400° F for 35-40 minutes or until the casserole is bubbling all the way through. Allow the dish to rest for 5 minutes before serving.

128. Loaded Quinoa Veggie Sliders

Serving: Makes 12 | Prep: | Cook: | Ready in:

Ingredients

- 1 cup Quinoa
- 1/3 cup Frozen Spinach
- 1/3 cup Frozen Broccoli
- 4 Garlic Cloves
- 1/3 cup Red Pepper (Chopped)
- 2 Large Eggs
- 1 cup Breadcrumbs
- 1/2 cup Cheddar Cheese
- 2 tablespoons Fresh Herbs (Basil, Cilantro or Parsley)

Direction

- Cook the quinoa according to package instructions. Let this cool before you work it into the rest of the dish.
- Cook the frozen spinach and broccoli according to package instructions. Then drain them and place them in a food processor with the garlic and red pepper and pulse until they are chopped thoroughly.
- Note: What you want is a sort of batter that you can press into patties that isn't too wet and sticky, but also doesn't fall apart. Add in more breadcrumbs as necessary to find this balance.
- When the burger mix is ready, take a handful and roll it into a round that's a little larger than a golf ball but smaller than a racket ball. Place each onto a sheet pan lined with parchment paper and gently press into slider shape. Leave them thicker than you want the finished product to be as you'll press them a bit more once they cook. Ideally you should refrigerate them for at least half an hour so they set nicely.
- Bring a large skillet up to medium high heat and add a small amount of olive oil. Place the sliders into the skillet and gently press them down. Cook for 4-5 minutes per side until browned and crispy. Remember that you're using raw eggs, so they need to be cooked all the way through.

129. Maple Mulberry Quinoa Oatmeal Bowl

Serving: Serves 1 | Prep: | Cook: | Ready in:

Ingredients

- 1/4 cup oats
- 1/4 cup quinoa
- 1 pinch salt
- 1 1/2 cups liquid (milk of choice/water)
- 1/4 teaspoon vanilla extract
- 1/2 teaspoon cinnamon
- 2 tablespoons maple syrup (or to taste)
- 1 bunch berries of choice
- 1/8 teaspoon orange zest
- Splash milk of choice (optional)

Direction

- In a pot on the stove, combine the oats, quinoa, salt, and 1 cup of liquid. Bring to a gentle simmer, and cook on low heat while stirring. Continue to cook so that the grains absorb the liquid, and begin to plump up.
- After about 5 minutes, most of the liquid will be gone, but the quinoa will still be hard. Add the rest of the liquid, vanilla, cinnamon, and maple syrup. Continue cooking, stirring occasionally, for about 5 minutes.
- You'll know the grains are done when the liquid is gone and the quinoa looks like a little spiral. You can cook more or less, depending on your preferred tenderness. Turn off the heat and toss in the berries, giving them a gentle stir, just enough so that the heat up and become a bit jammy.
- Transfer all to a bowl or dish. Top with orange zest, extra berries, a splash of milk, and/or maple syrup. Enjoy!

130. Maple Quinoa Granola

Serving: Makes 5 to 6 cups | Prep: 0hours7mins | Cook: 1hours0mins | Ready in:

Ingredients

- 2 cups whole rolled oats
- 1/3 cup pre-rinsed, uncooked quinoa
- 1/2 cup raw walnuts, in pieces or coarsely chopped
- 1/3 cup raw almonds, coarsely chopped
- 1/3 cup raw sunflower seeds
- 1/3 cup unsweetened coconut flakes (raw)
- 1/4 cup white raisins
- 1/4 cup dried sweetened cranberries
- 3 tablespoons split hemp seeds (optional)
- 1/3 cup coconut oil
- 1/3 cup grade B maple syrup
- 1 dash cinnamon
- 1 dash nutmeg

Direction

- Preheat your oven to 225°F.
- Mix all dry ingredients (excluding cinnamon and nutmeg) in a great big mixing bowl.
- In a small saucepan over really low heat (or just in a bowl if your coconut oil is liquid), combine oil, syrup, and a dash each of the spices. You only need to get it up to a temperature that melts the coconut oil, then turn it off immediately. Pour your syrup/oil over the mixing bowl, then stir it all up until you don't see any more dry oats. Mix it up good.
- Spread the mix onto a cookie sheet lined with parchment paper. Flatten it out so it's even; it should take up the whole sheet. Bake at 225° F for 60 minutes.
- Let cool completely. When cooled, lift the ends of the parchment and let it crumble to the center. I leave the big chunks big; they'll break up as you pour everything into your jar. You can also just grab them and eat them.
- Because of the coconut oil here, this needs to be kept in an airtight container in the fridge, or safely below 70°, otherwise it risks losing its crispy crunchy.

131. Mediterranean Toasted Quinoa Salad ~ Chickpeas, Roasted Red Peppers & Herbs

Serving: Makes a large bowl full | Prep: | Cook: | Ready in:

Ingredients

- 6 small cucumbers, chopped into small pieces. I use seedless Persian cucumbers.
- 6-8 scallions, diced
- 3 red bell peppers, sliced in half and seeded
- 1-2 lemons
- A large handful of dill, chopped
- A large handful of mint, chopped
- A large handful of parsley, chopped
- 1 15 ounce can of chickpeas, rinsed and drained, patted with a paper towel
- Drizzle of honey (optional)
- Olive oil
- Sea salt to taste
- Fresh cracked pepper to taste
- 1 1/2 cups of cooked quinoa
- Serving Suggestions: toasted pine nuts or almonds, pita bread, baguette, lemon wedges, drizzle of olive oil, flaky sea salt, grey celtic salt, crumbled feta, olives

Direction

- Instructions For Cooking The Toasted Quinoa: Rinse one cup of quinoa. In a small pot, over medium heat, toast the rinsed quinoa in a little olive oil until it's fragrant and starts to make a crackling sound, about 3-5 minutes. Carefully add two cups of water and salt to taste. Bring to a boil. Cover and reduce the heat to low. Simmer for about 15 minutes or until the quinoa is done. Toss 1 1/2 cups of cooked quinoa with a little salt, pepper and olive oil and set aside.
- Salad Instructions: Make the toasted quinoa and set aside. Roast the peppers by placing the sliced peppers, cut side down, on an oven safe baking sheet lined with tin foil. Broil on high until their skins are charred and blackened.

Remove from the oven, place the peppers in a covered bowl or wrap in more tin foil to steam. Once cool enough to handle, peel the skin and discard. Chop and set aside. In a large bowl, combine the cucumbers, scallions, roasted red peppers, mint, dill, parsley, rinsed and drained chickpeas, drizzle of honey, salt and pepper. Add a couple of good drizzles of olive oil and a squeeze or two from a juicy lemon. Toss and taste. Adjust salt, lemon and olive oil. Stir in the toasted quinoa. Taste again to adjust seasonings. Serve with suggestions and enjoy.

132. Mediterranean Vegetable Bowls With Quinoa, Toasted Chickpeas, And Harissa Tahini

Serving: Serves 4 | Prep: | Cook: |Ready in:

Ingredients

- For the bowls:
- 1 medium eggplant
- 2 large zucchini
- 1 tablespoon olive oil
- 3 cups cooked chickpeas (or 2 cans chickpeas, drained and rinsed)
- 1/2 teaspoon smoked paprika
- 3/4 teaspoon chili powder
- 1/2 teaspoon salt, plus more to season
- 1 tablespoon lemon juice
- 1 tablespoon olive oil
- 1 tablespoon fresh oregano leaves (or 1 teaspoon dried oregano)
- Pepper
- 1 cup dry quinoa
- 6 cups tightly packed, washed greens of choice (arugula, baby spinach, baby kale, mizuna, and/or mesclun would all be great)
- For the harissa tahini sauce:
- 1/2 cup tahini
- 2 tablespoons lemon juice
- 1 teaspoon red wine vinegar
- 1 large clove garlic, chopped
- 1 teaspoon maple syrup
- 3/4 teaspoon harissa paste or powder
- 1/2 teaspoon smoked paprika
- 1/2 teaspoon ground cumin
- 1/2 teaspoon salt
- 3/4 cup water

Direction

- Preheat the oven to 400° F. Trim the eggplant and cut it into 1-inch cubes. Place the eggplant cubes into a colander and sprinkle them liberally with salt. Allow them to sit for 20 to 30 minutes. Pat any moisture that collects on the eggplant dry with a paper towel. Meanwhile, trim the zucchini and cut it into 1/4-inch strips lengthwise.
- For the toasted chickpeas, mix the chickpeas, paprika, chili powder, salt, lemon juice, and olive oil in a mixing bowl. Transfer the coated chickpeas to a parchment-lined baking sheet.
- Lay both the zucchini and the eggplant onto parchment-lined baking sheets. Brush them with olive oil, and sprinkle them with oregano, salt, and pepper. Transfer all three pans—the chickpeas, the zucchini, and the eggplant—to the oven. Roast the vegetables for 20 to 25 minutes, stirring once through, or until they're golden and tender. Allow the chickpeas to cook for 30 to 35 minutes, or until they're well toasted and browning. Remove all roasted ingredients from the oven and set aside.
- Rinse the quinoa through a fine sieve for about a minute. Transfer it to a medium-sized pot. Add 2 cups of water and a pinch of salt and bring to a boil. Reduce the heat to a simmer. Simmer, covered, for 15 minutes, or until all of the water has been absorbed into the grain. Fluff the grain lightly with a fork, cover it again, and allow it to sit for ten minutes more.
- While the quinoa cooks, make the sauce. Blend the tahini, lemon, vinegar, garlic, maple syrup, harissa, paprika, cumin, salt, and water in a food processor or blender till smooth.

- To assemble the bowls, place 1 1/2 cups tightly packed greens at the bottom of each bowl. Layer one quarter each of the cooked quinoa, roasted vegetables, and chickpeas on top. Drizzle the entire bowl generously with harissa tahini sauce. Serve.

133. Millet And Quinoa Summer Squash Salad

Serving: Serves 4-6 people | Prep: | Cook: | Ready in:

Ingredients

- 1/2 cup millet
- 1/2 cup quinoa
- 2 cups water (for cooking quinoa and millet)
- 1 tablespoon rice vinegar
- 1 tablespoon soy sauce
- 3 tablespoons extra virgin olive oil
- 1/2 cup diced green onion
- 1/2 cup chopped cilantro
- Pinch fresh ground black pepper
- 1 small yellow squash
- 2 teaspoons vegetable oil, or other oil for sauteeing squash

Direction

- Chop the zucchini into about 1cm cubes and sauté in a skillet with vegetable oil until lightly browned.
- Put the millet, quinoa and water into a pot, bring to a boil, and simmer on low until all the water has absorbed.
- Mix together the pepper, rice vinegar, soy sauce, and extra virgin olive oil then pour over the cooked quinoa, and mix to distribute.
- When the grain mixture has cooled, mix in the squash, green onions and cilantro.
- This quinoa salad is tasty both warm and cold.

134. Miso Masala Kabocha & Cauliflower Quinoa Salad

Serving: Serves 4 | Prep: | Cook: | Ready in:

Ingredients

- 1 small kabocha squash, about 2 ½ pounds, peeled, seeded, and cut into 1" chunks
- 1/2 head of cauliflower, cut into bite-sized florets
- 1 bunch lacinato (or any) kale, destemmed and sliced into 1" ribbons
- 1/4 cup shiro miso
- 1/4 cup olive oil
- 1 teaspoon chaat masala (I used MDH brand)
- 1 teaspoon cumin
- 1/4 teaspoon cayenne (optional)
- 1 cup quinoa
- 2 cups broth or water (for the quinoa)
- 1/4 cup goat cheese crumbles (I think feta would also do well)
- 2 tablespoons pomegranate arils
- salt
- pepper

Direction

- Preheat the oven to 400F
- In a large bowl, whisk together the miso, olive oil, cumin, chaat masala and cayenne (if using). Reserve 2 tablespoons of the mixture for the dressing.
- Toss the squash and cauliflower in the miso-spice mixture, coating everything evenly.
- Spread the squash and cauliflower onto a baking sheet in a single layer and roast in the oven for 30 minutes, or until vegetables are tender. Remove from oven and let cool for 10 minutes.
- Rinse and cook the quinoa according to package directions. (Generally, it's cooked in a 1:2 ratio of quinoa to broth or water.)
- Pour the 2 tablespoons of the reserved miso-spice mixture back into the large bowl and whisk in the lemon juice. Add a pinch of salt and pepper. Add the kale to the bowl and

slowly toss it in the dressing, gently massaging the dressed leaves.
- Add the quinoa, vegetables, mint, cheese and pistachios to the bowl and gently mix. Sprinkle pomegranate arils over the top and serve.

135. Miso Quinoa Pilaf With Grilled Cucumber, Eggplant, And Soy Dressing

Serving: Serves 4 to 6 as a side | Prep: 0hours15mins | Cook: 0hours25mins | Ready in:

Ingredients

- For the Pilaf
- 1 large English cucumber
- 2 small, long eggplants, about 5 to 6 inches (I used Gretel variety from my raised bed, Fairytale eggplants are comparable or 1 slender long eggplant of a larger variety)
- Olive oil for grilling
- 1 tablespoon unsalted butter (can sub vegan butter)
- 1 cup quinoa
- 1 cup 2 % milk (can sub nut milk, such as almond)
- 1 cup water
- 1 1/2 tablespoons white miso (we used barley miso, which is darker)
- 3 tablespoons chopped cilantro
- For the Soy Dressing
- 1/4 cup gluten-free tamari
- 1/4 cup balsamic vinegar
- Juice from 1/2 an orange (about 1/4 cup)
- 1/4 cup canola oil

Direction

- For the Pilaf
- Prepare a medium gas or charcoal grill.
- Trim ends off cucumber and eggplants. Slice eggplants in half lengthwise. Cut cucumber crosswise into thirds, then cut each piece in half lengthwise. Place vegetables in a baking pan and drizzle cut sides with olive oil, rubbing oil with your fingertip to cover the vegetables. Set aside until grill is hot.
- While you are waiting for your grill to heat up, start your quinoa by melting butter in a small saucepan. Add quinoa and cook over medium heat, stirring constantly to toast the grains. After about 5 minutes, quinoa should start to pop and smell nutty (a few grains will turn golden brown). At this point, add milk and water, and whisk in miso. Cover pot and adjust heat to maintain a simmer. Cook for 17 to 20 minutes until grains are tender and liquid has been absorbed. Remove pot from heat.
- Grill cucumber and eggplant pieces cut side down until lightly charred and tender, about 5 minutes for cucumber and 7 to 8 for eggplant. Flip and grill skin side down for 2 to 3 minutes more. Cucumber skin will start to wrinkle and eggplant flesh should yield easily when poked with a knife. Transfer to a cutting board and let cool slightly. Slice cucumbers and eggplants crosswise into half-moons.
- Fluff quinoa and transfer to a large mixing bowl. Add sliced cucumber, eggplant, and half of the cilantro. Whisk or shake dressing to re-emulsify and add to taste (note that tamari and miso can both vary widely in saltiness, so dress sparingly at first, then add more as you like). I use about half of the dressing. Using a spatula or wooden spoon, gently fold to combine components of pilaf. Taste and add more dressing if desired. Transfer to a serving platter. Sprinkle with remaining cilantro. Serve warm or at room temperature. Pilaf is also delicious cold, the next day. Enjoy!
- For the Soy Dressing
- Combine tamari and vinegar in a small saucepan. Bring mixture to a boil over medium heat. Lower heat to a simmer and cook until mixture is reduced to 1/4 cup, about 6 to 7 minutes. Remove from heat and whisk in orange juice and canola oil. Transfer to a glass jar with a lid.

- This will make more dressing than you need for this recipe. Use remaining as a dressing for other grilled vegetables or as a marinade for meat.

136. Moroccan Quinoa & Chickpea Salad With Dried Fruit

Serving: Serves 6-8 | Prep: | Cook: | Ready in:

Ingredients

- 1 tablespoon olive oil
- 1/2 cup sweet onion - diced
- 2 cloves garlic - minced
- 1 teaspoon Ras el Hanout plus:
- 1/2 teaspoon ground cinnamon
- 1/2 teaspoon ground cumin
- 1/2 teaspoon ground coriander
- 1/2 teaspoon ground ginger
- 1 cup chickpeas (cooked from dry or canned)
- 1/3 cup quinoa - uncooked
- 1/3 cup golden raisins
- 1/3 cup dried apricots - sliced
- 1 cup vegetable stock (preferably homemade)
- 1/2 cup fresh orange juice
- 1/3 cup fresh lemon juice
- 1 zest of 1 lemon
- salt and pepper
- 1/4 cup slivered almonds
- 3 tablespoons mint - chopped
- 3 tablespoons parsley - chopped

Direction

- Prepare chickpeas if using dried. Rinse thoroughly and drain if using canned. Rinse and drain quinoa.
- Heat oil over medium heat in a Dutch oven. Add onion and garlic. Sauté until translucent – about 4-5 minutes. Add dry spices and cook for 1 minute stirring constantly. Add quinoa, chickpeas and dried fruit. Stir to combine.
- Add stock, juices, and lemon zest. Season with salt and pepper. Raise heat to medium high and bring mixture to a light boil. Reduce heat to simmer and cook until the quinoa is tender and the liquids have been absorbed – about 15-20 minutes.
- When quinoa is tender and liquids have been absorbed turn off the heat, cover the pot, and let rest for 10 minutes. Remove lid, fluff with a fork, mix in slivered almonds, parsley, and mint…and transfer to a serving bowl. Enjoy!

137. Moroccan Tilapia With Red Pepper, Lemon And Quinoa

Serving: Serves 4-6 | Prep: | Cook: | Ready in:

Ingredients

- 2 pounds tilapia filets, fresh or frozen (defrosted)
- 1/4 cup olive oil
- 1 whole head of garlic, cut in half and peeled
- 2 sweet red bell peppers, seeded, trimmed, and sliced into 1/2" strips
- 1 lemon with peel, washed well, cut into 1/4" dice
- 2 tablespoons harissa, or to taste*
- 1 tablespoon turmeric powder
- 1/2 teaspoon ground cumin
- 2 cups fresh cilantro or parsley leaves, including stems, roughly chopped
- 1/2 cup quinoa
- salt and pepper, to taste
- 3/4 cup water or chicken stock
- salt and pepper, to taste
- 1/2 cup quinoa

Direction

- You will need a large saute pan with a top. Over medium-high, heat oil.

- Stir in garlic, pepper slices, and lemon pieces, saute for about 30 seconds.
- Add harissa, turmeric, cumin, and chopped cilantro (or parsley) and again, saute for 30 seconds.
- Stir in quinoa and water -- stir to combine and bring to a simmer.
- Place filets over the vegetable mixture and reduce heat to medium. Cover and cook gently, undisturbed -- it should simmer not boil -- for 30-40 minutes until fish is cooked through, and the quinoa has "sprouted".
- Garnish with sprigs of fresh cilantro and lemon slices.
- Harissa is a North African chili paste available in many Mediterranean or Middle Eastern specialty shops, some Trader Joe's and Whole Foods. If you don't have harissa, you can substitute with a mixture of 1/4 teaspoon of hot chili pepper flakes, 1/2 teaspoon ground coriander, and 1/2 teaspoon ground cumin (in addition to the cumin already in the recipe). Note that this is not a recipe for harissa, which features garlic and red peppers that are already in this recipe.

138. Mung Bean, Lentil, And Quinoa Salad Stuffed Avocado

Serving: Serves 6 | Prep: | Cook: | Ready in:

Ingredients

- Salad
- 1/2 cup mung beans, uncooked
- 1/2 cup green (french) lentils, uncooked
- 1/2 cup quinoa, uncooked
- 1/2 cup cucumber, chopped
- 1/2 cup bell pepper, chopped
- 1/4 cup red onion, finely chopped
- 3 tablespoons cilantro, finely chopped
- 1 pinch sea salt
- 1 pinch freshly ground black pepper
- 3 avocados
- Dressing
- 2 tablespoons lemon juice
- 4 tablespoons extra virgin olive oil
- 1/4 teaspoon Dijon mustard
- 1 pinch cumin
- 1 dash chili powder
- 1 dash sea salt

Direction

- 1. Prepare beans, lentils, and quinoa, separately, according to package instructions.
- 2. Once beans, lentils, and quinoa cool slightly, combine in a medium-sized bowl. Add the rest of the salad ingredients and combine.
- 3. To prepare the vinaigrette, combine ingredients in a small bowl and whisk until a uniform consistency forms. Taste, and add additional salt and pepper to taste.
- 4. Dress the salad with half of the vinaigrette, taste, and add more according to preference. Let sit to marinate in the refrigerator for at least 15 minutes.
- 5. Slice avocados lengthwise and remove pits. To serve, stuff the salad into the center of the avocado. Serve cold.

139. Mushroom Quinoa Soup

Serving: Serves 4 | Prep: 0hours10mins | Cook: 0hours30mins | Ready in:

Ingredients

- 2 tablespoons olive oil
- 1 large onion, chopped
- 1 head of garlic, cloves separated and peeled
- 1 pound button or cremini mushrooms, sliced
- 4 carrots, peeled and sliced
- 4 cups low sodium vegetable stock
- 2 cups water
- 1/2 cup uncooked quinoa
- 2 cups packed kale leaves
- 1/2 teaspoon black pepper
- 1/2 teaspoon kosher salt

Direction

- Preheat a large pot over medium high heat. Once hot add the oil. Allow to heat for 1 minute. Add the onion, garlic, and mushrooms, and sauté 5-10 minutes, until the mushrooms are beginning to caramelize.
- Add the carrots and sauté a minute or two more. Add the stock and water and bring to a boil. Reduce to a simmer and add the quinoa. Cook for about 15 minutes, until the quinoa is tender. Add the kale and cook just until it starts to wilt. Season with pepper and salt.
- Serve immediately. Soup may be stored in an airtight container in the refrigerator for up to 2 days. Reheat in the microwave for 1-2 minutes, until heated through.

140. Mushrooms & Quinoa

Serving: Serves one | Prep: | Cook: |Ready in:

Ingredients

- 3 handfuls chopped mushrooms
- 1 handful chopped onion
- 1/2 handful cooked quinoa
- 1 drop fat (coconut oil, ghee, or olive oil)
- 5 dashes yummy seasonings (herbs, spices, salt, pepper)

Direction

- COOKING TIP: Preheat your pan to high before sautéing, then reduce to medium-high. You can hold your hand over the pan and if you feel heat, it's ready.
- Sauté chopped onions in a small bit of fat a short time, until a bit tender.
- Add mushrooms and continue cooking until mushrooms at soft. (5 minutes?) Don't cook too long as they will turn into rubber. Yuck!
- Mix in cooked quinoa.
- Add seasonings.
- Plate and enjoy!

141. My Favorite Quinoa Breakfast Hash

Serving: Serves 4 | Prep: | Cook: |Ready in:

Ingredients

- 2 sweet potatoes, chopped and roasted
- 1 small cauliflower, chopped and roasted
- 1 red pepper, chopped
- 1/2 bunch of kale or spinach, chopped
- 1 sweet onion, chopped
- 1/2 cup dry quinoa, rinsed and cooked
- 1/2 teaspoon smoked paprika
- 1/2 teaspoon cumin
- a few dashes of cinnamon
- salt and pepper, to taste
- 4 eggs, cooked to your preference
- olive oil
- chopped parsley, cilantro or basil to top

Direction

- First chop both the sweet potato and cauliflower. Place each on their own rimmed baking sheet in a single layer and toss each liberally with olive oil and sea salt. Roast them at 400° for about 25 minutes or until they are tender and starting to brown.
- While the potatoes and cauliflower are roasting, rinse and cook the quinoa. Set aside.
- In a large pan (you'll be adding everything to it), sauté chopped onion in a bit of olive oil until translucent and starting to brown - about 5 minutes. Season with a dash of salt.
- Add chopped red pepper and kale or spinach. Season again with a few dashes of salt. Sauté until kale wilts a bit and pepper starts to soften -about 3 minutes. (Kale will hold up better if you're making extra for the week)
- Add sweet potatoes and cauliflower to the pan.

- Toss with spices....cumin, paprika and cinnamon. Sometimes I add a dash of olive oil here as well.
- Mix in the cooked quinoa and cook until everything is warm and ready to eat!
- Adjust seasonings to taste along with more salt and pepper to taste. I like extra cinnamon!
- In a separate pan cook your eggs to your preference.
- Place a serving of quinoa/veggie mixture into a bowl. Top with cooked egg. Sprinkle with parsley.

142. Nectarine Quinoa

Serving: Serves 1 | Prep: | Cook: | Ready in:

Ingredients

- 2 Nectarines
- 1 tablespoon butter
- 1 tablespoon brown sugar
- 1/2 teaspoon ground nutmeg
- 1/2 cup almond slices
- 1 cup quinoa, cooked

Direction

- In a pan, heat the butter over medium to low heat until melted.
- Add the nectarines and sauté until warmed through.
- Sprinkle with the brown sugar and the nutmeg, stir and allow the nectarines to bubble and caramelize for a few minutes.
- Serve over the quinoa and garnish with almond slices.

143. Nectarine Quinoa Salad

Serving: Serves 4 as light lunch or side dish | Prep: | Cook: | Ready in:

Ingredients

- 2 candy beetroot
- 100 grams quinoa
- 1 tablespoon olive oil
- 1/2 juice lime
- 30 grams mint, roughly chopped
- 20 grams parsley, chopped
- 1 nectarine
- 25 grams pistachio, roasted
- 100 grams watercress, washed & roughly chopped
- 50-70 milliliters dressing
- salt & pepper to taste
- Dressing
- 60 milliliters lime juice
- 60 milliliters olive oil
- 1 teaspoon dijon mustard
- 1 tablespoon nutritional yeast
- Pinch salt & pepper

Direction

- Steam the beetroot in a pan with about 2 inches of water. Cook for about 30-40 minutes depending on the size of the beetroot. I cooked the beetroot so it still had bite rather than being totally soft. While the beetroot is cooking prepare the rest of your ingredients.
- Cook the quinoa with a pinch of salt and the 200ml water by steaming in a pan with the lid on until the water is absorbed, about 10 minutes. Once the liquid is absorbed, leave the lid on for a further few minutes. Fluff with a fork and dress with a tablespoon of olive oil and the juice of half a lime.
- To make the dressing, blitz all the ingredients in a high-speed blender. If you don't have one, whisk the ingredients together and slowly drizzle the oil in until the dressing is emulsified and creamy. Any extra dressing you can save for another day.
- Roughly chop your herbs and pistachio. Peel your beetroot, cut into 1 cm pieces, along with your nectarine. Once the quinoa has cooled a little, mix these through with your herbs, nuts, 50ml of dressings, adding more if needed. Mix

through the watercress, taste for seasoning and serve.

144. No Bake Quinoa Breakfast Bar

Serving: Serves 6 | Prep: | Cook: |Ready in:

Ingredients

- 150g quinoa flakes
- 50g flaked almond
- 25g coconut flakes
- 6 dried apple rings
- 25g dried cranberries or sultanas
- 2 tablespoons pumpkin seeds
- 1 tablespoon chia seeds
- 3 dried figs
- Small piece fresh ginger
- 100ml Fresh orange or apple juice (you may need slightly more)

Direction

- Place quinoa flakes, almonds and coconut into a nonstick frying pan and lightly toast over a medium heat
- Leave to cool and then place into a food processor with all ingredients except the juice
- Shred for a few minutes and then slowly incorporate the juice until you have a thick sticky dough
- Place the dough into a lined dish or silicone mold and flatten with down with the back of a fork
- You can sprinkle the top with additional seeds or dried fruit if you like
- Cover with cling film and place into the freezer for two hours before transferring to the fridge

145. Nutty Cherry Lentil Quinoa Salad

Serving: Serves 2 | Prep: | Cook: |Ready in:

Ingredients

- 1/2 cup French Lentils
- 1/2 cup Red Quinoa
- 1/2 cup Fresh sweet cherries
- 3/4 cup Fresh sweet cherries
- 1/2 cup pistachios
- 1 Shallot
- 1/2 teaspoon cumin
- 1/2 tablespoon Red wine vinegar
- 1 tablespoon Extra Virgin olive oil
- 1/2 tablespoon Cranberry juice
- butter

Direction

- Cook the French Lentils to package instructions and drain
- Cook the Red Quinoa to package instructions and drain
- Mince and Sauté the large shallot in a pan with a little butter
- In a food processor pulse the pistachios until they are in small pieces
- Add the cooked French lentils and pulse until blended
- Add the cooked Red Quinoa and pulse until blended
- Add the first 1/2 cup of fresh sweet cherries and pulse until blended. Do not over process
- Place this mix in bowl and add the cumin, olive oil, red wine vinegar, cranberry juice, and sauté shallot.
- Cut the 3/4 cup of fresh sweet cherries until quarters and add to mix. Stir together and enjoy this healthy dish.

146. Nutty Quinoa Salmon Burgers

Serving: Makes 6 medium patties | Prep: | Cook: | Ready in:

Ingredients

- 2 cups tinned salmon, well drained, and small bones removed (or lightly poached salmon, flaked)
- 2 tablespoons ground flaxseed
- ½ cup cooked quinoa
- ½ cup pecan pieces (or walnuts, though pecans seem more flavorful)
- 1 tablespoon quinoa flakes (or quick oats)
- 1 egg
- 1 teaspoon Worcestershire sauce
- ½ teaspoon Dijon or similar mustard
- 1 scallion, finely chopped
- 2 tablespoons finely diced celery
- 3 tablespoons finely chopped parsley
- 1-2 tablespoons chopped dill or sweet pickle (to taste)
- Zest of one lemon, grated or finely chopped
- Salt
- Grapeseed or olive oil for frying
- Phulka roti or other flatbread, or brioche or other buns for serving
- Garnishes such as arugula or watercress, and tomatoes
- FOR THE SAUCE
- 3 tablespoons tahini
- 1 tablespoon fruity olive oil
- Juice of one lemon
- 2 tablespoons chopped dill or sweet pickle
- 1 tablespoon finely chopped parsley
- Pinch of salt

Direction

- In a large bowl, mix together the salmon and flaxseed, mashing the salmon somewhat. Add the cooked quinoa and stir to combine.
- In a food processor, gently pulse the nuts four or five times to break down into small bits. (Or, chop them with a knife.) Add to the bowl with the salmon.
- Lightly beat the egg with the Worcestershire sauce and the mustard.
- Add the quinoa flakes or oats to the bowl with the salmon, along with the beaten egg, scallion, celery, chopped parsley, chopped pickle, lemon zest and a generous pinch of salt. Stir well to combine.
- Form into patties – you'll need to squeeze it together tightly with your hands -- and set aside, lightly covered, for 5-10 minutes.
- While the patties are resting, make the sauce by combining all of the sauce ingredients. Test for salt and correct if necessary.
- Heat a skillet to medium, and add about a tablespoon of oil. When the oil is hot (4 or 5 seconds), fry the patties for 5 minutes. Reduce the heat, cover and cook for about 3 minutes. Remove the cover, gently flip the burgers over and cook for another 3 minutes over medium heat.
- Serve in wraps using phulka roti or other flatbread, or on light buns, lightly toasted, with a generous dollop of sauce and tomatoes, salad greens, etc.
- Enjoy!! ;o)

147. Oats And Quinoa Breakfast Bars

Serving: Serves 16 bars | Prep: | Cook: | Ready in:

Ingredients

- 2 tablespoons canola oil
- 3/4 cup quinoa, rinsed
- 2 cups old fashioned oats
- 1 cup roasted, salted cashews, chopped
- 1/3 cup roasted sunflower seeds
- 1 cup dried fruit, chopped (cranberries, raisins, apricots, etc)
- 1/2 cup dark chocolate chips (optional)
- 1 1/2 cups Multigrain Cheerios

- 1 cup sugar
- 1/3 cup water
- 1 teaspoon vanilla
- 1/4 cup half and half
- 1/4 cup peanut butter

Direction

- Line a 9x13 inch baking pan with foil so that the foil hangs over the sides. Spray with cooking spray and set pan aside.
- Heat oil in a large sauté pan. Add quinoa and oats, toss to coat with oil, and toast lightly. Remove from heat and let cool.
- Put oat mixture into a large mixing bowl, then add cashews, sunflower seeds, fruit, chocolate chips (if desired), and Cheerios. Stir well to combine.
- Pour sugar and water into a medium saucepan, stir lightly to combine, and bring to a boil. Cook over medium-high heat, without stirring, until sugar turns a light golden color, about 6 minutes. Reduce heat to medium low and continue to boil until sugar is a dark amber color (another 1 to 3 minutes). Stir only as needed.
- Immediately remove from heat, then whisk half and half, vanilla, and peanut butter into the sugar. The mixture will bubble vigorously, so be careful. Work quickly because caramel will start to thicken.
- Pour caramel over the oat mixture and stir well to combine. Immediately transfer granola mixture into the prepared pan and press and pack well into a flat layer. Be sure to press very tightly, or the bars will break apart.
- Refrigerate for at least 3 hours. Remove from pan by lifting the foil, and then cut into 16 bars. Wrap bars in wax or parchment paper, to keep them from sticking together.
- Refrigerate extra bars in an airtight container, or freeze.

148. Okra And Tomato Quinoa

Serving: Serves 4-6 | Prep: | Cook: | Ready in:

Ingredients

- 16 ounces okra
- 14.5 ounces can Hunt's® Diced Tomatoes with Basil, Garlic & Oregano
- 1 cup raw quinoa
- 2 cups vegetable broth
- 1/2 cup parmesan cheese
- additional basil & oregano to taste (if desired)

Direction

- Preheat oven to 375 degrees.
- Pour vegetable broth, quinoa, okra and tomatoes (with juice) in 9x9 baking dish.
- Grate parmesan. Mix with additional spices if you choose to do so and then sprinkle mixture on top.
- Bake for 30-40 minutes, or until quinoa is cooked.

149. Olive Oil Fried Chicken With Pesto Quinoa And Heirloom Tomatoes

Serving: Serves 2 | Prep: | Cook: | Ready in:

Ingredients

- 2 boneless, skinless chicken thighs
- 2 small heirloom tomatoes
- 3 tablespoons olive oil
- 1/2 cup quinoa
- 1 small bunch parsley
- 1 small bunch basil
- 2 cloves garlic
- 1 lemon, juiced
- 2 tablespoons pine nuts
- salt

- pepper

Direction

- Preheat oven to 250 F. Lay pine nuts flat on a baking sheet and toast for 5-7 minutes. Make sure they don't burn! Remove as soon as they turn golden and begin to smell toasty. They'll continue to cook on the baking sheet.
- Then, prepare your chicken. Heat up 3 tablespoons olive oil over high heat until hot but not smoking. Season chicken thighs heavily with salt and pepper. Fry each side in olive oil over high heat for 2 minutes, until browned. Cover pan, turn heat to medium-low and cook for additional 8-10 minutes, or until cooked through. Should have a golden-brown crust, and be irresistibly crispy. Remove from heat.
- Next, make the pesto quinoa. Cook the quinoa over the stove according to the package directions. Remove from heat and put into a blender or food processor. Add additional 6 tablespoons olive oil, parsley, basil, and lemon juice. Peel and smash garlic cloves and throw those in too. Add 1/4 teaspoon salt and pepper and blend, until blended but not soupy. Taste and add additional salt as needed. Remove from blender.
- Chop up heirloom tomatoes into big chunks.
- Now assemble your bowls: Cut chicken breasts into slices or large pieces, and place in bowls with tomatoes and a big dollop of pesto quinoa. Add a bit of additional salt and pepper to tomatoes. Garnish with toasted pine nuts and grated parmesan.

150. One Pot Corn, Tomato & Quinoa Pilaf

Serving: Serves 2 to 4 | Prep: 0hours15mins | Cook: 0hours20mins | Ready in:

Ingredients

- 2 cups water
- 1/2 teaspoon kosher salt, plus more to taste
- 1 cup quinoa
- 1 cup fresh corn kernels
- 1 cup halved cherry tomatoes
- 1 tablespoon lemon zest (about 1 large lemon)
- 3 scallions, thinly sliced
- 1/3 cup crumbled feta
- 1 tablespoon olive oil
- 3 tablespoons sunflower seeds, toasted, plus more to top
- 1/2 cup roughly mint, plus more to top
- 1 pinch crushed red pepper flakes

Direction

- Add the water to a pot and bring to a boil. Add the salt and quinoa. Stir, cover, and lower the heat until it's at a simmer. Cook for 10 minutes, covered. Uncover, top with the corn and tomatoes, then re-cover. Cook another 5 minutes, then turn off the heat and allow to steam for 5 more minutes.
- While the quinoa is cooking, combine the lemon zest, scallions, feta, and olive oil in a big bowl.
- After the quinoa has steamed for 5 minutes, check how it's doing. The water should have absorbed. If it hasn't, cover and cook on the lowest-possible heat for another few minutes until it has.
- When it's done, fluff the pilaf and transfer to the waiting bowl with the remaining ingredients. Add the sunflower seeds and mint on top and toss. Season with salt and red pepper flakes to taste.

151. Orange Basil Quinoa Salad

Serving: Serves 6 | Prep: | Cook: | Ready in:

Ingredients

- Dressing

- 1/2 cup Orange Muscat vinegar or 1/4 c champagne vinegar & 1/4 C oj
- 3/4 teaspoon Ground Ginger
- 3/4 teaspoon Chipotle powder or smoked paprika if you don't like heat
- 1/2 teaspoon Salt
- 1/2 teaspoon Pepper
- 1/3 cup Extra virgin olive oil
- Salad
- 1 cup Quinoa, any color, rinsed well
- 1/2 cup Red lentils, picked over & rinsed
- 1 cup Low sodium veggie stock
- 4 ounces Baby spinach
- 1 cup Diced zucchini, 1 small
- 1 1/2 cups Roasted corn kernels
- 1 1/2 cups Diced tomato or halved cherry tomatoes
- 3/4 cup Diced sweet onion
- 2 tablespoons Basil, sliced thin (chiffonade)
- 2 tablespoons Flat leaf parsley chopped
- Basil for garnish

Direction

- Make the dressing – combine the vinegar, spices, salt and pepper. Slowly whisk in the olive oil. This makes a wonderful marinade for salmon too.
- Toast the quinoa in a heavy bottomed pan until it starts to pop and smell nutty. Carefully add the veggie stock and 2¼ C water to the pan. Bring to a simmer, add the lentils and cook for 15 min or until you see the tails come out of the quinoa. Drain remaining liquid, if any. Add the spinach to the hot quinoa mixture and stir to wilt it. Add the onion, zucchini, corn, tomato. Stir to combine. Drizzle in enough dressing to moisten well. Let cool. Mix in the parsley & basil chiffonade. Adjust seasonings to taste remembering that if it will be served cold a little more seasoning will be necessary. Garnish with the basil. Delicious at any temperature.

152. Orange And Strawberry Quinoa Salad

Serving: Serves 4 | Prep: | Cook: | Ready in:

Ingredients

- 2 handfuls of baby salad leaves
- 2.6 ounces cooked quinoa
- 1 orange peeled, pith removed and sliced
- 8 strawberries quartered
- 1.8 ounces cubed feta
- 2 tablespoons chopped toasted nuts
- 6 tablespoons olive oil
- 2 tablespoons balsamic vinegar
- 1 teaspoon 1 grainy mustard
- Pinch salt
- Pinch ground black pepper

Direction

- Mix all the ingredients from the salad leaves to the chopped nuts together.
- Whisk all the ingredients for the balsamic vinaigrette (from the oil to the pepper) together until combined.
- Adjust seasoning and drizzle on as much dressing as you would like onto your salad.
- Serve with fresh crusty bread and grilled fish, meats or vegetables.
- You can keep the rest of the vinaigrette on your counter top for another salad.
- You can easily double or triple the recipe to feed a crowd.

153. Oven Roasted Brussels Sprouts With Bacon, Chestnuts & Quinoa

Serving: Serves 4 | Prep: | Cook: | Ready in:

Ingredients

- 200 grams brussels sprouts
- 1 cup quinoa, uncooked

- 100 grams whole chestnuts
- 6 thick smoked bacon rashers, cubed
- 2 organic gluten-free stock cubes
- 2 tablespoons extra virgin olive oil
- 1 tablespoon butter
- 1 pinch salt
- 1 pinch pepper
- 1 handful fresh parsley

Direction

- Rinse and prepare the Brussel sprouts by removing the first few layers (if necessary) and using a knife to make two slight indents in the bottom of each sprout to produce an 'x'.
- Sprinkle on a little sea salt, pepper and oil over the Brussels sprouts and place in a tray and in the oven for approximately twenty minutes or until tender and golden in places.
- Fry the bacon and set aside.
- Add the cooked quinoa to the Brussels sprouts and carefully mix together. Add a bit more salt and pepper, if needed
- Add the bacon, chestnuts and parsley to the quinoa and sprouts and serve.

154. Overnight Toasted Oat And Quinoa Bowl

Serving: Serves 3-4 | Prep: | Cook: |Ready in:

Ingredients

- 1/2 cup thick rolled whole grain oats, I used Bob's Red Mill (gluten free if desired)
- 1/4 cup quinoa
- 1 3/4 cups almond milk
- 1/2 ripe banana, sliced (unless you have an apple banana, in which case use the whole thing)
- 1 whole dried date, pitted, chopped
- 1/4 teaspoon cinnamon
- pinch of ground ginger
- pinch of ground cardamom
- pinch of salt
- 1 tablespoon chia seeds
- 1/2 cup frozen blueberries (or other fruit of choice)

Direction

- DO THE NIGHT BEFORE: In a dry skillet, toast oats and quinoa over medium heat until fragrant and golden. Stir to prevent burning. Quinoa will start to pop.
- Add toasted grains to an assembled blender jar (with blade attached at bottom). Add all of the remaining ingredients except the blueberries. Place blender lid on blender jar and refrigerate overnight.
- IN THE MORNING: Place blender jar on base and puree mixture for 10 second intervals until combined. Add contents of blender to a small pot, add blueberries and heat until mixture bubbles. Divide into bowls and serve. Alternatively, divide blender contents into 4 microwaveable bowls, add blueberries to each bowl and nuke each bowl for 1 minute and 20 seconds. I used the microwave and was pleased with the results. Quick and delicious!

155. Paula Shoyer's Chocolate Quinoa Cake

Serving: Serves 12 | Prep: 0hours40mins | Cook: 1hours15mins |Ready in:

Ingredients

- Chocolate Cake
- 3/4 cup (130g) quinoa (enough to make 2 1/4 cups cooked quinoa)
- 1 1/2 cups (360ml) water
- 1 splash cooking spray or melted coconut oil, for greasing the pan
- 2 tablespoons potato starch or dark unsweetened cocoa, for dusting the pan
- 1/3 cup (80ml) orange juice (from 1 orange)
- 4 large eggs

- 2 teaspoons pure vanilla extract (or other vanilla if for Passover)
- 3/4 cup (180ml) melted coconut oil
- 1 1/2 cups (300g) sugar
- 1 cup (80g) dark unsweetened cocoa
- 2 teaspoons baking powder
- 1/2 teaspoon kosher salt
- 2 ounces (55g) bittersweet chocolate
- Glaze (optional)
- 5 ounces (140g) bittersweet chocolate
- 1 tablespoon sunflower or safflower oil
- 1 teaspoon pure vanilla extract (or other vanilla if for Passover)

Direction

- Place the quinoa and water into a small saucepan and bring it to a boil over medium heat. Reduce the heat to low, cover the saucepan, and cook the quinoa for 15 minutes, or until all the liquid has been absorbed. The quinoa should be fully cooked at this point—taste a little to make sure it's not crunchy (if it is, add a little more water to the pan and keep cooking till it's softened). Set the pan aside. The quinoa may be made 1 day or more in advance.
- Heat the oven to 350°F (180°C). Grease a 12-cup (2.8L) Bundt pan, sprinkle the potato starch over the greased pan, then shake the pan to remove any excess starch.
- Place the quinoa in the bowl of a food processor or blender. Add the orange juice, eggs, vanilla, oil, sugar, cocoa, baking powder, and salt and process until the mixture is very smooth.
- Melt the chocolate over a double boiler, or place in a medium microwave-safe bowl, and put in a microwave for 45 seconds, stirring and then heating the chocolate for another 30 seconds, until it is melted. Add the chocolate to the quinoa batter and process until well mixed. Pour the batter into the prepared Bundt pan and bake it for 50 minutes, or until a skewer inserted into the cake comes out clean.
- Let the cake cool for 10 minutes and then gently turn it out of the pan onto a wire cooling rack. Let it cool on the rack.
- To make the glaze, melt the chocolate in a large microwave-safe bowl in the microwave (see above) or over a double boiler. Add the oil and vanilla and whisk well. Let the glaze sit for 5 minutes and then whisk it again. Use a silicone spatula to spread the glaze over the top of the cake, letting it drip down the sides. Serve at room temperature and store any leftovers airtight at room temperature.

156. Perfect Long Grain Brown Rice With Black Or Red Quinoa

Serving: Serves 3-4 | Prep: | Cook: | Ready in:

Ingredients

- 1/4 cup black or red quinoa
- 1 cup long grain brown rice
- 5 cups boiling water
- 1/2 teaspoon sea salt
- 1 tablespoon extra virgin olive oil
- 1 tablespoon lemon juice (Meyer preferred) or hot water
- 1/2 teaspoon Maldon salt flakes or other artisan salt

Direction

- Preheat the oven to 350 degrees. Soak the quinoa in water for 5 minutes, then drain. Rinse the brown rice under tap water in a fine mesh colander for a few minutes. Boil 5 cups of water.
- In a casserole dish (which has a cover) add the quinoa, rice and sea salt. Mix evenly. Pour the boiling rice to cover completely the grains. Bake uncovered for 45 minutes. Then remove from the oven and drain most all the liquid off. Keep the oven on.

- Add the olive oil, lemon juice (or hot water), and Maldon sea flakes. Cover and return to the oven to bake for 15 minutes. Remove from the oven and let sit covered for another 15 minutes. Fluff and serve.

157. Peruvian Quinoa Lettuce Roll Ups

Serving: Serves 12 | Prep: | Cook: | Ready in:

Ingredients

- 1 cup quinoa, rinsed
- 2 cups vegetable broth or water
- 1 tablespoon olive oil
- 1/2 cup diced onion
- 1 cup diced red bell pepper
- 1 small chile, minced
- 1 cup diced potato (purple, if you can find them, or Yukon gold)
- 1-1/2 cups diced calabaza or butternut squash
- 3/4 cup diced tomato
- 1 teaspoon garlic powder
- 1-1/2 teaspoons kosher salt
- 1/4 cup minced cilantro
- 12 large romaine lettuce leaves
- 1 avocado, diced

Direction

- After you rinse the quinoa, drain well. Heat a medium saucepan; add the quinoa and toast over medium heat until quinoa is dry and starts to brown. Pour in the vegetable broth or water; bring to a boil. Lower the heat and simmer, covered, until liquid is absorbed, about 10 minutes. Fluff the quinoa and set aside.
- Heat the oil in a wide skillet. Add onion, red pepper, and chile and sauté until vegetables have softened. Add the potato, squash, tomato, garlic powder, and salt. Mix well and continue cooking until all vegetables are tender, about 20 minutes. Stir frequently. Mix in the cilantro and remove from the heat.
- Cut the ribs from the lettuce leaves just until the point where you can roll them. Lay a lettuce leaf flat. Place 1 cup filling at the bottom end of the leaf and roll it up, tucking in the leaf as needed. Repeat with remaining crepes and filling. Place the rolls on a plate and garnish with the diced avocado.

158. Peruvian Tri Color Quinoa Salad

Serving: Serves 6-8 | Prep: | Cook: | Ready in:

Ingredients

- 1 lb tri-color quinoa (also works with plain quinoa)
- 4-5 cups water
- 2 chicken bouillion cubes/OR 3 TBSP powdered chicken broth
- 2 TBSP FRESH minced garlic
- 1 tsp Adobo seasoning (if u like)
- 1/2 purple onion, chopped small
- 2 cups small seedless red grapes
- 2 ripe avocados, peeled and chopped
- 2 TBSP olive oil
- 4 TBSP fresh lime/lemon juice
- Salt and pepper to taste

Direction

- Put the water on the boil in a large soup pot and add the chicken bouillon, salt to taste, and fresh garlic (garlic powder will do if you don't have fresh garlic). Put the lid on and bring to a boil on High, then pour in the quinoa, stir well. Make sure the pot lid is fastened securely because you want it to work something like a rice steamer. Bring the heat down to a Medium simmer; keep covered! Cook quinoa for 30 minutes, stirring occasionally so it doesn't stick.

- Reserve a few grapes and 2 slices of avocado for garnish. Add the chopped purple onion, chopped avocado, and red grapes to a large mixing bowl and toss well--I have also added chopped fresh cilantro to the mix for an even fresher taste! When the quinoa is done, drain it in a strainer then pour the hot quinoa over the ingredients and toss gently to mix.
- Pour the olive oil and lemon/lime juice (either works well) over the mix and toss gently. Garnish with fresh red grapes and two slices of avocado. This salad can be served warm or cold and it's delicious either way. NOTE: If you cannot find seedless red grapes, cut the larger round seeded grapes in half and pick out the seeds before using.

159. Pesto Quinoa Veggie Bowl

Serving: Serves 3+ | Prep: | Cook: |Ready in:

Ingredients

- Pesto
- 1.5 tablespoons olive oil
- 1 garlic clove
- 2 handfuls basil leaves
- 1 pinch red pepper flakes
- 1.5 tablespoons lemon or lime juice
- 1/4 cup sliced almonds
- salt and pepper
- Quinoa and Veggies
- 1 cup red quinoa, rinsed and drained
- 1 2/3 cups water or chicken broth
- 1 teaspoon olive oil
- 1/2 onion, diced
- 3/4 cup carrots, sliced
- 2 small zucchini, halved and sliced into half moons
- 1 garlic clove, minced
- 1/4 cup pepitas, toasted
- 2 handfuls baby arugula
- 2 eggs (OPTIONAL)
- 2 tablespoons white vinegar

Direction

- Pesto
- Combine ingredients in a small food processor or blender (I used my immersion blender in a pinch). Blend till smooth, adding water till you reach a consistency like thick soup. Set aside.
- Quinoa and Veggies
- Combine quinoa and water or broth in a medium saucepan. Bring to a boil, cover, lower heat to simmer and cook 15 minutes. Drain quinoa and set aside.
- Meanwhile, heat olive oil in a medium-large skillet on medium heat till shimmering. Add onion and carrot, cook 5 minutes. Add garlic and zucchini, cook 3 minutes longer. Season with salt and pepper. Add quinoa, pepitas, and pesto to veggie skillet and stir to combine.
- Wash quinoa saucepan (I like efficiency) and fill with at least 3 inches water. Add white vinegar. Bring to a boil. Swirl water and poach eggs one by one, 2-3 minutes each.
- To serve, plate quinoa and veggies with a handful of arugula and top with a poached egg. Season with salt and pepper and serve.
- For a great next-day lunch or side dish, mix another handful of arugula into leftover quinoa, and pop into the microwave for about 45 seconds.

160. Pesto Quinoa Pilaf

Serving: Serves 4-6 | Prep: | Cook: |Ready in:

Ingredients

- 2 cups cooked quinoa, still warm, any variety
- 1/2 cup pesto, use homemade or just your favorite from a jar
- 1/2 sweet onion, diced small
- 2 cloves of fresh garlic, minced
- 2 medium zucchini, diced small
- 1/4 cup pine nuts

- 1/3 cup freshly grated Parmesan cheese
- 1 cup fresh basil, in a chiffonade (or more if you love basil as much as I do)
- olive oil

Direction

- In a large serving bowl, mix the pesto in with the warm quinoa. Set aside.
- Sauté the veggies in a little olive oil until the zucchini is just tender and the onions are just soft. Keep an eye on the garlic so it doesn't get too brown.
- Push the veggies off to the side and then quickly toast the pine nuts in the middle of the pan.
- Add about 1/4 cup of the fresh basil and stir to mix the veggies and pine nuts well and wilt the herbs.
- Add the veggie and herb mix to the quinoa and mix well. Add the cheese and mix well to melt thoroughly.
- Garnish with the rest of the fresh basil chiffonade just before serving. Pass more cheese when serving, if desired. Can be served warm or at room temp.

161. Pickled Shrimp With Tzatzki Quinoa

Serving: Serves 4 | Prep: | Cook: | Ready in:

Ingredients

- 1 pound Fresh shrimp, cleaned and tails removed
- 1 Small white onion, thinly sliced into wedges
- 3 Garlic cloves, thinly sliced
- 1 Fresh jalapeño, thinly sliced (almost shaved into paper-thin sliced)
- 3 sprigs Fresh oregano
- 1/2 cup Fresh lemon juice
- 1/3 cup Apple cider vinegar
- 1 cup Water
- 2 tablespoons Coarse ground salt
- 3 tablespoons Cracked black peppercorns
- 2 cups Cooked quinoa
- 1/2 pint Grape tomatoes, halved
- 1 cup Pitted Greek black olives, halved
- 1 cup Plain Greek yogurt
- 1/2 cup Sour cream
- 2 Garlic cloves, finely minced
- 1/4 cup Fresh chopped flat-leaf parsley
- 2 tablespoons Fresh chopped dill, plus extra for garnish
- 1 tablespoon Coarse ground salt
- 1 tablespoon Coarse ground black pepper
- 2 tablespoons Fresh lemon juice
- 1 cup Crumbled feta cheese
- Extra virgin olive oil, for drizzling [garnish]
- Lemon wedges [garnish]
- Warm pita bread, cut into wedges [garnish]

Direction

- In a non-aluminum Dutch oven, combine shrimp, onion, garlic, jalapeño, oregano, lemon juice, vinegar, water, salt and peppercorns. Bring to simmer over medium high heat and simmer for 5-6 minutes, or just until shrimp turn opaque and pinkish in color. Remove from heat allow to cool to room temperature. [It is recommended that you complete this step 1 day ahead to allow shrimp to marinate in pickling liquid overnight.]
- In a large mixing bowl, toss together cooked quinoa, grape tomatoes and olives.
- In a small mixing bowl, whisk together yogurt, sour cream, garlic, parsley, dill, salt, pepper, and lemon juice. Pour over quinoa mixture and toss gently to coat. [Tzatziki can be made up to 2 days ahead. Store in a tightly covered container in the refrigerator. Stir well before adding to quinoa.]
- Place approximately 1/2 cup quinoa salad in bottom of shallow bowl and top with 4-6 shrimp and sprinkle crumbled feta cheese over shrimp. Drizzle with a bit of pickling liquid and olive oil. Sprinkle with extra dill. Serve with lemon wedges and warm pita bread.

162. Poblano Stuffed Quinoa With Honey Lime Vinaigrette

Serving: Serves 6 | Prep: | Cook: | Ready in:

Ingredients

- Quinoa Ingredients
- 6 Medium poblano chiles
- 3 ears of corn in husks, soaked in water for 10 minutes
- Extra-virgin olive oil
- 1 cup red quinoa, rinsed and drained in a mesh strainer (or white, or a mixture of the two—whatever you have on hand is fine!)
- 1 2/3 cups water
- 1/2 cup pumpkin seeds, toasted
- 1/2 cup cilantro, chopped, plus more for garnish
- 1/2 cup queso fresco, crumbled (feta or goat cheese would also work)
- Honey-Lime Vinaigrette (recipe follows)
- Honey-Lime Vinaigrette Ingredients
- 2 tablespoons lime juice
- 2 tablespoons extra-virgin olive oil
- 1 tablespoon white wine vinegar
- 1 teaspoon honey
- 1 clove of garlic, minced

Direction

- To grill the poblanos and corn: Light grill. While grill heats, rub the poblanos with oil. Grill over high heat until poblanos are charred all over, approximately 5 minutes. Remove from grill and place in a bowl covered with plastic wrap for at least 5 minutes. When heat cools to medium, grill corn until tender, turning every 5 minutes for approximately 15 – 20 minutes. Set corn aside to cool.
- To cook the quinoa: Add the rinsed quinoa to a saucepan and turn heat to high. Allow some of the residual water to cook off, then add 1 2/3 cups water to the pan. Bring to a boil, then reduce heat to medium-low, cover, and simmer until quinoa has absorbed all of the water, about 15 minutes. Let stand off of heat, covered, for 5 minutes. Then remove lid and fluff in pan with a fork.
- To make the vinaigrette: While the quinoa cooks, combine all of the ingredients for the vinaigrette in a small bowl and whisk to combine.
- To finish the poblanos and corn: Use paper towels or a kitchen towel to rub the skin off of the poblanos. Remove the stems and the seeds, chop the peppers, and set aside in a mixing bowl. Remove the husks and silks from the corn. Cut the kernels from the cobs and add them to the bowl of chopped poblano.
- Assemble the quinoa: Mix the quinoa with the poblanos and corn. Add the pumpkin seeds, cilantro, queso fresco and vinaigrette and toss until all ingredients are well-combined. Garnish with extra cilantro and serve.

163. Pork With Peaches & Quinoa

Serving: Serves 2 | Prep: | Cook: | Ready in:

Ingredients

- 4 Organic Pork Chops
- 4 tablespoons Extra Virgin Olive Oil
- 1 Red Onion
- 2 Cloves of Garlic
- 1 pinch Salt
- 1 pinch Black Pepper
- 1 pinch Mixed Herbs
- 1 pinch Chilli Flakes
- 2 Fresh Peaches
- 1 handful Chives

Direction

- Grate the onion and garlic and add to the pork chops, along with the salt, pepper and mixed herbs.

- Heat a griddle pan and add the oil.
- Place the chops on the pan and fry on a high heat for several minutes, turning over, before lowering the heat to a medium heat.
- Continue frying the pork chops for approximately 10-15 minutes (or until cooked), turning over a couple more times and remove from the pan.
- Half the peaches, remove the stones and fry in the pan - on a high heat - for a few minutes.
- Serve with warm quinoa and vegetables and garnish with the peaches and chives.

164. Preseved Lemon Quinoa

Serving: Serves 2 to 4 | Prep: | Cook: |Ready in:

Ingredients

- 1/2 of a whole preserved lemon
- 1 handful dried cherries or cranberries
- 1 cup beef broth
- 1 &1/2 cups water
- 1 cup quinoa
- 1 handful toasted slivered almonds

Direction

- Discard pulp of preserved lemon, rinse well and fine chop peel
- Put chopped lemon, broth, water and quinoa in saucepan and bring to a boil over medium high heat (make sure you have a nice tight lid fit).
- Place cover on pan and reduce heat to simmer for about twenty minutes until liquid is absorbed.
- After twenty minutes, remove from heat and toss in dried cherries (or dried cranberries). toasted almonds and fluff all together with fork. Place the lid back on and let stand at least ten minutes. This can be served hot, warm or even room temperature.

165. Quinoa "Fried Rice"

Serving: Serves 6 | Prep: | Cook: |Ready in:

Ingredients

- 1/4 pound Sweet Pork Sausage, casings removed
- 4 cups Quinoa, cooked
- Extra Virgin Olive Oil
- 6 pieces Farm Eggs
- 3 cups Arugula, chopped
- 1/4 cup Dill, chopped
- 3 pieces Persian Cucumber, diced
- Sriracha for serving, optional

Direction

- Put a cast iron pan on the stove top on medium high heat and cook your pork sausage, breaking it up as you go. When cooked, remove from pan with a slotted spoon and place into a mixing bowl.
- Toast cooked quinoa in the rendered fat from the sausage so that the quinoa gets a little crispy. Season with salt and pepper to taste and add quinoa to mixing bowl. (Note: If you have just cooked your quinoa before doing this, allow it to cool first so that it doesn't just absorb the fat and become mushy)
- Lower the temperature of the pan to medium low. Add some extra virgin olive oil to the pan just to coat the bottom and crack your six eggs into the pan. Season the eggs with salt & pepper. Let the eggs cook for a minute as if you were to make sunny side up eggs, then crack the yolks and begin to move the eggs around in the pan so that you get a scramble that shows both the white and yellow of the egg. Cook to your liking (soft and fluffy or uber crispy!) Add your eggs to your mixing bowl
- Add arugula, dill, and cucumbers to your bowl. Drizzle the ingredients with extra virgin olive oil and sprinkle with salt and pepper. Toss ingredients to combine. Taste and adjust

seasoning/oil if necessary. Serve with Sriracha on the side. For fun, try serving out of Chinese takeout containers!

166. Quinoa & Mango Salad With Lemony Ginger Dressing

Serving: Serves serves 4-6 as a main course, 6-8 as a starter | Prep: 0hours25mins | Cook: 0hours50mins | Ready in:

Ingredients

- Quinoa and Mango Salad
- 1 cup regular, red or black quinoa, rinsed well in a strainer
- 2 cups water
- 3 mangoes
- 1 large red onion, halved stem to root and slivered
- 1 can black beans, rinsed and drained
- 2 cups micro greens (I used a rainbow blend package from Whole Foods herb section: mizuna, curly cress, red and yellow beet, arugula, cabbage) – if not available, mesclun, spring or baby greens are fine, rinsed and dried
- 3 tablespoons chopped cilantro
- 2 avocados, halved, pitted and sliced
- 1 tablespoon olive oil
- 1 pinch salt and pepper, to taste
- Lemony-Ginger Dressing
- 3 teaspoons lemon juice, plus more to taste
- 3 tablespoons olive oil, plus more to taste
- 1/2 teaspoon freshly grated ginger (or 1 tsp ground ginger)
- 1 pinch salt and pepper, plus more to taste

Direction

- Preheat oven to 400 degrees.
- Cook the quinoa: In a saucepan, bring quinoa and water to a boil. Reduce the heat to a simmer, cover, and cook until most or all of the water is absorbed, about 12-15 minutes. The little "tails" should pop free from the grain and it should still be pretty chewy. If any liquid remains, strain the quinoa. I usually add it to a strainer either way and rinse it under cold water to stop the cooking process, then continue to fluff it every so often as I'm preparing the other ingredients.
- Toss onion slivers with 1 tablespoon olive oil, salt and pepper. Roast for about 30 minutes. Resist stirring until they begin to brown, then stir occasionally; not too much or they will not brown as nicely. Remove when they are soft and nicely colored. Let cool.
- Pit and dice mangoes. Try to squeeze out some of the juices from the fibrous part surrounding the pit before discarding it – there's often a lot of juice in that section. Add it to the diced mangoes
- Make the dressing: Whisk the olive oil into the lemon juice. Whisk in the ginger and add salt and pepper to taste.
- Assemble the salad: Mix the quinoa, mango (and juices), black beans, and cilantro together. Spread the micro greens on a large plate and layer the quinoa mixture over the greens. Top with the roasted onions and the avocado slices. Drizzle the dressing over the salad and serve.

167. Quinoa & Pine Nut Salad

Serving: Serves 3-4 | Prep: | Cook: | Ready in:

Ingredients

- 2 cups Cooked Quinoa (I used multi colored)
- 3 tablespoons Raw Pine Nuts
- 2 Chopped Large Tomatoes (or 8 cherry tomatoes, halved)
- 1 Diced Avocado
- 2-3 tablespoons Olive Oil

Direction

- Place cooked Quinoa in the fridge to cool.
- Heat a small skillet on medium high heat.

- Add the Pine Nuts and cook until golden brown (about 2 minutes), making sure to stir often)
- Put chopped Tomatoes, Avocado, and Olive Oil in a medium size bowl.
- Add Pine Nuts and Quinoa and season with Salt and Pepper. Enjoy!

168. Quinoa & Roasted Sweet Potato Superfood Salad

Serving: Serves 4 | Prep: | Cook: | Ready in:

Ingredients

- salad
- 1/2 cup quinoa
- 1 sweet potato
- 1/3 cup walnuts or pumpkin seeds
- 1 avocado
- 3 cups hearty mixed greens
- 2 pinches salt and pepper
- chili lime vinaigrette
- 1 lime juiced
- 1/2 cup olive oil
- 1/2 teaspoon chili powder
- 1 teaspoon honey

Direction

- Prepare quinoa per package instructions.
- Preheat oven to 350. Peel your sweet potato and cut into 1-inch chunks. Toss the sweet potato with olive oil and salt and pepper. Place on parchment-lined cookie sheet and roast for about 25 minutes, flipping them over once in the middle of roasting.
- Slice avocado.
- Prepare the dressing. Then combine the warm ingredients (quinoa and sweet potato) and add half of your dressing to those ingredients.
- Toss the remaining ingredients with the dressing and compose your salad.

169. Quinoa & Bulgur Salad With Spinach, Chards, Radishes, Soft Boiled Eggs And Cappe

Serving: Makes 2 salads | Prep: | Cook: | Ready in:

Ingredients

- For the salad :
- 1/2 cup bulgur
- 1/2 cup quinoa
- 3 handfuls of spinach
- 6-8 pieces chards
- 4 quail eggs (or 2 normal eggs)
- 6 red radishes
- For the pesto: salt and freshly ground pepper
- 2 handfuls of basil leaves
- 2 clove of garlic
- 2 teaspoons of capers
- 2 tablespoons virgin olive oil
- some raisins (optional)
- oregano and parsley
- salt and freshly ground pepper

Direction

- In boiling salted water add the quinoa and the bulgur, sweet paprika, salt and pepper and let them boil. Meanwhile sauté the garlic and add the chopped chards, spinach, oregano and parsley and stir until they become tender, but without losing their bright green color. Once ready, remove the pan from the fire and let it aside.
- Then boil the eggs for 1 minute (for the quail eggs) or for 2.5 minutes (for the normal eggs). Remember that the times are relative and depend on the power of your cook.
- For the pesto, chop all ingredients together until they create a nice omiogenic mixture. Many people create pesto by putting everything in the blender, but I like to keep some textures intact.

- To serve, in a dish put peripherally the quinoa and the bulgur with the sauté vegetables (all together or separate, to define what goes in each bite) Add a big scoop of pesto in the middle and fresh olive oil, some chopped radishes and soft-boiled eggs. Bon appetit.

170. Quinoa 'Mac' And Cauliflower Chard Cheese Sauce

Serving: Serves 6-8 | Prep: | Cook: | Ready in:

Ingredients

- 3 cups cooked quinoa
- 1 tablespoon olive oil
- 1/4 cup diced yellow onion
- 1 minced garlic clove
- 3 cups chopped cauliflower florets
- 1 teaspoon salt, divided, plus more to taste
- 1/2 teaspoon black pepper
- 3/4 teaspoon onion powder
- 1/2 teaspoon dry mustard powder
- 1 small, dried bay leaf
- 2 cups water
- 1/4 cup unsweetened almond milk
- 15 scrapes of a nutmeg seed
- 2 cups chopped rainbow chard (or another dark leafy green)
- 6 ounces grated cheddar cheese
- 1/2 cup grated parmesan
- 1/3 cup walnut meal
- 1 mist of olive oil

Direction

- Heat the oil in a large saucepan (one that has a fitted lid).
- Add the onions to the pan, and sauté for about three minutes.
- Add the garlic to the pan, and sauté for 30 seconds, just until fragrant.
- Next, add the cauliflower to the pan along with 1/2 teaspoon of salt, the black pepper, onion powder, mustard powder, and bay leaf.
- Stir and sauté the mix for 1-2 minutes, just until you smell the cauliflower.
- Add in the water and bring the mix up to a boil.
- Reduce the heat to a low simmer, and cover the pan for 10 minutes.
- Let the mix simmer (uncovered) for another 10 minutes.
- Remove the pan from the heat, and stir in the milk.
- Remove and discard the bay leaf.
- At this time, preheat the oven to 350 degrees.
- Using an immersion blender, blend the mix until smooth and creamy.
- Stir in the fresh nutmeg and six ounces of cheese (not the parmesan) while the cauliflower puree is still warm.
- Stir the mix until the cheese is melted or nearly so.
- Oil an 8 x 8 baking dish.
- To the cauliflower cheese mix, add the cooked quinoa, remaining 1/2 teaspoon of salt, and chopped greens.
- Gently stir the mix until well combined.
- Taste the mix and add extra salt if desired.
- Pour the contents of the saucepan into the oiled baking dish.
- Top evenly with the parmesan and walnut meal.
- Spray the top with a bit of olive oil from a Misto or cooking spray (this helps give the top a nice golden crust).
- Bake 20-25 minutes until top is lightly golden.
- Broil on high for another 2-3 minutes (watch it carefully so it doesn't burn) to get a nice brown crust.
- Cool for about 10 minute before cutting into squares and serving.

171. Quinoa (Sort Of) Diane

Serving: Serves 2, or 1 with leftover for lunch | Prep: | Cook: | Ready in:

Ingredients

- 1/2 cup quinoa of any color
- 1 cup chicken or vegetable stock
- 6 stalks nice thin spring asparagus, trimmed, bias cut 1/2 "
- 1/2 red bell pepper, small dice
- Good fruity olive oil to generously film the bottom of the skillet or wok
- 1 medium shallot, small dice
- 12 button mushrooms, stems removed and saved for stock, gently wiped with a damp towel, 1/4" slice
- 4 ounces white vermouth
- Juice of 1/2 lemon
- Sea or kosher salt to taste
- Fresh chives, snipped with scissors

Direction

- Measure quinoa of your choice (red would be very dramatic, though I used white) into a strainer and rinse under cold water. Bring stock to a boil, add quinoa, cover pot, reduce to a simmer, and set a timer for 10 minutes. When time is up, add asparagus and red pepper, and steam for 5 minutes. Remove from heat when time is up. Season to taste with salt and pepper, and put the lid back on the pot.
- Meanwhile, back at the mushroom venue, be sure to wipe the caps gently with a damp towel to clean, and save the stems for stock. I find them to be different enough in texture from the caps that I separate them. Generously film the bottom of a wide skillet or a wok with a nicely fruity olive oil. I know, olive oil is pressed in the fall, but work with me here. Heat the pan over medium-high heat. When the oil shimmers, add the shallot and a pinch of salt to encourage it to shed its water rapidly. When just softened and fragrant, add the mushrooms and a few pinches of salt. They want to shed their water quickly without overcooking. Salt has a great love of water, and heaven knows mushrooms contain a lot of it. When you can see that they've stopped shedding water into the bottom of the pan, add the white vermouth. Let it come to a good boil, then flame it off with a match or a fire starter. After flames subside, let liquid reduce by about half. Remove from heat and add lemon juice. Stir in, and season to taste with sea or kosher salt to taste.
- Light a candle. Pour a glass of your favorite wine. If you love it, it will go with this dinner. Set place settings.
- Spoon some of the quinoa mixture into a bowl. Spoon some mushrooms over it. Snip some fresh chives over, pick up a fork, and savor the taste of spring.

172. Quinoa Black Bean Burgers

Serving: Serves 6 | Prep: | Cook: | Ready in:

Ingredients

- 2/3 cup quinoa
- 1 cup Raw Black Beans soaked overnight or 1 can Black beans
- 1 piece Celery diced
- 1 Carrot diced
- 2 Mushrooms Diced
- 1/2 Yellow Onion diced
- 1 Shallot Diced
- 3 Garlic cloves, mashed, minced, or however you prefer your garlic
- 1 Red Bell Pepper, Roasted
- 8-15 Sun-Dried Tomatoes chopped
- 1/2 cup Oatmeal (give or take depending on the amount of moisture)
- 3 tablespoons Quinoa Flour
- 3 tablespoons Toasted Pine Nuts
- 1 tablespoon Dijon Mustard
- 1 tablespoon Dried Oregeno
- 1 tablespoon Braggs Liquid Aminos
- Pepper To Taste
- Olive Oil to cook Veggies and Burgers in

Direction

- After soaking beans overnight boil until completely cooked. Strain
- Toast the quinoa in pan and add 1 and 1/3 cup water. Simmer until water is absorbed (about 25 minutes)
- Roast bell pepper in 400-degree oven for 30 minutes.
- Caramelize celery, carrot, onion, mushroom, shallots, garlic and oregano in a small amount of Olive Oil
- Blend sun dried tomatoes a small amount of hot water until it is a smooth paste. If using already re hydrated sun dried tomatoes you can blend them without the hot water. Combine with caramelized Veggies
- Smash Half the black beans
- Combine smashed black beans, whole black beans, quinoa, oatmeal, quinoa flour, veggies, pine nuts, chopped and roasted bell pepper, Dijon, and braggs. Mix Until oatmeal is evenly moist. If there is remaining liquid on the bottom add more quinoa flour or oatmeal until it is absorbed.
- Use a half-cup measuring cup to press mixture into. Once half cup is full press firmly down. Burger mixture will pop out of the measuring cup, once in your hands continue to press until about ½ inch thick. Continue process for all mixture.
- Heat oil for frying. Place however many burgers you can in pan without them touching. Cook on each side for about 4 minutes, medium heat and burger is dark brown.

173. Quinoa Black Bean Summer Salad With Tahini Dressing

Serving: Serves 4-6 | Prep: 0hours10mins | Cook: 0hours15mins | Ready in:

Ingredients

- For the Salad
- 1 red bell pepper
- 1 yellow bell pepper
- 1/4 cup fresh cilantro
- 1 15-oz. can low-sodium black beans
- 3/4 cup fresh or frozen corn
- 3 cups cooked and cooled quinoa
- 1 5-oz bag spring mix salad greens
- For the Dressing
- 1/4 cup tahini
- 1/4 cup water
- 2 teaspoons apple cider vinegar
- 1 teaspoon chili powder
- 1/2 teaspoon onion powder
- 1/2 teaspoon garlic powder
- salt to taste

Direction

- Make dressing by adding all ingredients to a small and stirring well to combine. If you need it a little thinner, add a Tbsp. of water at a time. Set aside.
- Dice bell peppers and onion and add to large bowl.
- Roughly chop cilantro and add to peppers and onions.
- Add black beans and corn and mix well.
- Add in your salad greens and toss well.
- Finally, add the quinoa and toss once more.
- When you're ready to eat, drizzle with Southwest Tahini Sauce and enjoy!

174. Quinoa Burritos

Serving: Makes 4 10 inch burritos | Prep: | Cook: | Ready in:

Ingredients

- 1/2 cup quinoa, cook according to package directions
- 1 tablespoon vegetable oil

- 1/2 red onion, diced
- 1/2 bell pepper, diced (red, orange or yellow)
- 1/2 teaspoon chili powder
- 1/4 teaspoon ground cumin
- 2 ounces raw shrimp, chopped
- juice of 1 lime
- 1 tablespoon chopped cilantro
- salt and pepper to taste
- 4 10 inch flour tortillas
- sour cream, Monterey Jack cheese, hot sauce, avocado, salsa or other taco toppings to taste

Direction

- Heat oil in a sauté pan over medium high heat. Sauté onions and peppers until slightly softened.
- Add chili powder and cumin and cook till fragrant - about 30 seconds. Add in garlic and cook another 30 seconds.
- Season chopped shrimp with salt and pepper. Add shrimp to pan and cook till almost cooked through - about 90 seconds.
- Deglaze with lime juice (use half of juice to start out, add more to taste if needed). Reduce heat to low, and stir in cooked quinoa.
- Taste and adjust seasoning as necessary - adding more lime, salt or pepper. To adjust heat, add hot sauce. Stir in cilantro.
- Heat tortillas. And fill as you would with your favorite burrito toppings.

175. Quinoa Confetti Salad

Serving: Serves 8-12 | Prep: | Cook: |Ready in:

Ingredients

- Dressing
- 1/3 cup olive oil
- 1/4 cup lime juice
- 2 teaspoons red wine vinegar
- 1 teaspoon cumin
- Salad
- 3 cups quinoa, cooked
- 1 cup frozen roasted corn, thawed
- 2 cups cherry tomatoes, halved
- 7 green onions, chopped
- 3 cups canned black beans, rinsed (approx. 2 cans)
- 1/4 cup avocado, chopped
- salt and pepper, to taste

Direction

- Dressing
- Add ingredients to a jar with fitted lid.
- Shake to combine.
- Salad
- Mix quinoa, corn, tomatoes, onions, black beans, and cilantro with half of the dressing.
- Refrigerate overnight.
- Just before serving, toss salad with the remaining dressing and chopped avocado.
- Serve chilled or at room temperature.

176. Quinoa Cookies With Coconut & Chocolate Chunks

Serving: Makes about 24 cookies | Prep: 0hours10mins | Cook: 0hours15mins | Ready in:

Ingredients

- 1 1/2 cups whole wheat flour
- 1 teaspoon salt
- 1/2 teaspoon baking powder
- 1/2 teaspoon baking soda
- 1/2 cup unsalted butter, at room temperature
- 1/4 cup sugar
- 1/4 cup light brown sugar
- 1/4 cup honey
- 2 large eggs
- 1 teaspoon vanilla
- 1/2 teaspoon almond extract
- 1 cup cooked quinoa, cooled
- 1/2 cup dessicated coconut (unsweetened)
- 1 cup dark chocolate chunks or chips

Direction

- Preheat oven to 375° F and line 2 baking sheets with parchment paper.
- Whisk together the flour, salt, baking powder, and baking soda.
- With a stand or electric mixer, cream butter, sugars, and honey until light and fluffy. Add eggs, vanilla, and almond extract, and mix until pale and fluffy, about 2 more minutes.
- Mix in flour mixture, 1/2 cup at a time. Stir in quinoa, coconut, and chocolate.
- Plop spoon size balls of dough onto sheets an inch or so apart, and bake until golden, 12 to 15 minutes. Cool on wire rack.

177. Quinoa Couscous Salad

Serving: Serves 2-4 | Prep: | Cook: |Ready in:

Ingredients

- 1 Small Boston Lettuce, Chopped
- 1 Large Honeycrisp Apple, Diced
- 2 ounces Feta Cheese, Diced
- 1 cup Quinoa Couscous Pilaf
- 5 tablespoons Newman's Own Roasted Garlic Dressing

Direction

- Toss together chopped lettuce, diced apple, diced feta, pilaf and dressing in a large bowl. Serve!!!
- I like to use a ready mixed store bought pilaf but if you can't find one you can make your own. 1/2 cup black quinoa cooked. 1 cup couscous cooked with veggie stock, pinch onion powder, pinch garlic powder, salt and white pepper. After both are cooked mix together and fluff with fork. This can be made ahead and stored in the fridge for 1-2 weeks.

178. Quinoa Cranberry Chocolate Chip Cookies

Serving: Makes approximately 40 | Prep: | Cook: |Ready in:

Ingredients

- 3/4 cup Bob's Red Mill GF All Purpose Baking Flour Mix
- 3/4 cup Baking Blend Flour Mix*
- 2 tablespoons Coconut Flour
- 1/4 cup Golden Flax Meal
- 1 teaspoon Baking Soda
- 1 teaspoon Salt
- 1 1/2 teaspoons Xanthan Gum
- 1 teaspoon Ground Cinnamon
- 1 cup Coconut Oil (I use expellar pressed, which has no taste)
- 3/4 cup Granulated Sugar
- 3/4 cup packed Dark Brown Sugar
- 6 tablespoons Unsweetened Applesauce
- 1 tablespoon Pure Vanilla Extract
- 3 cups Quinoa Flakes
- 1 cup Semi Sweet Chocolate Chips (I like Tropical Source, owned by Sunspire)
- 1 1/2 cups Dried Cranberries

Direction

- Preheat oven to 350° F. In a large bowl, mix the first 8 ingredients (all the dry ingredients).
- In a separate bowl mix the coconut oil, granulated sugar & brown sugar until well combined (I use a stand mixer, but you can do this by hand).
- Add the applesauce & vanilla extract and continue mixing.
- Using a rubber spatula carefully add the dry ingredients (in the large bowl) to the wet mixture and stir until a grainy dough is formed.
- Stir in quinoa, cranberries, and chocolate chips (If using a mixer, do this step by hand).
- Using a large melon baller or an ice cream scoop, place the dough onto the prepared baking sheets spacing them 1" apart.

- Gently press each with the heel of your hand to help them spread.
- Bake on the center rack for 15 minutes – rotating 180 degrees after 9 minutes. Cool on baking sheets for 10 minutes; remove to wire racks to cool completely.
- *Baking Blend Flour Mix is 2 parts White Rice Flour; 1 part Tapioca Starch; 1 part Potato Starch.

179. Quinoa Crepes

Serving: Serves 12 (makes 12 - 6" crepes) | Prep: | Cook: | Ready in:

Ingredients

- 1/3 cup quinoa flour
- 1/4 cup brown rice flour
- 2 teaspoons cornstarch
- 2 large eggs
- 2 large egg whites
- 1 cup almond milk

Direction

- Combine the flours & cornstarch in a medium bowl. Add the eggs, egg whites and almond milk and whisk until smooth.
- Heat a lightly oiled, six-inch skillet, on medium-high heat. Pour two tablespoons of batter into the center of the pan, tilting in a circular motion to spread evenly over the bottom
- Flip the crepe when the edges begin to curl (about 30 to 45 seconds). Cook the other side for another 30 seconds, then remove from the pan.
- Place the hot crepe on a plate and cover with foil. Repeat with the remaining batter.

180. Quinoa Crisps

Serving: Serves 10 | Prep: | Cook: | Ready in:

Ingredients

- 2 cups cooked quinoa
- 1 tablespoon coconut oil
- non-stick cooking spray

Direction

- Preheat the oven to 350ºF.
- Stir coconut oil into cooked quinoa until evenly distributed. Spray sheet pan with non-stick cooking spray.
- Transfer quinoa to a baking sheet and spread out in an even layer. Bake for 30-40 minutes, stirring every 10 minutes to make sure it doesn't burn.
- Once golden brown and crispy, cool quinoa completely. Transfer to an airtight container and store on the counter for up to 1 week.
- Sprinkle on top of yogurt, salads, smoothies, anywhere you want a healthy crunch!

181. Quinoa Croquettes

Serving: Serves 4 | Prep: | Cook: | Ready in:

Ingredients

- 100 grams Quinoa
- 1 piece Celery
- 1 Carrot
- 1 tablespoon Parsley
- 2 Garlic cloves
- 1 Onion
- 2 Eggs
- 1 cup Dry bread crumbs

Direction

- Wash the quinoa and rub it in your hands until the fine film that contains it is released.

- Boil the quinoa with water (1 part of quinoa with 2 parts of water) in a covered pot for 10-15 minutes. The quinoa is cooked when it has doubled its volume. Add a pinch or two of salt only at the end of the cooking time.
- In the food processor, put the celery, carrot, parsley, garlic and onion and finely chop the vegetables.
- Put the vegetables in a pan with 2 tablespoons of hot oil and cook for half an hour, add water from time to time.
- Mix the vegetables with the cooked quinoa (the quinoa must have a dry consistency). Amalgamate the ingredients, add a raw egg, salt and pepper. You can add if you like a little grated ginger (optional).
- With the wet hands form the croquettes, roll them in flour, one egg and the breadcrumbs. Fry them in abundant oil until they start to color.

182. Quinoa Crêpes With Blackberry And Plum Compote

Serving: Serves 2 | Prep: | Cook: |Ready in:

Ingredients

- For the compote
- 150 grams Plums
- 150 grams Blackberries
- 150 grams Honey
- For the pancake
- 120 grams Quinoa Flour
- 250 milliliters Almond Milk
- 1 tablespoon Coconut Oil
- 1 pinch Salt

Direction

- De-stone the plums and cut them into quarters.
- Place the plums, berries and honey in a pan on a medium heat and let this caramelize for 5 minutes (add in 100ml of water gradually as you go so nothing burns).
- When all the water has been added, place a lid over the top and let this simmer for 10 minutes. Place the crepe mix ingredients in a bowl, whisk well and let this sit in the fridge for half an hour.
- Heat a large pan with coconut oil on a medium heat, poor out a scoop of the batter and let it cook for few minutes until golden brown then flip.
- Start small then make your crepes bigger as you feel more confident. I often fold them in half like an omelette as they don't fall apart, this makes them still taste divine.

183. Quinoa Eetch (Red Quinoa Tabouli)

Serving: Serves a crowd | Prep: | Cook: |Ready in:

Ingredients

- 1 cup Quinoa
- 2 cups Tomato sauce
- 1/2 bunch Parsley, chopped
- 4 Scallions, chopped
- 1 Large onion, diced fine
- 1 Large green bell pepper, diced fine
- 1/4 cup Fresh lemon juice
- Drizzle of olive oil
- Dash of cayenne pepper
- Salt and Pepper to taste

Direction

- Bring tomato sauce and quinoa to a boil;
- Reduce to a simmer until quinoa blooms (tendrils uncurl);
- Remove from heat and cool to room temperature;
- Stir in remaining ingredients;
- Chill until sauce is absorbed and flavors have a chance to meld;

- If a looser consistency is desired, add a little more tomato sauce - no need to cook;
- Serve with crackers, celery sticks, bagel chips, pita chips, tortilla chips, etc.

184. Quinoa Fried Rice Recipe

Serving: Serves 4 | Prep: 0hours10mins | Cook: 0hours15mins | Ready in:

Ingredients

- 1 teaspoon olive oil.
- 2 eggs, whisked.
- 2 medium carrots, peeled and diced.
- 1 small white onion, diced.
- 3 cloves garlic, minced.
- 4 cups cooked quinoa
- 3 green onions, thinly sliced.
- 3-4 tablespoons soy sauce, or more to taste.
- 2 teaspoons oyster sauce (optional).
- 1/2 teaspoon toasted sesame oil.

Direction

- In a pan over medium heat, add ½ tsp olive oil. Add the eggs and scramble slightly with a pinch of salt and pepper (optional), until barely cooked. Remove from a pan and put it into a bowl. Set aside.
- Pour ½ tsp olive oil in medium heat. Add onion, carrots, peas, and garlic. Sauté for about 5 minutes or until the onion, peas, and carrots are soft. Then, add the cooked quinoa (how to cook Quinoa), green onions, soy sauce, and oyster sauce and stir-fry until incorporated, about 2 minutes.
- Add in the eggs and stir to combine. Finally, add the sesame oil, and remove from heat.

185. Quinoa Fried Rice With Tomatoes

Serving: Serves 8 | Prep: | Cook: | Ready in:

Ingredients

- 1 14 ounce can of Muir Glen tomatoes
- 1 onion, peeled and quartered
- 2 jalapeno peppers
- 2 cups quinoa, rinsed
- 2 tablespoons canola oil
- 4 cloves garlic, minced
- 2 cups low-sodium chicken broth
- 1 tablespoon tomato paste
- 1 chipotle pepper in adobo sauce plus 1 teaspoon adobo sauce
- 1 tablespoon kosher salt
- 1/2 cup minced cilantro
- 1 teaspoon lime zest
- 1 tablespoon lime juice

Direction

- Prepare Tomatoes: Process tomatoes and onions in food processor until smooth and thoroughly pureed, about 15 seconds, scraping sides of bowl if needed. Transfer mixture to liquid measuring cup. There should be 2 cups. If more, pour some out until it equals 2 cups.
- Prepare Jalapenos: Remove seeds and ribs from jalapeno peppers and discard insides. Mince peppers and set aside.
- Prepare Quinoa: Place quinoa in fine-mesh strainer and rinse under cold water, about 1-2 minutes. Shake briskly to remove excess water. (If you don't rinse, quinoa will be very bitter).
- Make Fried Rice: Heat oil in large skillet or Dutch oven with tight fitting lid, over medium-high heat, 1 minute. Add quinoa and fry, stirring constantly, until golden and translucent, 1-2 minutes. Reduce heat to medium, add garlic and seeded jalapenos. Cook, stirring frequently, until fragrant, 1 minute. Stir in pureed tomatoes and onions, chicken broth, tomato paste, chipotle pepper

and adobo and kosher salt. Increase heat to medium-high and bring to boil. Reduce to simmer, cover and cook 15-20 minutes or until liquid is absorbed. Remove from heat, cover with a clean towel and lid and let stand covered until ready to serve. (The towel absorbs the excess water).

- Serve: Right before ready to serve, add cilantro, lime juice and zest. Fluff quinoa with wet fork or rice paddle.

186. Quinoa Granola

Serving: Makes 950g | Prep: | Cook: | Ready in:

Ingredients

- 250 grams quinoa flakes
- 150 grams nuts of choice
- 150 grams mix of sunflower & pumpkin seeds
- 50 grams buckwheat
- 50 grams coconut oil, melted
- 1.5 teaspoons ground cinnamon
- 1 teaspoon good quality vanilla extract
- 100g grams coconut flakes
- 50 grams chia seeds
- 50 grams goji berries

Direction

- Preheat over 170C. In a large mixing bowl, place your quinoa flakes. Lightly crush your nuts, keeping them chunky. Add to the quinoa with your seeds, buckwheat, maple syrup, melted coconut oil, vanilla and cinnamon. Mix together well, making sure everything is coated with the coconut and maple syrup.
- Spread onto a baking sheet lined with parchment and bake for 10 minutes. At this point take the baking tray out of the oven. Add your coconut flakes and chia flakes, mix and cook for another 10 minutes until your ingredients are a healthy brown color, delicious and toasted. Mix through the goji berries. Let cool and serve with your choice of yoghurt or milk, along with some fresh or cooked fruit. Or just munch as a snack!

187. Quinoa Lettuce Wraps

Serving: Makes a lot | Prep: | Cook: | Ready in:

Ingredients

- Quinoa Salad
- 1 cup Quinoa
- 1 handful Cherry tomatoes, quartered
- 1/2 Cucumber
- 1/2 cup Feta cheese, cubed
- 2 tablespoons Red onion, diced
- 1 handful Olives, chopped
- 1/2 Yellow pepper
- 1 Head of boston lettuce
- Lemon-Tahini Sauce
- 1/2 cup Tahini
- 1/4 cup Olive oil
- 1/4 cup Apple cider vinegar
- 1 Garlic clove, minced
- 1 pinch Cayenne
- 1 Lemon, juiced
- 2 tablespoons Water

Direction

- Use the vegetables and cheese in amounts that are suitable for your tastes. My only note here is to dice them fairly finely, so that the wraps roll easily and so that you get as many flavors as possible in each spectacular bite. Substitute vegetables and cheese at your own discretion, depending on what you have on hand. Keep lettuce aside, for assembling wraps.
- Mix all ingredients for the Lemon-Tahini Sauce together and process with an immersion blender.
- Assemble the wraps. Smear some Lemon-Tahini Sauce on a leaf of lettuce. Spoon on some Quinoa Salad. Roll the lettuce leaf around the salad and eat with your fingers.

188. Quinoa Minestrone With Kale Pesto

Serving: Serves 6 | Prep: | Cook: |Ready in:

Ingredients

- minestrone
- 2 cloves garlic, diced
- 1 leek, sliced
- 4 tomatoes, diced
- 1 cup green beans, chopped
- 2 sticks celery, diced
- 1/4 cabbage, shredded
- 2 cups kale leaves
- 1 bay leaf
- 1 teaspoon dried thyme
- 2 1/2 liters vegetable stock
- 1/2 cup red quinoa
- 1/2 cup quinoa
- 1/2 cup celery leaves
- pesto
- 1 cup kale leaves
- 1 cup celery leaves
- 1/2 cup almonds
- 1 clove garlic
- 3/4 cup olive oil

Direction

- Heat a little olive oil in a large casserole pot over med heat. Cook the garlic and leek for 2 minutes until translucent. Add the tomatoes, carrots, beans, celery, cabbage, kale, bay leaf, thyme, stock and bring to the boil, then turn heat down, cover and gently simmer for 1 hour.
- Add the quinoa and celery leaves and cook a further 20 minutes.
- Place all pesto ingredients into a food processor along with salt and pepper and pulse until desired consistency is reached.
- Serve soup topped with a drizzle of pesto and parmesan. For the kids blend in a food processor until smooth and use as a pasta sauce.

189. Quinoa Patties

Serving: Serves a crowd | Prep: | Cook: |Ready in:

Ingredients

- Patties
- 1/2 cup quinoa – uncooked (cook as directed on the box. Usually 1/2 c uncooked quinoa is cooked in 1 c salted water)
- 3/4 cup Cannellini beans (or chickpeas)- canned
- 1/2 potato – boiled (instead of using egg)
- 1/4 small red onion
- 1/4 cup cilantro
- 1 Serrano peppers (depending on your spice level tolerance)
- 2 cloves of garlic
- 2 teaspoons lemon juice
- 1 1/2 teaspoons ground cumin
- Salt, to taste
- Yogurt Sauce
- 1 cup plain non-far Greek yogurt
- 1 teaspoon Lime zest (optional)
- A drizzle of honey if the yogurt is too tart
- Salt, to taste
- Pepper, to taste

Direction

- Patties
- Pulse onions, garlic, green chilies.
- Add Cannellini beans, cilantro, lemon juice, salt, ground cumin, and pulse for 30-45 seconds (until the beans have just broken down).
- Add boiled potato, cooked quinoa, and pulse until everything is mixed. Don't over-pulse the mixture or it will get too mushy.
- Make 1 inch balls and flatten them.
- Heat a non-stick or a ceramic pan on medium heat.

- Drizzle vegetable or extra virgin olive oil on the pan and carefully place the patties on the pan.
- Cook the patties for ~5 minutes on each side or until they reach a beautiful brown toasted color.
- These patties can be served at room temperature so let the patties cool off on a wire rack while you make the yogurt sauce.
- Yogurt Sauce
- Mix everything in a bowl and refrigerate until ready to serve.
- Slice ~10 cherry tomatoes in halves or thin slices, whatever you prefer.
- Assemble
- Place patties on a serving platter.
- You can either dollop a small amount of yogurt on each patty (this could get messy) or use the sandwich bag technique. Transfer the yogurt mixture in a sandwich bag and cut a small piece at one of the corners and pipe the yogurt onto each patty. This made the dish mess-free and pretty at the same time.
- Place sliced cherry tomatoes on each patty.

190. Quinoa Pilaf

Serving: Serves 4 | Prep: | Cook: |Ready in:

Ingredients

- 3 tablespoons extra-virgin olive oil
- 4 small shallots – chopped (or use 1/4 cup chopped red onions if you don't have shallots)
- 1 small red pepper
- 1/4 cup edamame or peas
- 1 teaspoon salt
- 1/2 teaspoon black pepper
- 1 1/2 cups quinoa
- 2 cups vegetable broth
- 1 teaspoon lemon zest
- 1/2 cup toasted slivered almonds

Direction

- In a large saucepan, heat the oil on medium heat.
- Add shallots and saute for 1-2 minutes.
- Add the chopped red pepper, salt and pepper and cook for about 3-4 minutes, or until they're soft.
- Add spinach and edamame, and cook for 1-2 minutes.
- And quinoa and stir for 1-2 minutes, until coated with oil.
- Add vegetable broth, cover the saucepan and simmer for about 10 minutes or until the quinoa is cooked. The original recipe called for 1 1/2 cup of broth but I ended up added 1/2 cup more because the quinoa was not fully cooked.
- Using a fork, fluff the quinoa once it's cooked.
- Add lemon zest and additional salt and pepper if needed.
- Serve with toasted almonds.

191. Quinoa Pilaf With Citrus Soy Dressing

Serving: Serves 4-6 | Prep: | Cook: |Ready in:

Ingredients

- Citrus-Soy Dressing
- 1/2 cup extra-virgin olive oil
- 1/4 cup fresh orange juice
- 3 tablespoons fresh lemon juice (about 1 lemon)
- 2 tablespoons low-sodium tamari soy sauce
- 1 tablespoon raw honey
- sea salt and freshly ground black pepper
- Quinoa Pilaf
- 1 cup cooked quinoa (or brown rice)
- 2 cups water
- 1 pinch sea salt
- 1 bunch asparagus or broccoli
- 1 cup slivered almonds
- 1 cup grated carrots
- zest of 1 lemon

Direction

- Snap off ends of asparagus spears and cut into 2-inch pieces.
- Steam asparagus or broccoli until still bright green and crisp-tender, about 5 minutes.
- Toast almonds on a baking sheet in oven or toaster until lightly browned.
- Make Citrus Dressing: whisk together olive oil, orange juice, lemon juice, soy sauce, honey, and salt and pepper.
- Grate carrots and lemon zest.
- Place quinoa, asparagus or broccoli, toasted almonds, zest of 1 lemon, 1 cup of shredded carrots in a large serving bowl. Pour dressing over the pilaf and gently toss.

192. Quinoa Pilaf With Curry Powder

Serving: Serves 3 | Prep: | Cook: | Ready in:

Ingredients

- 1 cup Quinoa
- 2 cups water
- 1 large onion cut in half and sliced into thin semi circular slices
- 1 red bell pepper finely diced
- 1 green bell pepper, finely diced
- 1 - 1.5 teaspoons curry powder
- 1/4 teaspoon turmeric
- 1/4 - 1/2 teaspoons cayenne or paprika powder, as per taste
- 2-4 tablespoons Olive oil (dependign on how well done you want your onions)
- Salt to taste
- chopped Cilantro for garnish
- Lemon wedges for serving
- 1/2 cup Walnuts

Direction

- Bring the 2 cups of water to a boil. In the meantime, rinse the quinoa several times, drain, and add it to the water. Lower the heat and cover the pan. Cook for 10 - 12 minutes until the water is absorbed and the seeds have sprouted a tail. Cover and set aside.
- Toast the walnuts lightly, break into pieces and set aside
- Heat the oil in a wide pan and add the onions. Sauté on low heat and allow the onion to turn a light caramelized brown. Add the peppers at this point along with the turmeric, cayenne and curry powder. Once the peppers wilt, add salt as per your preference (remember, you need to account for the quinoa as well).
- Cook down until most of the water from the peppers have evaporated and then add the cooked quinoa. Fold gently to combine the vegetables. Taste and Adjust for seasoning. Garnish with cilantro and sprinkle the walnuts as per taste. Serve warm with a side of Raita, tsatziki, or plain sour cream. Spritz some lemon juice on the quinoa if you prefer.

193. Quinoa Pilau

Serving: Serves 2 | Prep: | Cook: | Ready in:

Ingredients

- 1 cup quinoa (washed and drained)
- 2 cups water
- 1/2 teaspoon sea salt
- 3 tablespoons olive oil or 50/50 blend flax seed oil
- 1 finely chopped onion, small/medium, depending on onion heat
- 1 piece fresh ginger, approx 2" sq, finely chopped
- 2 tablespoons fresh mint, finely chopped
- 2 tablespoons fresh coriander (cilantro), finely chopped
- 1/2 teaspoon ground cinnamon
- 1/2 teaspoon ground cloves
- 1 dash ground black pepper
- 1 pinch chopped blanched almonds (optional)

Direction

- In medium saucepan, boil quinoa in water and salt approximately 15-20 minutes over medium heat, until water is absorbed.
- For efficiency, while quinoa is cooking, finely chop onion, ginger, mint, and coriander.
- Heat oil in large stir-fry pan. Add ginger and onion, lightly brown. Add cinnamon and cloves, stir well. Add cooked quinoa, stir ingredients well. Remove from heat. Add black pepper and any additional salt to taste.
- Note: Dairy consumers may choose to add 1/2 cup plain yogurt to mixture when adding cooked quinoa.
- Allow to cool and fluff with fork. If desired, serve topped with chopped blanched almonds.

194. Quinoa Pizza Dough

Serving: Makes 2 12-13 inch pizzas | Prep: | Cook: | Ready in:

Ingredients

- Dry Ingredients
- 1 1/2 cups any GF flour blend (I like Gluten Free Pantry brand)
- 1 1/2 cups Quinoa Flakes
- 1/2 teaspoon salt
- 2 1/2 teaspoons yeast granules
- Wet Ingredients
- 3 tablespoons Flax meal
- 9 tablespoons water
- 6 tablespoons olive oil
- 1 tablespoon sugar
- 1/2 cup warm water

Direction

- In a stand mixer, mix together all wet ingredients except for the 1/2 cup warm water. Let sit until flax meal thickens the mixture (5 min or so).
- In a separate bowl thoroughly combine all dry ingredients.
- With the mixer on low speed slowly add the flour into the wet mixture, adding a bit of water as you go. The dough should resemble a traditional pizza dough. Very thick, but not crumbly. Turn your mixer speed to a medium speed for a few minutes to agitate the dough.
- Turn out the dough into a medium to large size bowl. Immediately freeze half if you want to only make one pizza. Cover the bowl with a damp tea or hand towel and place in the fridge overnight until ready to use. Take out the dough 1-2 hours prior to baking to let it continue to rise and come to room temperature.
- Bake in a 450 preheated oven until edges are browned and any toppings and cheese melted. We use a preheated pizza stone to bake on. If you do not have a pizza stone, depending on your desired level of crispiness, you may want to pre bake the dough for 5-10 min on a greased and floured baking sheet before adding toppings.

195. Quinoa Pizza With Tomato And Mushrooms

Serving: Serves 6 | Prep: | Cook: | Ready in:

Ingredients

- 120 grams Kinoa
- 1 pinch Salt
- 1 tablespoon olive oil
- 4 Mushrooms
- 1 pinch Oregano and thyme

Direction

- Quinoa soaked in water for 6-8 hours (or overnight) .Grease with olive oil, a frying pan that can go in the oven
- Pass the quinoa by plenty of water and drain it. Place in blender and grind it with salt and

olive oil, until a thick but creamy paste. Pour the batter into the pan and smooth it out so as to be uniform and bake for about 15 minutes. Remove, turn the dough and again to the oven for another 10-15 minutes until golden brown and the edges are crisp.

- Cover the base of quinoa pizza with tomato sauce, the sliced mushrooms, and cheese and bake for 12-15 minutes, until the cheese has melted and is lightly browned. Serve immediately!

196. Quinoa Ranch Casserole

Serving: Serves 6 | Prep: | Cook: | Ready in:

Ingredients

- 3 cups Cooked, plain quinoa
- 4 Cooked, diced chicken breasts (seasoned to taste)
- 1.5 cups Sautéed summer squash, zucchini and mushrooms
- 1/2 cup Shredded cheddar cheese
- 1/4 cup Bacon bits
- Ranch dressing

Direction

- Spray clay casserole dish with olive oil.
- Preheat oven to 375.
- Spread the cooked quinoa evenly in your casserole dish.
- Sprinkle the bacon bits atop the quinoa.
- Drizzle ranch dressing over the bacon bits.
- Spread the shredded cheddar evenly over the ranch.
- Layer your sauteed squash/zucchini/mushroom on the casserole.
- Top with diced, cooked chicken.
- Cover with clay lid or foil and cook 25 minutes or until heated through.

197. Quinoa Salad With Strawberries, Goat Cheese & Crispy Kale

Serving: Serves 2-3 | Prep: | Cook: | Ready in:

Ingredients

- 1 cup Rinsed Quinoa
- 2-3 cups Kale, Rinsed, Dried and Thinly Sliced
- 1-2 cups Strawberries, Cleaned and Quartered
- 1/4 cup Pomegranate Seeds
- 1-2 ounces Herbed Goat Cheese
- 2 tablespoons Olive Oil
- Salt and Pepper To Taste

Direction

- Bring quinoa and 2 cups of salted water to a boil. Reduce to a simmer and cover, cook about 15 minutes or until all water is absorbed.
- Lay kale out on a baking sheet and sprinkle with salt, pepper, and a few drops of olive oil. Mix to coat well. Cook at approximately 10-15 minutes at 350 degrees, until crispy.
- Combine, kale, quinoa, goat cheese, strawberries and pomegranate seeds. Toss with olive oil and season with salt and pepper to taste.

198. Quinoa Salad With Currants, Pistachios, Red Onion And Mint

Serving: Serves 4 | Prep: | Cook: | Ready in:

Ingredients

- 1 cup quinoa
- 2 cups water
- 1/4 cup dried currants
- 1 medium red onion
- 1/4 cup toasted pistachios

- 1 tablespoon fresh mint, chopped or chiffonade
- generous pinches of salt to taste
- 2-3 tablespoons extra virgin olive oil

Direction

- Combine water, quinoa and currants and a pinch of salt in a small saucepan. Bring to a boil, uncovered. Once at a boil, turn down to a simmer and cover with a slight opening for air to leave. Cook until the water is fully absorbed, approximately 15 minutes.
- Meanwhile, peel and cut the red onion, small dice. In a large sauté pan, sweat onion over a low heat until tender and translucent in a generous amount of olive oil 1-2 tablespoons, about 10 minutes. Add more olive oil if needed to prevent the onions from developing any browning.
- Roughly chop pistachios. Add to onions once they are fully sweated.
- When the quinoa is done, add to sauté pan with onions and pistachios. Mix well. Season with salt to taste. Toss in mint and serve!

199. Quinoa Salad With Feta, Blood Oranges And Mint

Serving: Serves 4 | Prep: | Cook: | Ready in:

Ingredients

- 1 cup quinoa
- 1.25 cups water
- 3 blood oranges
- 1 shallot, finely chopped
- 1/3 cup pine nuts, toasted
- 1/4 cup chopped mint
- 3 tablespoons olive oil
- 3 ounces feta cheese
- salt and pepper

Direction

- Make the quinoa: Rinse the quinoa in a mesh strainer. Bring the water and a pinch of salt to a boil in a small saucepan. Add the quinoa and reduce heat to a simmer. Cover and simmer for 15 minutes until quinoa is tender.
- While the quinoa is cooking, prepare the oranges. Cut the peel off of two of the oranges and then cut them into bite-sized sections, removing any really fibrous bits. (If you know how to supreme an orange - do that.)
- Combine the cooked quinoa, chopped or supreme oranges, shallots, pine nuts, and mint. Squeeze the juice of the other orange over the salad and drizzle it with olive oil (about 2-3 tablespoons). Gently stir in the feta cheese. Taste the salad and add salt and pepper to taste.

200. Quinoa Salad With Roasted Tomatoes And Fried Leeks

Serving: Serves 10 | Prep: | Cook: | Ready in:

Ingredients

- 2 cups quinoa
- 1/2 cup olive oil, more for frying and serving
- 1/4 cup lemon juice
- 1/4 cup pomegranate molasses, more for serving
- 1 leek, trimmed, halved, and sliced thinly
- 1 pint cherry tomatoes, halved
- 1/3 cup pumpkin seeds
- 6 ounces arugula
- salt and pepper to taste

Direction

- Lightly toast the pumpkin seeds. Add them to a pan over medium heat, stirring often, until golden-brown and fragrant. Set aside.
- Preheat the oven to 400 degrees. Toss the cherry tomato halves in olive oil, salt and pepper until coated. Roast the tomatoes in the

oven until slightly shriveled, about 25-30 minutes. Add the tomatoes to a large bowl when finished roasting.
- Meanwhile, fry the leeks. Put enough oil at the bottom of a pan to cover the leeks. Add the leeks in batches, and remove with a slotted spoon when brown and crispy. Place them on a paper towel-lined plate.
- Place the quinoa in a mesh strainer and rinse. Add the quinoa to 2.5 cups boiling salted water. Simmer covered until water is completely absorbed, about 20 minutes.
- Add the quinoa and the toasted pumpkin seeds to the bowl of roasted tomatoes. Stir to combine.
- Combine the pomegranate molasses and lemon juice with 1 tsp of salt and a pinch of pepper. Whisk in the olive oil.
- Add the dressing to the quinoa, tomato and pumpkin seed mixture. Stir to combine.
- Place arugula on a platter, top with quinoa and frizzled leeks, and drizzle olive oil and pomegranate molasses just before serving. Can be served warm or cold. If serving cold, refrigerate up to 3 days. Keep arugula, quinoa mixture and leeks separate and assemble just before serving.

201. Quinoa Salad With Spinach, Strawberries And Goat Cheese

Serving: Serves 4 | Prep: | Cook: | Ready in:

Ingredients

- Quinoa Salad
- 1 cup quinoa, rinsed (I used red quinoa)
- kosher salt and black pepper
- 2 cups baby spinach leaves
- 2 tablespoons fresh basil, cut into chiffonade (ribbons)
- 2/3 cup sliced strawberries
- 1 ounce goat cheese, crumbled
- 1 1/2 tablespoons sliced almonds, toasted
- Balsamic Dressing
- 2 tablespoons balsamic vinegar
- 1 teaspoon Dijon mustard
- 1/2 teaspoon honey or agave nectar
- 2 tablespoons extra virgin olive oil
- Kosher salt and black pepper

Direction

- Place the quinoa in a medium saucepan along with 2 cups water and ¼ teaspoon salt. Bring to a boil then cover with a lid and reduce to a simmer. Simmer the quinoa about 15 minutes until cooked. Remove the lid and cook another 2-3 minutes until all of the water has evaporated. Remove from the heat and fluff with a fork. Let the quinoa cool to room temperature.
- Meanwhile, make the balsamic dressing. Whisk the vinegar, mustard and honey together in a small bowl. Slowly pour in the olive oil while you continue to whisk. Season the dressing with salt and pepper.
- Place the quinoa in a salad bowl along with the spinach, basil, strawberries, goat cheese and almonds. Add the dressing and toss to combine all ingredients well. Serve the salad alone or if desired, topped with slices of grilled chicken breast.

202. Quinoa Salad With Tangerine Balsamic Tofu And Cinnamon Vinaigrette

Serving: Serves 4-6 | Prep: | Cook: | Ready in:

Ingredients

- 4 tablespoons balsamic vinegar, divided
- 1 tablespoon soy sauce
- 2 tablespoons olive oil, divided
- 1 tablespoon honey
- 1 teaspoon water
- 1/4 teaspoon freshly ground black pepper

- 1 tangerine, cut in half
- 1 (14-ounce) container of extra-firm tofu, pressed, drained, and cut into small cubes
- 1 teaspoon cinnamon
- 3 cups cooked quinoa (about 1 cup dry)
- 1 Granny Smith apple, chopped into bite-sized pieces
- 1/2 cup dried cranberries
- 1/3 cup sunflower kernels

Direction

- In a small bowl, whisk together 3 tablespoons of the balsamic vinegar, soy sauce, 1 tablespoon of the olive oil, honey, water, black pepper, and the juice of half the tangerine. Put the marinade and the tofu into a shallow dish or container and gently toss the tofu until it becomes coated. Refrigerate for at least 30 minutes.
- Preheat the oven to 350 degrees Fahrenheit. Line a baking sheet with parchment paper and arrange the marinated tofu pieces in a single layer, making sure they don't touch. Bake for 20 minutes, or until the tofu turns golden brown and slightly puffy.
- In a small bowl, whisk together the remaining tablespoon of olive oil, the remaining tablespoon of balsamic vinegar, cinnamon, and the juice of the other tangerine half. Set aside.
- In a large bowl, toss together the marinated tofu, quinoa, apple, cranberries, and sunflower kernels. Drizzle the dressing over the salad and toss once more. Serve cold.

203. Quinoa Salad With Toasted Pine Nuts, Raisins And Lime

Serving: Serves 8 | Prep: | Cook: | Ready in:

Ingredients

- 3 cups quinoa
- 4 ounces pine nuts
- 1/2 cup lime juice (or up to taste)
- Grated zest of two limes
- 2 garlic cloves, crushed
- 1 tablespoon cumin
- 1 generous cup of raisins
- 1/4 cup good quality extra virgin olive oil
- 1 cup parsley, minced
- Salt and freshly ground pepper

Direction

- Toast the pine nuts in a dry skillet over medium-low heat. Shake the skillet frequently to ensure even browning. When the nuts are fragrant and gently browned, take the pan off the heat and transfer the pine nuts to a plate to cool.
- Combine the quinoa with six cups of water and bring to a boil. Reduce the heat to medium-low, cover with lid and simmer for about 15 minutes, until the grains are translucent and the germ has spiraled out from each grain. Drain the quinoa and let it cool.
- In a bowl, mix the quinoa with all the ingredients except the pine nuts. Let the flavors combine for about an hour or two. Add the pine nuts, mix well, taste, adjust acidity if needed and serve.

204. Quinoa Salad With Roasted Grapes

Serving: Serves 4-6 | Prep: | Cook: | Ready in:

Ingredients

- 1/2 pound Red seedless grapes
- 1 cup Quinoa, rinsed
- 1 Lemon
- 1/4 cup Fresh basil chiffonade
- 3 tablespoons Extra virgin olive oil
- 1/4 cup Slivered blanched almonds

- 2 Small onions or shallots, halved and sliced thinly
- 1/4 pound Goat Tomme cheese

Direction

- Preheat oven to 350 degrees Fahrenheit. Combine grapes and 1 tablespoon oil in a baking sheet and toss to combine. Roast in oven for 10-15 minutes.
- Combine quinoa with 2 cups water and bring to a boil. Turn down heat and let simmer for 15 minutes.
- Heat a small skillet over medium heat. Add almonds and toast until nutty and fragrant. Set aside.
- Add 1 tablespoon oil to skillet and return to medium heat. Add onions and sauté, stirring every 5 minutes, until lightly brown, about 20-30 minutes.
- Combine the juice of one lemon with basil, 1 tablespoon oil, and salt and pepper to taste. When quinoa is cooked, add almonds, grapes, onions, and vinaigrette and stir to combine. Set aside to cool.
- Cut cheese into 1/2 inch cubes. When salad has cooled, add cheese.

205. Quinoa Salsa Egg Muffins

Serving: Serves 6 | Prep: | Cook: | Ready in:

Ingredients

- 1 cup cooked quinoa (1/4 cup dry)
- 3 large egg whites
- 1 large egg yolk
- 1/2 teaspoon cumin
- 1/2 tablespoon garlic powder
- Pinch of salt & pepper
- 6 tablespoons store bought or homemade salsa* per egg muffin

Direction

- Preheat oven to 325 degrees
- Generously spray a muffin tin with cooking spray
- In a large bowl, whisk together egg whites, egg yolk, garlic powder, cumin, salt & pepper until eggs are frothy
- Add cooked quinoa to the egg mixture to combine
- Divide the mixture among 6 muffin cavities, filling each cavity 3/4 of the way full
- To each cavity, add 1-2 tbsp. salsa stirring the salsa into the egg/quinoa mixture to disperse
- Bake muffins 20-25 minutes until edges are slightly browned

206. Quinoa Shakshuka With Feta And Kale

Serving: Serves 2-3 | Prep: | Cook: | Ready in:

Ingredients

- 2 Red bell peppers - julienned
- 2 Garlic cloves - chopped
- 3 Eggs
- 1 cup Kale - chopped and rinsed
- 10 ounces Marinara sauce
- 2 tablespoons Extra virgin olive oil
- 8 ounces Brown Rice and Red Quinoa Medley
- 3 tablespoons Fetta cheese
- 1/2 teaspoon Salt and pepper

Direction

- Preheat oven to 350 degrees.
- Heat olive oil in cast iron skillet over medium-high heat. Add chopped garlic and sweat for one minute.
- Add julienned red bell peppers and sweat until soft. Approximately 5 minutes.
- Add marinara sauce and quinoa & brown rice. Stir until incorporated. Adjust seasonings with salt and pepper.

- Crack eggs one at a time over top of marinara mixture, allowing plenty of room in between each egg.
- Transfer skillet to finish in the oven for 15 minutes.
- Serve over a bed of kale, garnished with desired amount of feta cheese on top.

207. Quinoa Soup

Serving: Serves http://www.queensquinoa.com/ | Prep: | Cook: | Ready in:

Ingredients

- 1/2 cup washed and drained
- 4 cups Broth/Stock/water
- 2 cups Mixed Vegetables (tomatoes, beans, carrots, peas, cabbage, zucchini, mushroom)

Direction

- Green Chilies – to taste, slit
- 1 small, chopped
- Salt – to taste, Black Pepper – to taste. Cilantro (Coriander) – for garnishing, finely chopped. Lime Juice – to taste for garnishing
- Method: Place washed Quinoa, Onions, Mixed Vegetables, Green Chilies, Broth and Salt in a pressure cooker.2. Cover and pressure cook for 1 whistle and switch off stove.3. Once pressure is gone from the cooker, open lid and add Cilantro, Black Pepper and Lime Juice to taste.4. Serve hot.

208. Quinoa Spinach Salad With Peanut Ginger Dressing

Serving: Serves 2 | Prep: | Cook: | Ready in:

Ingredients

- Peanut-Ginger Dressing
- 2 tablespoons soy sauce
- 1 tablespoon sesame oil
- 1/2 tablespoon garlic
- 1/2 cup unsalted peanut butter
- 1/2 tablespoon fresh ginger
- 3 tablespoons water (as needed)
- Salad Veggies
- 2 cups cooked quinoa
- 1/2 cup diced cucumber
- 1 diced red bell pepper
- 1 carrot, julienned or shredded
- 1/4 cup diced green onions
- 4 cups fresh spinach
- 1/4 cup fresh diced cilantro
- 1 tablespoon sesame seeds
- 1 tablespoon fresh chopped basil leaves (optional)

Direction

- Peanut-Ginger Dressing
- Blend all ingredients in a food processor or blender until smooth.
- Add water (or more soy sauce – just make sure you taste as you go so you can gauge the saltyness) until you get the consistency you want.
- Salad Veggies
- Chop up all of the veggies and toss into a large mixing bowl with the cooled cooked quinoa.
- Add dressing to the veggies and stir until everything is coated.
- Divide evenly onto serving dishes and sprinkle with sesame seeds.

209. Quinoa Springtime Salad

Serving: Serves about 10 people +/- | Prep: | Cook: | Ready in:

Ingredients

- 1 1/2 cups regular quinoa (not red quinoa)
- 1/2 teaspoon cayenne pepper
- 2 teaspoons garlic powder
- 2 teaspoons ground cardamom

- 1 1/2 cups light coconut milk
- 1 cup water
- 4 tablespoons balsamic vinegar
- 2 tablespoons fresh lemon juice
- 2 tablespoons extra virgin olive oil
- 2 garlic cloves, crushed and minced
- 1 pound green peas; fresh or frozen (if frozen, thaw in room temp water)
- 1 pound chopped strawberries
- 2 cups thinly sliced green onions
- 20-30 medium fresh mint leaves, thinly shredded
- 3 tablespoons lemon zest (I prefer Meyer lemons)

Direction

- After rinsing the quinoa, place it in a medium sized pot and mix with the spices, then add the coconut milk and water. Bring mixture to a boil, then reduce to a simmer and cook until done; about 20 minutes.
- Place the cooked quinoa in a large mixing bowl and add the vinegar, lemon juice, olive oil and garlic; mix to combine. Set aside and cool to room temperature.
- Once the quinoa has cooled down, add the remaining ingredients to the large mixing bowl, one at a time, adding each one only when the previous ingredient is mix in well enough. I suggest using a mixing spatula, so the ingredients mix, but don't get mashed together.

210. Quinoa Stuffed Bell Peppers

Serving: Serves 4 | Prep: | Cook: | Ready in:

Ingredients

- 4 bell peppers
- 1 cup uncooked quinoa
- 1/2 onion, chopped
- 2 cloves garlic, minced
- 1 can black beans, rinsed and drained
- 1 cup shredded cheese (cheddar or mexican style)
- 1 1/2 tablespoons lime juice
- 3/4 teaspoon cumin
- 1/2 teaspoon chili powder
- 1/2 teaspoon kosher salt
- 1/4 teaspoon pepper
- 3 teaspoons hot sauce

Direction

- Cut tops off of bell peppers and scoop out insides. Place in a microwavable and oven safe dish deep enough to fit peppers. Fill dish with about a cup or so of water depending on dish size (there should be about an inch of water). Cover dish tightly with plastic wrap and poke a few holes in it. Microwave on high for about 5 minutes or until peppers are softened. Remove peppers from dish, discard water, and place peppers back in.
- Cook quinoa according to package directions. Cook onions and garlic in a little olive oil for about 5 minutes. Mix onions, garlic, and rest of the ingredients into the cooked quinoa. Stuff each pepper with a couple spoonful of the mixture and top with cheese. Bake at 350 for about 25 minutes or until cheese is melted. Serve with sour cream, jalapeno slices, and extra hot sauce if desired.

211. Quinoa Stuffed Grape Leaves

Serving: Makes about 36 rolls | Prep: | Cook: | Ready in:

Ingredients

- 2 cups red wine vinegar
- 1 cup sugar
- 1.5 cups quinoa (white)
- 1/2 teaspoon kosher salt or sea salt
- 1/4 cup neutral vegetable oil
- 1.5 cups finely chopped yellow onion

- 1/4 cup pine nuts
- 1 cup white raisins
- 1 cup barberries or dried currents
- 2 tablespoons sour salt (citric acid) OR lemon juice
- 1 16oz jar grapeleaves, rinse, remove stems
- 1 cup dried apricots
- 1 cup small pitted prunes

Direction

- Make a syrup with the vinegar and sugar. Heat the combination in a heavy pan over very low heat. Ventilate the room, the heated vinegar is very strong smelling. Simmer and stir and until the mixture becomes syrupy (it will stick to the mixing spoon and drizzle off in a thick slow stream). Cool.
- Prepare the quinoa according to the package directions.
- Prepare the filling: In a skillet, heat the oil, saute the onions until translucent. Add the pine nuts, saute another minute or two. Add the raisins and barberries, saute for a few minutes. Add the cooked quinoa, salt, sour salt and 3-4 TBSP of the prepared syrup. Taste the mixture, you may want a bit more syrup, but you must be careful, the filling cannot be "soupy."
- Pour 1/2 c water into a heavy saucepan, line the bottom of the pan with several grape leaves to prevent the rolls from sticking.
- On a work surface: place a grape leaf, dull side facing you, place about 1 TBSP filling close to the stem end, fold sides of the leaf toward the center, over the filling and roll tightly. Place the roll on top of the leaves in the saucepan. Continue rolling, packing the leaves side by side in a single layer. Once you have filled the bottom of the pan with a layer, scatter some of the apricots and prunes on top of the rolls, then lay leaves on top of the fruit/ rolls and continue making rolls and forming a second layer. Scatter fruit on the 2nd layer. Cover with leaves. You should have enough filling to make approximately 36 rolls that will form 2 or 3 layers.
- Cover the top layer with leaves. Combine the remaining syrup with a scant 1/4c water, pour over the layered stuffed rolls. Place a small plate on top of the layers of rolls (I use a bread and butter size plate). Cover the pot and bring to a boil.
- Lower to a simmer and cook the stuffed rolls for about an hour. Cool before removing the plate or the rolls. They will firm up as they cool and will be easier to handle.
- Remove the rolls from the saucepan. They store well in a container for 2-3 days in the refrigerator. Serve on a platter, scattering the apricots, prunes and syrup around the stuffed rolls or alternately, serve as individual appetizers on a bed of lettuce, garnished with a few apricots, prunes and olives.
- These stuffed grape leaves also freeze well. Layer them in a single layer in a freezer container, cover with syrup and a layer of grape leaves and freeze for up to 2 months.

212.   Quinoa Stuffed Peppers

Serving: Serves 6 | Prep: | Cook: |Ready in:

Ingredients

- Quinoa
- 3 cups vegetable or chicken stock
- 1.5 cups Quinoa
- 2 each Red, yellow, green bell peppers. Tops cut off and seeded
- vegetable oil for casserole dish and outside of peppers
- salt to taste
- .5 teaspoons cayenne pepper
- The Stuffing
- 2.5 tablespoons olive oil
- 1 medium onion, diced
- 2 cups butternut squash, finely diced
- 1 bunch spinach, blanched for 2 minutes, dried and chopped

- .5 cups shelled pumpkin seeds and more for garnish
- 2 cloves garlic, minced
- 6 ounces feta, crumbled
- 1/8 cup chopped fresh oregano
- 1/8 cup finely chopped thyme
- salt
- lemon juice
- .5 cups water

Direction

- Quinoa
- In a medium heavy saucepan, bring the 3 Cups stock to a boil and add quinoa. Cover and simmer until liquid is absorbed and quinoa is very tender. About 30 minutes. Set aside
- Preheat oven to 400. Oil the outside of the peppers and season the inside with salt and the cayenne pepper. Trim bottom of peppers so they stand up in the casserole dish. Oil the casserole dish
- The Stuffing
- Heat the olive oil in a large pan. Sauté the onion, garlic, squash, and pumpkin seeds until they begin to get tender. Add the quinoa, spinach, and herbs and continue to sauté until blended. Add feta and mix well. Add a squeeze of lemon and Salt to taste. Fill each pepper with the stuffing mixture and top with a few crumbles of feta and a few pumpkin seeds.
- Place filled peppers in the prepared pan. Ad ½ C water or stock to pan and cover with foil. Bake 20-25 minutes until peppers are tender.

213. Quinoa Stuffed Squash

Serving: Serves 4-6 | Prep: | Cook: | Ready in:

Ingredients

- 4- 1 pounds Winter squash such as Amber Cup or Golden Nugget
- 8 ounces Sausage, any kind you like but if you use pork be sure to drain all but 1 tablespoon of the fat left behind after cooking
- 1/2 cup carrot, roughly chopped
- 1/2 cup onion, finely chopped
- 2 cloves garlic, minced
- 1 large portabella mushroom, roughly chopped
- 1 cup uncooked quinoa
- 2 cups water
- 2 tablespoons fresh flat-leaf parsley
- 1 teaspoon fresh thyme
- 1/4 teaspoon salt
- 1/4 teaspoon freshly ground black pepper
- 4 ounces cheddar or Monterey Jack cheese, shredded

Direction

- Prepare the squash. Cut off the top of each squash about a quarter of the way down. Scoop out the seeds and scrape the inside of the squash. Place two of the squash in a microwave safe dish. I used an 11 x 7-inch dish. Fill the dish with 1-inch of water. Microwave on high for 15 minutes. Remove squash from the dish and place on a plate to cool. If you are using 4 squash, repeat the process with the remaining two squash.
- Preheat oven to 375.
- Cook the quinoa. In a medium saucepan bring 1 cup quinoa and 2 cups water to a boil. Turn the heat down, cover and simmer for 10-15 minutes until the quinoa is soft and grains appear translucent.
- While the squash and quinoa are cooking, prepare the filling. Heat a large skillet with a swirl of olive oil over medium-high heat. Remove the casings from the sausage and add to the pan. Sauté the sausage for about 5 minutes, stirring and crumbling with a wooden spoon. Add the carrot, onion, garlic, and mushroom. Cook, stirring often, until the mushroom releases its juices and the carrot it soft.

- Remove the skillet from the heat. Mix in the quinoa, parsley, thyme, salt, pepper and a ½ cup of shredded cheese.
- Place the squash on one or two baking sheets, depending on how many squash you used. Also place the squash tops on the baking sheet(s). Fill the squash with the quinoa mixture. Top each with 1-2 tablespoons of shredded cheese. Bake for 20 minutes or until thoroughly heated.

214. Quinoa Stuffed With Everything Good

Serving: Serves 2, with leftovers | Prep: | Cook: | Ready in:

Ingredients

- 12 ounces cubed butternut squash (or sugar pie pumpkin)
- 1 cup quinoa
- 2 stalks green onion
- 1 large clove of garlic
- 1 tablespoon minced fresh sage
- 3 ounces feta cheese
- 1 bunch lacinato kale, stems removed, chopped into bite-size pieces
- 4 pieces high quality bacon, cooked and diced
- 3/4 tablespoon olive oil
- salt and pepper

Direction

- Preheat oven to 425. If your squash isn't pre-cubed, cube it now. Place squash on heavy-rimmed baking sheet with olive oil, salt, and pepper. Roast for 30-35 minutes (maybe less if your squash is cubed on the smaller side), checking occasionally and shaking the pan if any pieces look stuck. Remove from oven and set aside; your squash should be dark brown on some sides but not burnt.
- While the squash is roasting, rinse quinoa and add it to a medium saucepan with 2 cups water. Bring to a boil uncovered, then reduce to a simmer, cover, and let cook 10 minutes. Add kale on top and recover, simmering for 5 minutes longer. Then, turn your burner off and let the kale continue to steam, covered, for 5 additional minutes.
- While the quinoa is cooking, mince your sage and garlic; chop your green onions. I like to use the entire onion, from the dark green parts all the way down until just before the onion bulb. Place sage, garlic, green onion, and feta in the bottom of a large bowl with a sealable lid (if you don't have one of these, a large pot would work in a pinch). Mash the feta with a fork or spoon to break up any large crumbles, and top with some freshly ground black pepper.
- Once the quinoa and kale are done steaming, quickly fluff the mixture and toss it on top of the feta mash. Mix to incorporate and seal the lid onto your bowl. I try to do this as quickly as possible, as the steam will very lightly "cook" your garlic and melt your feta, distributing the flavors wonderfully. Let sit 5 minutes to allow flavors to meld.
- By now, your squash should be cooked. If it's not, that's fine-- the quinoa mixture can continue to steam until it's ready. Add it to the bowl, smashing the cubes into the quinoa as you incorporate it. Stir in bacon bits and diced celery. Finish with a healthy pinch of salt, stir once more to combine, and enjoy!

215. Quinoa Tabbouleh

Serving: Makes 8 - 10 cups | Prep: | Cook: | Ready in:

Ingredients

- 1 cup Quinoa
- 2 bunches Italian Parsley, coarsely chopped
- 1/2 English Cucumber, diced
- 4 Green Spring Onion, minced
- 4 sprigs Celery, thinly sliced
- 8 Radishes, thinly sliced

- 1/2 cup Fresh Mint, minced
- Juice from 2 Lemons
- 1/2 cup Olive Oil
- Salt & Pepper (to taste)

Direction

- In a medium saucepan, bring 2 cups water to boil. Add quinoa and simmer over low heat for 15 minutes.
- While the quinoa is cooking, add remaining ingredients in large mixing bowl and mix well. When quinoa is cooked, add (either warm or cooled) to the salad and mix well.
- Serve at room temperature or chilled. Keeps for 2 days.

216. Quinoa Tabbouleh Chickpea Burger With Beet Ketchup & Roasted Peaches

Serving: Serves 8-10 | Prep: | Cook: |Ready in:

Ingredients

- 3 cups canned chickpeas, drained and rinsed
- 3/4 cup quinoa tabbouleh
- 1 teaspoon paprika
- 1 teaspoon cayenne
- 2/3 cup chickpea flour
- 1 large egg, lightly beaten (eliminate to make recipe vegan)
- 6 cloves garlic, finely minced
- 1/2 small onion, peeled and roughly chopped
- 1/2 teaspoon ground black pepper
- large handful fresh mint, chopped
- grapeseed oil for frying
- salt to taste
- 3 large ripe peaches
- 1-2 tablespoons coconut oil
- 1 teaspoon cinnamon

Direction

- In a large bowl, mash the chickpeas. You want some large-ish pieces in there for texture, but nothing so big that the patty won't hold.
- Add the quinoa tabbouleh, chickpea flour, egg, paprika, cayenne, garlic, onion, and mint. Add salt to taste.
- Divide the mixture into eight, and pat each portion into a round, flat patty.
- Heat a cast-iron or non-stick skillet. Spray with some oil and, when hot, place the burger patties on it, at least an inch apart.
- Cook for a few minutes until the underside is golden brown, then flip over and continue cooking the other side.
- For the roasted peaches, Pit peaches and thinly slice cross-wise into 8-10 pieces each. Spread across a coconut-oil-brushed baking sheet. Sprinkle with cinnamon and bake at 400 degrees Fahrenheit for 8-10 minutes, until softened and delicately browned.
- To assemble: Spread bottom half of a toasted bun with beet ketchup. Top with chickpea patty, a handful of fresh microgreens, a few roasted peaches, and a few Gordy's Pickle Jar Sweet Pickle Chips. Top with top half of toasted bun.
- Enjoy!

217. Quinoa Tabbouleh Stuffing With Roasted Squash And Mushrooms

Serving: Serves 4-6 | Prep: | Cook: |Ready in:

Ingredients

- 1 large loaf challah, cut into large cubes and dried out overnight (alternatively, you can toast the bread at 100 degrees Fahrenheit until lightly crispy)
- 1 1/2 cups yellow onion, diced
- 1 1/2 cups celery, diced
- 2 cups wild mushrooms, diced
- 2 acorn squash, sliced

- 3 cloves garlic, minced
- 2 tablespoons fresh thyme, finely chopped
- 1 tablespoon fresh rosemary, finely chopped
- 1-1/2 teaspoons salt
- 1 teaspoon ground black pepper
- 3 cups low sodium vegetable broth
- 6 tablespoons butter, melted
- 1 package Cava Quinoa Tabbouleh

Direction

- Preheat the oven to 400 degrees Fahrenheit. Lightly grease a 9×13 inch baking dish or a large cast-iron skillet.
- Slice the ends off of each squash and cut in half. Scoop the seeds out of the center with a spoon. Slice each half into 3/4-inch thick half-moons. Toss the squash with olive oil and sea salt, and arrange in a single layer on a baking sheet. Roast for 15 minutes, flipping halfway, until the squash is lightly browned. Remove from heat and set aside. Reduce oven temperature to 300 degrees Fahrenheit.
- Heat a large skillet over medium-high heat. Add the olive oil, onion, and celery. Cook, stirring often, until the onions are fragrant, about 5 minutes. Stir in the mushrooms and squash (cut squash rings into smaller pieces if desired), and cook until the squash is fork tender and the mushrooms have caramelized, about 10 minutes. Stir in the garlic, thyme, rosemary, and sage. Cook another minute or so, then season generously with salt and pepper. Remove from the heat and set aside to cool slightly.
- In a very large mixing bowl, gently toss the bread and the broth to coat. Add the squash/mushroom mixture and 4 tablespoons of butter to the pan. Gently toss to combine with the bread cubes. Pour the mixture into your prepared baking dish.
- Cover the dish with foil and bake for 40 to 45 minutes. Remove the foil, sprinkle evenly with a layer of quinoa tabbouleh, and dot with a few pats of butter. Continue baking for another 10 to 15 minutes, until the stuffing is golden on top. Serve warm. Enjoy!

218. Quinoa Tabbouleh With Kale

Serving: Serves 6 | Prep: | Cook: | Ready in:

Ingredients

- 1 cup rinsed quinoa
- 4 tablespoons fresh lemon juice
- 2 teaspoons lemon zest
- 1 teaspoon garlic chopped
- 1/2 cup olive oil
- 1 cup Persian cucumbers thinly sliced
- 1 pint Komato, cherry or grape tomatoes, cut in half
- 1 cup flat leaf parsley, chopped small
- 1 cup kale, chopped small
- 1/2 cup basil and tomato flavored feta

Direction

- Cook quinoa according to package directions adding salt to water. Do not forget to fluff with a fork after the quinoa rests for five minutes. This will prevent it from getting sticky.
- Make the dressing by whisking the juice, zests and olive oil. Salt and pepper to taste.
- After quinoa has cooled add the dressing, cucumbers, tomatoes, parsley, kale and feta. Add salt and pepper to taste.

219. Quinoa Tabouli

Serving: Serves 4-6 | Prep: | Cook: | Ready in:

Ingredients

- 1 cup Quinoa, cooked
- 1 Whole Lemon
- 1 tablespoon Tahini
- 3 tablespoons Extra Virgin Olive Oil

- 1 Small English Cucumber(The seedless kind)
- 1 pint of plum/cherry tomatoes, roasted
- 1 Heirloom tomato, diced (optional)
- 4 Green Onions
- 1 Handful, Fresh Spinach
- 2 tablespoons Each, Fresh Mint, Dill, Parsley
- 1 Salt and Pepper, to taste

Direction

- Zest lemon and add to plum tomatoes. Place on sheet pan. Roast tomatoes on 325 for about 30 minutes
- Cook quinoa according to package. Let cool slightly.
- Chop onion, cucumber, herbs and spinach
- Add olive oil, tahini, juice from the lemon, and salt and pepper to a medium bowl.
- Add quinoa, then veggies to the olive oil mix. Stir to combine. Chop fresh tomato and add if desired.
- Taste for seasoning and add more olive/salt/pepper as needed

220. Quinoa And Apple Muffins

Serving: Serves 24 | Prep: | Cook: | Ready in:

Ingredients

- Muffin Ingredients
- 1 cup all purpose flour
- 1 cup whole wheat flour
- 1 cup sugar
- 1 tablespoon baking powder
- 1 teaspoon baking soda
- 1 teaspoon salt
- 2 teaspoons cinnamon
- 1.25 cups fat free yogurt
- 2 tablespoons milk
- .25 cups canola oil
- 2 large eggs
- 1 teaspoon vanilla extract
- 2 cups diced apple
- 1 cup quinoa cooked with 2 cups of water for 15 minutes, cooled
- Oatmeal and Cinnamon Topping Ingredients
- .5 cups old fashioned oatmeal
- 2 tablespoons brown sugar
- 2 tablespoons butter, melted
- 1 teaspoon cinnamon
- 1 teaspoon all-purpose flour

Direction

- Cook 1 cup of quinoa according to package instruction. Set aside to cool.
- Preheat oven to 400 degrees F. In a large bowl mix together the all-purpose flour, whole wheat flour, sugar, baking soda, baking powder, cinnamon and salt.
- In another bowl, combine yogurt, milk, oil, vanilla, and eggs, stirring with a whisk.
- Add yogurt mixture to the flour mixture, and stir just until moist.
- Fold in cooled quinoa and diced apple.
- To make the topping, combine together in a small mixing bowl, ½ cup of the old-fashion oatmeal, brown sugar, butter, cinnamon, and flour.
- Fill muffin pans with liners. Spoon 1/4 cup of batter into each liner. Sprinkle evenly with oatmeal and cinnamon topping.
- Bake at 400 degrees F for 15 to 16 minutes.
- Cool in pan for 10 minutes on a wire rack.
- Remove muffins from pan, and serve warm or at room temperature. This recipe makes 24 muffins.

221. Quinoa And Carrot Tabbouleh Salad

Serving: Serves 6 to 8 as a side dish | Prep: | Cook: | Ready in:

Ingredients

- 1 1/2 cups red or white quinoa (I used half and half)
- Salt
- 1 tablespoon extra-virgin olive oil
- 3 green onions, white and green parts thinly sliced
- 1 large carrot, peeled, finely grated
- 1 medium red bell pepper, stemmed and seeded, finely diced
- 1 jalapeno pepper, stemmed and seeded, minced
- 1 garlic clove, minced
- Juice of 1/2 lemon
- 1 teaspoon Tabasco sauce
- 1 teaspoon ground cumin
- 1 teaspoon freshly ground black pepper
- 1/2 teaspoon sweet paprika
- 1/2 cup chopped fresh cilantro
- 1/4 cup chopped fresh Italian parsley
- 1/4 cup chopped fresh mint

Direction

- Place quinoa, 2 1/2 cups water and 1 teaspoon salt in a medium saucepan. Bring to a boil. Reduce heat to low, cover and simmer until water is absorbed and the grains release their germ, about 20 minutes. Transfer quinoa to a large bowl. Add the olive oil and stir to coat. Cool to room temperature.
- Stir all of the remaining ingredients except the fresh herbs into the quinoa. Taste for seasoning and add more salt if desired. (The tabbouleh may be prepared in advance to this point. Cover and refrigerate for up to 6 hours). Before serving, fold in the fresh herbs. Serve chilled or at room temperature.

222. Quinoa And Chickpea Flour Falafel With Romesco Sauce

Serving: Makes 32 falafels | Prep: | Cook: | Ready in:

Ingredients

- For the romesco sauce:
- 2 bell peppers
- 1 garlic clove, roughly chopped
- 1/4 cup olive oil
- 2 tablespoons hazelnuts, toasted and skins removed
- 1 tablespoon tahini paste
- 2 teaspoons apple cider vinegar
- 3/4 teaspoon paprika
- 1/4 teaspoon sea salt
- 1/4 teaspoon cayenne pepper (optional)
- For the falafel:
- 1/2 cup quinoa, rinsed
- 1 cup plus 3 tablespoons water
- 1/2 cup whole mung beans
- 1 tablespoon ground flaxseed meal
- 1/2 cup parsley, plus extra for serving
- 1/4 cup chickpea flour, toasted*
- 1 shallot, roughly chopped
- 2 garlic cloves, roughly chopped
- 1 tablespoon fresh lemon juice
- 2 teaspoons sea sat
- 1 1/2 teaspoons ground cumin
- 1 1/2 teaspoons ground nutmeg
- 1 teaspoon paprika
- 1/4 teaspoon ground turmeric
- 1 tablespoon black sesame seeds
- Extra-virgin olive oil, for brushing

Direction

- For the romesco sauce:
- Turn oven to broil and line a rimmed baking sheet with parchment paper.
- Place the peppers on the baking sheet and broil, turning over every 30 seconds, until skins are blackened in spots. Place the peppers in a large bowl and cover tightly with plastic wrap for 10 minutes. Peel the peppers' skins with your fingers.
- Cut the peppers, removing the white ribs and seeds; then rinse and pat dry. Place the peppers, garlic, oil, hazelnuts, tahini, vinegar, paprika, salt, and cayenne (if using) in a food processor. Blend until smooth and creamy.

Transfer the sauce to a bowl and cover with plastic wrap until ready to use. (Rinse food processor and set aside.)
- For the falafel:
- Cook the quinoa with 1 cup of water for 12 to 14 minutes, until cooked and water has evaporated; set aside. Meanwhile, fill a small saucepan three-quarters of the way with water, add the mung beans and bring to a boil, turn heat down to a simmer and cook for 25 to 30 minutes, until tender and doubled in size; drain any remaining water and set aside.
- In a small bowl, whisk together the flaxseed and 3 tablespoons of water; let mixture sit for 10 minutes, until thick.
- In the food processor, add the cooked quinoa, mung beans, flaxseed mixture, parsley, flour, shallots, garlic, lemon juice, salt, and spices. Blend until thoroughly combined; taste for salt and lemon and adjust if necessary. Transfer to a large bowl and stir in the sesame seeds; cover with plastic wrap and refrigerate for 1 hour or overnight.
- Preheat oven to 375° F (190° C) and line two baking sheets with parchment paper; set aside.
- Pinch off golf ball–size pieces of mixture and roll between palms to shape into a ball. Place on prepared baking sheets and repeat.
- Lightly brush the tops and bottoms of the falafel with oil. Bake for 20 to 25 minutes, rotating the baking sheets and flipping falafels over halfway through the baking time.
- Serve warm with romesco sauce and garnish with parsley.
- *To toast the chickpea flour. Place 1 cup of chickpea flour in a large skillet, turn the heat to medium, and stir. Keep stirring for 5 to 7 minutes, until the flour is lightly browned and has a nutty fragrance. Place in a bowl or on a plate and let it cool at room temperature. Store toasted chickpea flour in an airtight container at room temperature if not using right away.

223. Quinoa And Corn Patties

Serving: Makes about 35 | Prep: | Cook: | Ready in:

Ingredients

- 3 cups cooked quinoa, make with 1/2 teaspoon Adobo powder in the water
- 1 small onion, small diced
- 3 cobs of corn, cooked and taken off the cob
- 1 red pepper, small diced
- 1 bag frozen spinach, defrosted and drained of water
- 1 cup whole wheat breadcrumbs
- 1/2 cup fresh grated Parmesan cheese
- 6 eggs, beaten
- 1/4 cup canola or olive oil for frying

Direction

- Mix all the ingredients together in a large bowl, except for the olive oil. Form small patties by hand with all the mixture.
- Heat a tablespoon of the oil in a large non-stick skillet over medium heat. When hot, begin frying the patties in batches. Add more oil as needed. Don't over-crowd the pan as this can lead to soggy patties. Serve hot.

224. Quinoa And Edamame Salad With Basil, Mint, And Lemon

Serving: Serves 3-4 people as a main | Prep: | Cook: | Ready in:

Ingredients

- Quinoa and Edamame Salad with Basil, Mint, and Lemon
- 1 cup quinoa
- 1 1/2 cups water
- 1 cup frozen shelled edamame
- 1/4 cup finely chopped pickled red onions, recipe below

- 1 lemon, zested and juiced
- 3 tablespoons extra-virgin olive oil
- 1 teaspoon Dijon mustard
- 3/4 teaspoon salt
- 1/2 cucumber, washed, unpeeled and diced into 1-cm cubes
- 1 cup loosely packed fresh basil in chiffonade
- 1/2 cup finely chopped fresh mint
- 3 tablespoons sunflower seeds, raw or already roasted and salted
- 1/2 avocado, peeled, pitted, and sliced
- Pickled Onions
- 1 red onion, peeled and thinly sliced
- 1/2 cup apple cider vinegar
- 1/2 cup water, microwaved for about a minute to heat
- 1 tablespoon honey
- 1 1/2 teaspoons salt

Direction

- Quinoa and Edamame Salad with Basil, Mint, and Lemon
- Prepare the quinoa. Combine 1 cup quinoa and 1 1/2 cups water in a pot. Bring to boil, reduce the heat to low, and cover. Cook for 25 minutes on low. Allow to rest, covered for 10 minutes.
- In the meantime, cook the edamame. Combine the frozen edamame and enough water to cover by an inch in a small pot. Bring to a boil and then reduce heat to a simmer and cook edamame for 5 minutes or until just tender. Drain and set aside.
- Prepare the rest of the ingredients. If you are using raw sunflower seeds, toast the sunflower seeds. Heat 1/2 teaspoon olive oil or coconut oil in a skillet over medium heat and add the sunflower seeds. Toast for 5-7 minutes, stirring often or until sunflower seeds are toasted. Remove and allow to cool on a paper towel. Sprinkle with 1/8 teaspoon of salt while still warm.
- When the quinoa has finished, add the quinoa to a large bowl. Add the edamame, pickled onions, lemon juice, lemon zest, extra-virgin olive oil, Dijon mustard, and salt. Mix to combine. Toss in the basil and mint. To serve, sprinkle each serving with the toasted sunflower seeds and sliced avocado.
- Pickled Onions
- Combine all of the ingredients in a bowl, stirring to coat evenly. Allow the onions to pickle and slightly wilt for at least 20 minutes, stirring occasionally. This makes a lot more than you need for these tacos, but these onions should last about a week in the fridge so you can find some new uses for them.

225. Quinoa And Farro Salad With Pickled Fennel

Serving: Serves 6 to 8 as a side dish | Prep: | Cook: | Ready in:

Ingredients

- For the Pickled Fennel:
- 1 medium fennel bulb, fronds removed but with stems trimmed, quartered and sliced lengthwise into 1/8-inch planks
- 1 hot dried chili (optional)
- 2 sprigs dill
- 1/2 teaspoon yellow mustard seeds
- 1/2 teaspoon fennel seeds
- 1/4 cup sugar
- 1 tablespoon kosher salt
- 3/4 cup apple cider vinegar
- 3/4 cup water
- For the Salad:
- 1 1/2 cups cooked and cooled farro
- 1 1/2 cups cooked and cooled quinoa
- 3 tablespoons olive oil
- 1/2 cup finely (1/4-inch) chopped pickled fennel
- 1 tablespoon fennel pickling liquid
- Salt and freshly ground black pepper to taste
- 1/4 cup roughly chopped dill leaves (or half dill, half fennel fronds if you saved them)

Direction

- For the Pickled Fennel:
- Put the fennel in a 1-quart jar. Add the chili (if using), dill, mustard and fennel seeds.
- In a small saucepan, combine the sugar, salt, vinegar and water. Bring to a boil over high heat and then pour into the jar with the fennel. Screw on the lid and refrigerate and serve once cool. The pickled fennel will keep in the fridge for at least 2 weeks.
- For the Salad:
- In a serving bowl, combine all of the ingredients and fold gently to combine. Taste and add more salt and pepper, pickling juices or olive oil if you'd like. Serve right away or let the salad sit at room temperature for up to an hour before serving. It will also keep in the fridge for a couple of days.

226. Quinoa And Grilled Marinated Vegetable Salad

Serving: Serves 6-8 people | Prep: | Cook: |Ready in:

Ingredients

- Vinaigrette and Salad Ingredients
- Juice from 2 lemons
- 4 garlic cloves, minced
- 1 tablespoon sea salt
- 1 teaspoon ground pepper
- 2 tablespoons tahini
- 3 tablespoons balsamic vinegar
- 1/4 cup red wine vinegar
- 1 teaspoon oregano, chopped
- 1 teaspoon basil, chopped
- 1 teaspoon parsley, chopped
- 1/2 teaspoon crushed red pepper
- 1/2 cup extra virgin olive oil
- 3 cups grilled vegetables (see directions below)
- 2 teaspoons olive oil
- 2 cups quinoa, rinsed
- 6 cloves garlic, chopped
- 2 cups chicken stock
- 1/2 teaspoon kosher salt
- 4 green onions, chopped
- 1/2 cup roasted almonds, chopped
- 1/2 cup sunflower seeds
- 1 cup grape tomatoes, cut in half
- 1/4 cup basil, chopped
- 1/4 cup thyme, chopped
- 1/4 cup parsley, chopped
- Grilled Marinated Vegetables
- 2 red bell peppers, seeds and pulp removed
- 2 yellow bell peppers, seeds and pulp removed
- 2 zucchinis
- 2 large Portobello mushrooms
- 2 yellow onions
- The above are suggested vegetables. Please substitute with your choice of seasonal vegetables.

Direction

- Vinaigrette and Salad Ingredients
- To Make Vinaigrette: In a food processor, blend lemon juice, garlic, sea salt, ground pepper, tahini, balsamic vinegar, red wine vinegar, oregano, basil, parsley and crushed red pepper. Slowly drizzle in oil to emulsify. Set aside.
- To Make Salad: Heat olive oil in a small saucepan over low heat. Add the rinsed quinoa. Salute for 2 minutes, then add the garlic and chicken stock.
- Bring to a boil, cover and reduce heat to a simmer. Cook for about 20 minutes.
- Turn off heat and let sit for about 5 minutes. Fluff quinoa with a fork.
- In a large serving bowl, combine cooked quinoa with salt, onions, almonds, sunflower seeds, tomatoes, basil, thyme, parsley and marinated grilled vegetables. Toss with dressing and serve hot or cold. Taste and adjust seasoning as needed.
- Grilled Marinated Vegetables
- Slice bell peppers and Portobello mushrooms in equal size wedges, about 1/4 to 1/2 inch thick. Slice zucchini diagonally, about 1/4-inch thick. Set aside.

- In a large bowl, add equal parts balsamic vinegar and olive oil. Mix to combine. Add vegetables to the marinade and toss to coat. Transfer mixture to a baking dish, cover and marinate at room temperature for at least 3 hours or refrigerate up to 1 day.
- Prepare the grill for medium-high heat. Remove vegetables from marinade and pat with paper towels. Sprinkle with salt and pepper. Grill in batches, letting vegetables rest on the grill for about 3 minutes at the start to caramelize and create grill marks. Grill until they are crisp-tender and brown, about 6-8 minutes. Brush with the reserved marinade as the vegetables grill and put in a bowl.

227. Quinoa And Kale Crustless Quiche

Serving: Makes about 8 slices | Prep: | Cook: | Ready in:

Ingredients

- 1/2 cup Quinoa
- 1 cup water
- 2 tablespoons Olive Oil
- 1 bunch Kale, stems removed and cut into ribbons
- 1 Vidalia Onion, thinly sliced
- 2 cloves of garlic, minced
- 1/2 cup white cheddar cheese
- 3 ounces cream cheese, cubed
- 4 eggs
- salt and pepper to taste

Direction

- Preheat the oven to 350°F and prepare a 9" pie dish (either butter the dish thoroughly or spray with baking spray). Rinse the quinoa. Combine the quinoa and water in a pan. Bring to a boil on medium-high heat and then reduce to a simmer. This will take about twenty minutes. Set aside.
- Meanwhile, start to caramelize the onions. Heat the olive oil in a large sauté on medium heat. When the oil is shimmering, add the onions. Slowly cook until the onions are soft and browned.
- Remove the onions from the pan, and place them in a large mixing bowl. Add the kale into the hot onion pan. On medium heat, cook until the kale is wilted and bright green, about two minutes.
- Allow the greens to cool. Squeeze out any extra liquid using a sieve or a clean dish towel.
- Add the kale, quinoa, garlic, cream cheese and cheddar to the mixing bowl with the onions. Stir the ingredients so that they are evenly distributed.
- In a small bowl, whisk the eggs so that they are well combined. Pour over the quinoa/kale mixture. Stir until the egg clings to the greens. Add salt and pepper.
- Pour the mixture in the prepared pie dish. Bake for about 45 minutes, until the top is golden and the pie has started to pull away from the edge of the baking dish. This dish is delightful hot, but even better at room temperature.

228. Quinoa And Oat Breakfast Porridge

Serving: Serves 2 generously | Prep: | Cook: | Ready in:

Ingredients

- 2 cups unsweetened almond milk, divided, see notes above
- 1 cardamom pod, crushed with the flat side of a knife
- 1/2 a bay leaf, fresh is best
- 1/2 cup quinoa, red is nice for color
- 3/4 cup rolled oats, extra-thick if you can find them, see notes above
- 1 teaspoon coconut oil
- 2 tablespoons maple syrup

- 1/4 teaspoon kosher salt, plust more to taste
- toasted coconut, toasted almonds, fresh berries such as strawberries and blueberries, for garnish

Direction

- Place 1 cup of the almond milk, the lightly crushed cardamom pod, and the 1/2 bay leaf in a small pot. Bring to a simmer, reduce heat to low, and keep warm.
- In a medium pot, combine the quinoa with 1 cup of water. Add a pinch of salt. Bring to a boil, turn heat to low, cover, and cook until tender, about 20 minutes. Remove from heat, and let stand covered.
- In another medium pot, combine the oats, remaining 1 cup almond milk, ¼ cup water, coconut oil, maple syrup, and salt. Bring to a simmer, then turn heat to low and cook until oats are tender, about 10 minutes. Taste. Add more salt to taste if necessary.
- Add ½ cup of the cooked quinoa to the oats along with ½ cup of the infused almond milk, taking care to leave the bay leaf and cardamom pod (and any seeds) behind. Stir to combine. Taste. Add more salt if necessary. Add more quinoa to taste (or save extra quinoa in the fridge in an airtight container for porridge on a future morning).
- To serve, pour ¼ cup of the warm, cardamom-infused almond milk into each bowl. Spoon porridge over top. Top with toasted coconut, almonds, and berries if using.

229. Quinoa And Salmon Breakfast Torte

Serving: Serves 4 | Prep: | Cook: | Ready in:

Ingredients

- 4 eggs
- 1 cup cooked quinoa
- 6 ounces cooked salmon
- 2 scallions, thinly sliced
- Salt
- 2 tablespoons olive oil

Direction

- In a medium sized bowl, crack and beat the eggs. Add the cooked quinoa and mix. Flake the salmon into small pieces and add it to the egg mixture. Add the scallions and season with a bit of salt. Mix well.
- Heat the oil in a small, non-stick saute pan. Turn the heat to high. Add the egg mixture, cook 1 minute and reduce the heat to low. This will give you a nice brown color on the torte. Let the eggs cook for about 5-7 minutes on low heat. The sides will start firming up and just the center will remain wet. Using a plate, slide the torte out of the pan, top the plate with the saute pan, and invert so that the top of the torte is now on the bottom of the pan. Cook another 5 minutes on low heat. Cut and serve hot.
- * I've made this with 2 tablespoons of grated Parmesan cheese added to the egg mixture and it's also delicious. ** If you don't have leftover quinoa, take 1/2 cup dry quinoa, and a scant 1 cup of water or chicken broth, bring it to a boil, reduce heat, cover and simmer about 15 minutes.*** If you don't have cooked salmon, bake it in a 400 degree oven for about 10 minutes.

230. Quinoa And Vegetable Chorizo Salad

Serving: Serves 4 | Prep: | Cook: | Ready in:

Ingredients

- Vegetable chorizos
- 1/2 cup sundried tomatoes, rinsed
- 3/4 cup cashew nuts, toasted
- 1/2 red onion, coarsely chopped

- 1/2 small red chili, seeded and finely chopped
- 6 unsulphured dried apricots, coarsely chopped
- 2 sprigs fresh oregano, leaves picked and chopped
- 1 cup rice flour
- 1 tablespoon xanthan gum
- 1 tablespoon flax seeds, ground
- 1/4 cup extra virgin olive oil, for frying
- Quinoa salad and dressing
- 1 cup black quinoa
- 15 cherry tomatoes, halved
- 2 small red apples, diced
- 1/2 onion, sliced
- 2 cups cooked lima beans
- 1/3 cup extra virgin olive oil
- 1/2 lemon, juice and zest
- 3 tablespoons hot English mustard
- 1 pinch sea salt
- 2 sprigs fresh oregano, to garnish

Direction

- To prepare the chorizos, combine the sundried tomatoes, cashew nuts, onion, chili, and apricots in a food processor or blender.
- Pulse until finely chopped.
- Add the herbs, rice flour, xanthan gum, and flax seeds and pulse until everything is combined.
- Add the olive oil and 1/4 cup water and pulse until a dough is formed. It should be easy to handle and form into a sausage shape.
- Divide the dough into 5 equal parts. Roll each piece into a sausage, place on the cheese cloth, roll up and tie the twine firmly around both ends. Repeat with the rest of the sausages.
- Bring the vegetable stock to the boil in the widest frying pan you have. Lay the chorizos in it and let them boil for about 45 minutes.
- Next, carefully remove the cloths from the boiled chorizos. Heat the olive oil in a frying pan on a medium-high heat and fry them until they are nicely browned all over.
- Next prepare the quinoa salad. Place 2 1/4 cups water, the quinoa, and salt in a heavy-based saucepan. Bring to the boil, lower the heat, and gently simmer for 15 to 20 minutes.
- Drain any excess water and set aside to cool.
- Prepare the tomatoes, apples, and onion, and slice the fried chorizos.
- Whisk together olive oil, lemon, mustard, and sea salt in a small bowl.
- Put the quinoa, tomatoes, apples, onions, and lima beans into a large bowl. Add the chorizo slices, then pour the dressing over the salad and toss about to make sure all the ingredients are well coated.
- Garnish with oregano and serve.

231. Quinoa And Wild Rice Casserole With Kale, Leeks, And Gruyère Biscuit Crust

Serving: Serves 6 | Prep: | Cook: | Ready in:

Ingredients

- 2 bunches kale, de-ribbed and chopped
- 1 cup water
- 3 tablespoons olive oil, divided
- 2 large leeks (or 3 medium-sized leeks) white and light green parts only, cut into 1/4 inch rounds
- 2 large sweet onions
- 1 pound baby portabella (or cremini) mushrooms, sliced
- 3 garlic cloves, minced
- 1 teaspoon dried thyme
- 1 teaspoon dried rosemary
- 2 cups cooked wild rice
- 2 cups cooked quinoa
- 3 tablespoons unsalted butter
- 1/4 cup all-purpose flour
- 1 cup vegetable stock
- 1 cup milk
- 1/4 cup heavy cream
- 1/4 teaspoon nutmeg
- 4 ounces (about 1 cup) Gruyère cheese, shredded

- 2 cups all-purpose flour
- 2 teaspoons baking powder
- 1/2 teaspoon baking soda
- 1 tablespoon sugar
- 1/2 teaspoon salt
- 6 tablespoons cold unsalted butter, cut into small pieces
- 4 ounces (about 1 cup) Gruyère cheese, shredded
- 1 1/3 cups well-shaken buttermilk

Direction

- In a large skillet, heat the kale and water over medium-high heat, covered, for about 10 minutes, or until all the water is absorbed. Remove the kale from the skillet and set aside in a large mixing bowl.
- In the same large skillet, heat 2 tablespoons of the olive oil over medium-high heat. Add the leeks and onions and cook, stirring occasionally, for 15 minutes, until the onions are beginning to turn translucent and the leeks are starting to soften. Add the mushrooms and cook for 5 minutes. Season to taste with salt and pepper. Push some of the vegetables out from the middle of the skillet to expose the bottom of the pan. Add the remaining 1 tablespoon of olive oil, garlic, thyme, and rosemary, and cook for 30 seconds. Give it all a good stir and remove from the heat, adding the vegetable mixture to the kale in the large mixing bowl. Add the cooked rice and quinoa and mix together.
- In a medium-sized saucepan, heat the butter over medium heat. Once the butter is melted, whisk in the flour to form a paste. While whisking constantly, add the vegetable stock, milk, and heavy cream. Continue to whisk constantly, until the sauce starts to boil, about 7 minutes.
- Reduce the heat to low and simmer, stirring occasionally, until sauce begins to thicken, about 10 minutes.
- Remove the sauce from the heat and stir in the nutmeg and the Gruyère cheese until blended. Salt and pepper to taste. Pour the sauce in the large mixing bowl with the wild rice, quinoa, and vegetables, and mix together until blended. Transfer the mixture into a greased 13-by-9-inch baking dish.
- Preheat the oven to 400 degrees Fahrenheit.
- In a large bowl, whisk together the flour, baking powder, baking soda, sugar, and salt. Work the butter into the mixture with either a pastry cutter or your fingers until the butter is incorporated and the dough has pea-sized lumps.
- Stir in the Gruyère and the buttermilk just until the dough comes together. Drop the biscuit dough onto the casserole filling in 6-8 large mounds, leaving a bit of space between each biscuit.
- Bake the casserole for 35-40 minutes, until the biscuits are golden brown on top and the filling is bubbling. If your biscuits start to brown too quickly, cover the dish with foil and continue to cook. Let the casserole stand 10 minutes before serving.

232. Quinoa And Cold Sauce

Serving: Makes 2 cups of sauce | Prep: | Cook: | Ready in:

Ingredients

- 15 basil leaves
- 6 green inions, more if you like, adjust to taste
- 5 or 6 garlic cloves, again adjust to taste
- salt and pepper to taste
- 4 tablespoons Olive oil
- 2 cups grape or cherry tomatoes

Direction

- Everything goes in the food processor, process to your preferences, I like it a little chunky.
- I make the quinoa for me and hubby favorite pasta. Put sauce over cooked pasta or quinoa add cheese if you want, and left over quinoa and this sauce it wonderful!!!!

233. Quinoa Date Pudding

Serving: Serves 2-3 | Prep: | Cook: | Ready in:

Ingredients

- 3 cups whole milk
- 1/2 cup quinoa
- 4 green cardamom pods, slightly bruised
- 2 cinnamon sticks
- 2 tejpatta (often sold in Indian grocery stores as Indian bay leaf)
- 20 Medjool dates, pitted
- 2 cups water
- kosher salt, to taste
- handful of chopped pistachios

Direction

- Add the whole milk, quinoa, cardamom, cinnamon and tejpatta in a large saucepan on medium heat and bring it up to a gentle boil. Boil for 20 minutes, stirring occasionally.
- While the quinoa is boiling, let's make the date syrup! Add the dates and 2 cups of water to a microwave safe bowl. Make sure that the dates are completely submerged in the water. I used a 4 cup measure and it worked great for me! Microwave for 6 minutes. Using an immersion blender or a food processor, puree the date mixture really, really thoroughly. Strain the date mixture through a fine mesh sieve that is lined with a double layer of cheesecloth. Once the mixture has cooled enough, you should be able to really twist the cheesecloth and get most of the liquid out. In the end you should have about 1 1/2 cups of the date liquid.
- Once the quinoa has cooked for 20 minutes, add the date liquid along with a pinch of kosher salt and bring the whole mixture up to a gentle boil. Cook, stirring frequently for about 10 minutes or so, until the mixture has thickened to the desired consistency. It is going to thicken as it cools, so you might want to take it off the heat while it is still a little liquid-y. Fish out the tejpatta, cardamoms and the cinnamon sticks and taste for salt. You can have the pudding at room temperature or chilled, garnished with chopped pistachios. Enjoy!

234. Quinoa Pudding Paletas With Plums

Serving: Makes about 8 3oz. paletas | Prep: | Cook: | Ready in:

Ingredients

- The plums:
- 3 plums, semi-ripe (still a bit tart)
- 1 tablespoon sugar
- The quinoa pudding, and assembly of paletas:
- 1 cup quinoa
- 1 1/2 cups water, divided
- 1 14 oz. can evaporated milk
- 3 tablespoons sugar, or to taste
- 1 cinnamon stick
- 1/4 cup heavy cream
- the cooked and cooled plums, from above

Direction

- The plums:
- Start by peeling, pitting, and dicing the plums. You should end up with ~1.5 cups or so of chopped plum-material. Stir in the sugar and let it all macerate for about 15 minutes.
- Once it's good and macerated, throw it the plums a saucepan and cook it down until the plum chunks cease to be distinguishable and all is gooshy and delicious. Stir frequently, especially as it begins to cook down, to keep the bottom from burning. If it starts to get very thick before the plum chunks break down, add a splash or two of water to thin it out again and keep cooking. You should end up with about 1 cup of plum goo. Remove from heat

and chill until you're ready to make your paletas.
- The quinoa pudding, and assembly of paletas:
- Bring the quinoa and 1 cup of the water to a boil in a small pot. Boil gently, uncovered, for 4 minutes without stirring; then remove from the heat, cover, and let sit for at least 15 minutes. Go fold your laundry, or work on your lab report, or what have you-the quinoa has infinite patience. When you're ready, add the other 1/2 cup of water, the sugar, the evaporated milk and the cinnamon stick, and bring it all back to a boil. Then, turn down the heat and simmer it uncovered for about 30 minutes, or until most of the liquid is absorbed or evaporated away. You'll need to stir it pretty frequently to keep it from burning on the bottom. A skin may form on the surface; that's alright, just stir it right back in. Finally, stir in the cream, continue heating for another minute or two, and then take the pot off the stove. Let it cool.
- When the quinoa has cooled enough not to burn you, carefully extract the cinnamon stick with whatever utensil you please (in my kitchen, fingers may have been used for at least part of this process). If you taste the pudding now, it will taste very sweet, but fear not: when it's frozen you won't taste the sweet nearly as much. Anyway, to make the paletas: layer the pudding and the plum mixture into a popsicle mold, willy-nilly, any way you like. I found it surprisingly difficult to spoon stuff in neatly so I just went for broad stripes, but if you have mad paleta skills, you might try narrower bands, or swirls, or something. The number of paletas you make will depend on (a) your popsicle mold, and (b) your particular balance of plum to pudding. The ratio per paleta is very much to taste.
- Put the filled mold in the freezer for a couple hours or overnight, until the paletas are frozen solid. To serve, run the mold under hot water until you can extract the paletas, and eat!

235. Quinoa Salad With Avocado

Serving: Serves for 4 | Prep: | Cook: | Ready in:

Ingredients

- Salad
- 160 grams quinoa (or rice)
- 1 tablespoon olive oil
- 0,5 liters water
- 3 clove of gralic
- 2-3 avocado
- 3 tomato
- 1 tin of corn
- 1 jalapeño
- 5 green onion (or leeks onion, or both)
- Sauce
- 6 tablespoons olive oil
- 3 tablespoons jucie of lime
- 2 teaspoons cumin
- 1-2 teaspoons garlic powder
- 2 teaspoons cilantro
- 1 teaspoon honey
- 1 teaspoon salt

Direction

- Salad
- Add 1 tablespoon oil to pot, followed by 3 clove of garlic and the rice. Add the water and cook the quinoa (or the rice).
- While the quinoa (or the rice) boils, chop the vegetables.
- When the quinoa (or the rice) is fine, mix with the vegetables in a bowl.
- Sauce
- Get a bowl and mix the ingredients.
- Pour the sauce to the quinoa salad and mix it.

236. Quinoa Salad With Radishes, Avocado, And Citrus Vinaigrette

Serving: Serves 8 | Prep: | Cook: | Ready in:

Ingredients

- 2 cups Chicken stock
- 2 cups Water
- 2 cups Quinoa
- 2 Lemons, zested and juiced
- 1 Lime, zested and juiced
- 1 Orange, zested
- 1 Shallot, finely chopped
- 2 Garlic cloves, finely chopped
- Salt and pepper, to taste
- 2/3 cup Olive oil
- 1 Bunch radishes (about nine), trimmed and thinly sliced
- 2 Avocados, pitted, skinned and chopped
- 1/3 cup Chopped fresh parsley

Direction

- In a saucepan, bring the chicken stock and water to a boil. Add the quinoa, lower the heat to medium, and cover the pan. Simmer for about 18 minutes.
- Remove from heat and let the quinoa stand for 5 minutes. Transfer to a large bowl, fluff the quinoa with a fork, and set aside to cool.
- In another bowl, whisk together the lemon juice and rind, lime juice and rind, orange rind, shallot, garlic, salt, and pepper. Add the olive oil in a thin steady stream, whisking constantly.
- Add the radishes, avocado, and parsley to the quinoa. Pour the vinaigrette over the quinoa mixture, and toss gently to combine. Taste for seasoning and add more salt and pepper, if you like.

237. Quinoa With (Almost) Caramelized Onions And Shiitake Mushrooms Two Ways

Serving: Serves 4 | Prep: | Cook: | Ready in:

Ingredients

- 1 cup mixed red quinoa and cream colored quinoa (or even some black quinoa mixed with red), rinsed
- 2 1/2 cups low sodium vegetable stock (you can use chicken if you don't want it vegetarian)
- 1 large onion, peeled and halved and then thinly sliced
- 2 cloves garlic, minced
- 3 ounces shiitake mushrooms, stems removed and caps sliced thinly
- 1 small Napa cabbage or 1/2 of a larger one, sliced (about 2-3 cups). You can also use a bunch of asparagus, cut into two inch pieces on a bias and lightly steamed.
- 1-2 tablespoons soy sauce
- 1 teaspoon sesame oil

Direction

- Heat a sauté pan on medium heat. When pan is warm, add 2-3 tablespoons of olive oil to pan. Add the sliced onions and let them cook, stirring occasionally, about 10-15 minutes. You want them to get a little brown, but not actually caramelized.
- Meanwhile, put quinoa and stock or water in a saucepan and bring to a boil. Lower to a simmer and cover. I like to cook it on the shorter side to maintain a little more of a chewy mouth feel. After about 10 minutes, check the pot and see if the grain has become translucent. Taste it gingerly, as the stock or water is hot, and if it's still crunchy, leave it to simmer a couple of minutes more. When it is done, the individual grains should be translucent and you should be able to see a "ring" around the edge. That is the germ of the grain. You just don't want to let it get mushy. I

find that it takes less time than the packages instruct.
- When the quinoa is done, drain over a fine mesh strainer or colander if there is still liquid in the pan. You can reserve some of the stock if you are not using soy sauce.
- Lower the heat in the sauté pan to medium-low and add the garlic and mushrooms. Once they have softened, about 3 minutes, add the cabbage or asparagus. Add the soy sauce one tablespoon at a time (or water or stock) to moisten the pan. Add the other if needed. Let cook, stirring occasionally for about 3 more minutes.
- If you are using the soy sauce and sesame oil, take the pan off the heat and add the sesame oil and mix and serve. If you are omitting the soy sauce and sesame oil in favor of the pepper, add the cayenne or Aleppo pepper here and taste for salt.

238. Quinoa With Broccoli "Dust", Haloumi Cheese, And Mint

Serving: Serves 6 main course servings, 10-12 side servings | Prep: | Cook: | Ready in:

Ingredients

- 8 cups water
- 2 teaspoons sea salt, divided
- 1 pound broccoli crowns
- 2 cups quinoa
- 1/4 cup freshly squeezed lemon juice
- 1 tablespoon apple cider vinegar
- 2 cloves garlic, minced
- 1 tablespoon Dijon mustard
- 1/2 teaspoon freshly ground black pepper
- 1/2 cup extra-virgin olive oil
- 1/2 cup coarsely chopped fresh mint leaves, packed
- 1/2 coarsely chopped fresh parsley, packed
- 1 cup crumbled haloumi or feta cheese
- 4 medium, ripe tomatoes, seeded and diced, about 3/4 lb
- 4 green onions, thinly sliced
- 1/2 cup coarsely chopped walnuts

Direction

- Bring the water to a boil in a medium pot. Add 1 tsp (5 mL) salt and the broccoli. As soon as it turns bright green, remove it with tongs and cool under cold water. Drain in a sieve or colander and let sit while you prepare the other ingredients.
- Add the quinoa to the pot the broccoli was dunked in. Keep at a lively simmer for 10 minutes. Drain the quinoa well, return it to the pot, and cover with tightly with a lid. Let sit for 20 minutes off the heat. Transfer the quinoa to a large bowl.
- While the quinoa is cooking and resting, make the dressing. Whisk the lemon juice, vinegar, garlic, 1 tsp (5 mL) salt and pepper together. Slowly whisk in the olive oil. Toss with the quinoa and let cool.
- Holding the broccoli by the stem, grate the florets and stalks using the large holes of a box grater. Toss the broccoli "dust" with the quinoa. Add the remaining ingredients and toss well. Taste and adjust the seasoning, and serve.
- Note: Quinoa and grain salads will diminish in seasoning after refrigeration overnight. Check and correct the seasoning before serving.

239. Quinoa With Butternut Squash And Pumpkin Seeds

Serving: Serves 4 as veggie meal | Prep: | Cook: | Ready in:

Ingredients

- 1 cup quinoa
- 2 tablespoons olive oil
- 1/2 red onion, finely diced

- 3/4 teaspoon chili powder
- 1 2-pound butternut squash, cut into 3/4-inch cubes
- 1 3/4 cups water or vegetable stock
- 1 teaspoon salt
- 1/2 cup pumpkin seeds
- 2 large handfuls baby spinach
- 1/2 cup dried cranberries

Direction

- Put the quinoa in a bowl and cover it with cool water. Rub it between your hands and pour off most of the water. Add fresh water and repeat two or three times, until the water runs clear. Drain thoroughly in a fine-meshed strainer. Set the strainer over a bowl until you are ready to cook the quinoa.
- Heat the olive oil in a large (4 to 5-quart) pot. Add the onion and cook over medium heat for about 3 minutes, until it begins to soften. Stir in the chili powder and the squash and cook, stirring every so often, for 3 more minutes. Add the drained quinoa, water or stock and salt. Bring the liquid to a boil, adjust the heat to a simmer, and cook, covered, for 15 minutes.
- Meanwhile, set a small plate next to the stove. Pour a few drops (about 1/2 teaspoon) of olive oil into a small skillet. Heat the oil over medium heat and add the pumpkin seeds. Stir and shake the pan until the pumpkin seeds turn from green to olive to slightly golden brown. Sprinkle with a pinch of salt and immediately scrape them onto the awaiting plate.
- Remove the pot from the heat and add the spinach and cranberries. Cover the pot and let rest in a warm place for 10 minutes. Mix and fluff up the grains with a fork. Serve sprinkled with toasted pumpkin seeds.

240. Quinoa With Butternut Squash, Cinnamon And Mint

Serving: Serves 8 | Prep: | Cook: | Ready in:

Ingredients

- 1 1/2 cups quinoa
- 1 1/2 cups homemade chicken stock
- 3/4 teaspoon cumin seeds, toasted and ground
- 3/4 teaspoon coriander seeds, toasted and ground
- 1/4 teaspoon saffron threads
- 1/2 teaspoon ground cinnamon
- 3/4 teaspoon kosher salt
- 2 tablespoons pomegranate molasses
- 1 tablespoon extra virgin olive oil
- 1 cup butternut squash, cut into 1/2-inch dice
- 1/2 yellow onion, cut into 1/2-inch dice
- 2 large carrots, cut into 1/2-inch dice
- 1 1/4 teaspoons kosher salt
- 2 scallions, white and green parts, chopped
- 1/4 cup cilantro, chopped

Direction

- Prepare Quinoa: Rinse quinoa under running water for 2 minutes. (This step is very important or else it will taste bitter). Bring quinoa, stock, spices, saffron, cinnamon, salt to boil in a medium saucepan. Once boiling, turn down the heat. Cover and let simmer for about 20-25 minutes, until the liquid is fully absorbed and the quinoa is tender. Remove from heat and stir in the pomegranate molasses.
- Sauté Vegetables: Heat the oil in a very large sauté pan. Add the squash, onions and carrots, and salt. Cook until all vegetables are soft but not soggy, about 5 more minutes. Remove from heat, cool slightly and mix in with the quinoa.
- Serve: Just before serving, stir in the scallions and cilantro. Serve at warm or at room temperature.

241. Quinoa With Chard, Sausage, And Corn

Serving: Serves 2 (with leftovers for lunch) | Prep: | Cook: | Ready in:

Ingredients

- 1.5 cups quinoa
- 3 cups vegetable broth (my preference is Better than Bouillon - it makes everything so tasty)
- 1 tablespoon olive oil
- 2 cloves garlic, minced
- 1 bunch chard
- 4 large mushrooms, sliced
- 2 chicken sausages, sliced
- 2 ears corn, grilled or boiled, with the corn removed from the ears
- 1 handful grated Parmesan (optional)

Direction

- Bring vegetable broth to a boil in a medium pot. Add quinoa and turn heat down to low. Cover and cook for approx. 20 minutes until quinoa has absorbed all the liquid and is nice and fluffy.
- Meanwhile, separate the chard leaves from the stalks. Dice stalks and slice up leaves into bite-size pieces.
- Heat olive oil in a large saucepan over medium-high heat. (If chicken sausages are not pre-cooked, add to pan at this point and sauté until cooked. If they are pre-cooked, then begin with chard stalks.)
- Add chard stalks and sauté for a few minutes.
- Add garlic, mushrooms, and sausage (if pre-cooked) and sauté, stirring frequently, for a few more minutes until garlic is fragrant and the sausage is beginning to brown.
- Add chard leaves and corn and cook until chard is beginning to wilt.
- Turn off heat and add quinoa to pan, mixing everything together.
- Enjoy either as is or with a healthy sprinkle of cheese!

242. Quinoa With Curried Cauliflower & Potatoes

Serving: Serves 2 | Prep: | Cook: | Ready in:

Ingredients

- Curried Cauliflower & Potato
- 1 1/2 cups cauliflower florets
- 1 medium sized russet potato, cubed
- 1/2 cup frozen peas
- 1 teaspoon grated ginger
- 1 teaspoon cumin seeds
- 1/2 teaspoon asafetida powder (hing)
- 2 tablespoons coriander powder
- 1/2 teaspoon turmeric powder
- 1 green chili, finely chopped
- 4 tablespoons light olive oil
- Salt to taste
- Quinoa
- 1/2 cup quinoa
- 1/2 cup cherry tomatoes, halved
- 1/4 onion, diced
- 1 teaspoon light olive oil
- 1/2 teaspoon red pepper flakes
- Salt to taste

Direction

- First make the curried cauliflower. Heat 4 tsp oil in a non-stick pan.
- Add the cumin seeds and cook till they brown and begin to splutter.
- Add the ginger and green chili and cook for another 20 seconds.
- Now add all the dry spices, mix well and cook for a minute till they become fragrant.
- Stir in the cauliflower, potatoes, peas, along with ½ cup water and mix well. Cover and cook on medium heat for 10- 12 minutes, or till

the potato and cauliflower are soft and thoroughly cooked.
- Turn heat to high, and sauté for 4-5 minutes till any excess liquid is absorbed and the edges of the vegetables begin to get brown & crisp.
- Remove from heat, add fresh coriander and cool to room temperature.
- Cook the quinoa as per instructions on the packet.
- Heat 1 tsp oil from "Quinoa" ingredients in a nonstick pan.
- Add the onions and tomatoes and cook for a few minutes, just till the tomatoes start to wilt.
- Add the cooked quinoa and 1 cup of curried cauliflower. Mash the cauliflower slightly, mix well and sauté for another 2-3 minutes.
- Adjust salt and add red pepper flakes (if you like that kick!). Remove from heat and serve hot with pickle and yogurt.

243. Quinoa With Onions

Serving: Serves 4 | Prep: | Cook: | Ready in:

Ingredients

- 1 cup Quinoa, dry measure, rinsed
- 2 cups Water
- 1 teaspoon Better than Bouillon
- 1 Medium onion, diced
- 1/4 Cup fresh parsley, chopped

Direction

- Rinse the quinoa in cold water through a fine mesh strainer.
- In a small sauce pan, bring the water and Better then Bouillon to a boil. Add the quinoa
- Reduce the heat, cover and simmer for 15 minutes. Remove from heat and let sit for 5 minutes. Fluff gently with fork.
- In a large skillet, add the olive oil and heat over a medium heat. Add onion and sauté until onions are translucent and carrots are soft about 3-5 minutes, add the cooked quinoa

and mix to deglaze flavor. Toss in parsley. Serve and enjoy.

244. Quinoa With Roasted Beets And Pear

Serving: Serves 2 | Prep: | Cook: | Ready in:

Ingredients

- 2 cups cooked quinoa (I prefer red)
- 2 medium-sized beets, scrubbed (I like a mix of colors)
- 1/4 cup walnuts
- 1 large pear, cubed
- 3 ounces crumbled feta
- 1 splash olive oil
- 1 splash Balsamic vinegar
- 1 pinch salt and pepper, to taste

Direction

- Preheat your oven to 400° F.
- Slice off the leaves at the top of the beets. Drizzle with a little olive oil, and then wrap each individually and loosely in tin foil. Place on a baking sheet and roast for 40 to 50 minutes, or until soft enough that you can easily stab one with a fork and it doesn't give you any problems. Unwrap and set aside to let cool; once touchable, run the beets under water to slide the skin off. Cut beets into cubes.
- Lower your oven temperature to 350° F. Spread walnuts out in a single layer on a baking sheet and toast for 8 minutes. Allow the nuts to cool before giving them a rough chop.
- Assemble the salad by dumping everything together into a bowl because you, brilliant human, know that's how salads work. Quinoa, beet cubes, pear cubes, walnuts and feta, a.k.a. the dream team. Toss with a slight drizzle of balsamic, a little olive oil, and some coarse salt and freshly ground pepper. Did

you know this is awesome warm or cold? It is. Bring it to work for lunch the next day because it will be bitchin' straight from the fridge, and your coworkers will be like ughhhhhhh.

245. Quinoa With Walnuts, Goat Cheese, And Thyme

Serving: Serves four | Prep: | Cook: | Ready in:

Ingredients

- 1 cup white quinoa
- sea salt
- walnut oil or extra-virgin olive oil
- 1/2 cup coarsely chopped walnuts
- a few sprigs thyme (lemon thyme is nice, too)
- 1/2 cup coarsely chopped pitted green olives
- freshly ground black pepper
- red wine vinegar or fresh lemon juice
- 3/4 cup crumbled goat cheese

Direction

- Bring two cups of water to a boil in a small saucepan. Add your quinoa and a good pinch of salt. Give it a quick stir and cover the pan. Cook for around 12-20 minutes, or until the quinoa is done and most (or all) of the water is absorbed. Fluff with a fork, then cover the pan and let sit off the heat for five minutes to steam.
- In a medium skillet, heat about a tablespoon of your oil over medium-high heat. Once it's good and hot, and your walnuts and thyme leaves and cook until nuts are fragrant and lightly toasted, just a few minutes.
- Turn the heat down to low. Add the olives, cooked quinoa, and a splash of vinegar or lemon juice to the skillet. Season with fresh black pepper and toss with the cheese. Transfer to a serving bowl and tuck in!

246. Quinoa With Apricot And Pine Kernels

Serving: Serves 4-6 | Prep: | Cook: | Ready in:

Ingredients

- Quinoa, apricots, pine kernels
- 2 cups Cooked quinoa
- 3 Apricots, best fresh ones
- 2 Garlic cloves
- 1 tablespoon Olive oil (extra virgin)
- 1/2 cup Cranberries, chopped
- 1 teaspoon Cumin
- Salt and white pepper
- Pine kernels and mustard leaves
- 1/2 cup Toasted pine kernels
- 1 cup Mustard leaves, chopped

Direction

- I find that the quinoa after rinsing well in water, gets more fluffy, when I cook it for 12 min, and then leave it in the water for another 6-8 min., and save. I start cutting the apricots in very small cubes, and peel and shop the garlic.
- In a skillet, heat the olive oil, add the garlic, and fry until golden, then add the apricot cubes, mix and fry for 3-4 min.
- Then add the cooked quinoa, the cumin, and the chopped cranberries, mix and leave on low temperature for some min., before you add salt and pepper after taste.
- At the moment of serving, add the toasted pine kernels and the mustard leaves and mix. You can do it in advance, and just add these two ingredients when serving, I like it hot, but my daughter like it room temperature, and love it the following day.

247. Quinoa With Edamame And Sundried Tomatoes

Serving: Serves 4 | Prep: | Cook: | Ready in:

Ingredients

- 1 cup Quinoa
- 2 cups Chicken broth
- 2 tablespoons sundried tomatoes (not in oil)
- 1/2 cup Edamane
- Dash Salt
- Dash pepper
- 1 tablespoon Lemon juice
- 2 tablespoons Olive oil

Direction

- Cook quinoa with the broth according to package directions.
- When quinoa is done add edamanes and chopped sundried tomatoes stir then drizzle with olive oil, add salt and pepper to taste. Put lid on pot let sit for five minutes. Serve with a squeeze of lemon juice and a little more olive oil.

248. Quinoa, Beet And Chickpea Burgers

Serving: Makes 6 large burgers, or 12-18 small sliders | Prep: | Cook: | Ready in:

Ingredients

- 1/2 cup dried chickpeas, soaked overnight in cool water (or 1 [14 ounce] can cooked chickpeas, drained and rinsed)
- 1 bay leaf (if using dried chickpeas)
- 1/2 cup raw quinoa
- 3 medium-sized red beets (about 10 ounces by weight)
- 1 tablespoon olive oil
- 1 medium yellow onion, finely diced
- 2 cloves garlic, minced
- 2 tablespoons cider vinegar
- 2-4 tablespoons finely chopped parsley
- zest from half a medium lemon
- juice from 1 medium lemon
- 1 large egg
- 1/2 cup quick (baby) oats
- sunflower oil or coconut oil for frying the burgers
- For serving the burgers (optional): 6 buns (such as Honey Oat Beer Buns), halved and toasted, mustard, mayonnaise, avocado, thinly sliced red onion, sprouts

Direction

- If using dried chickpeas, cook the beans: Drain the soaked chickpeas and place them in a medium saucepan with the bay leaf. Cover with 3 inches of water, bring to a boil, then reduce the heat and simmer, partially covered, until the beans are almost tender. At this point, add 1/2 teaspoon of salt to the pot. Continue cooking until the beans are very tender. This can take anywhere from 30 minutes to over an hour total, depending on the size and age of the beans. Add water to the pan as needed. When the beans are done, let them cool in their water until needed. If you like, you can slip the loose skins off the beans, though this isn't necessary.
- Cook the quinoa: Place the quinoa in a very fine mesh strainer, place the strainer in a bowl or measuring cup, and fill with water to cover the quinoa. Let soak 5-10 minutes, swishing occasionally, to rinse off the bitter coating. The water will turn a beige-yellow. Drain the quinoa well, discard the soaking water, and place the quinoa in a small saucepan with 1 cup of water and 1/4 teaspoon salt. Bring the mixture to a boil, immediately reduce the heat to very low, cover the pot, and let the quinoa steam until tender and all the water is absorbed, 15-20 minutes. Remove from the heat and let sit, covered, until ready to use.
- Cook the veg: Peel the beets with a potato peeler, then grate them on the large holes of a box grater. The beets will spray, so wear an

apron and have your work area clear of things you don't want covered in tiny red specks. Heat the oil in a wide sauté pan (that has a lid that you will use later) over medium heat. When it shimmers, add the onion and cook, stirring occasionally, until tender, 5-10 minutes. Add the garlic, the grated beets, and a big pinch of salt. Give it a stir, then cover the pan and let the mixture cook, stirring occasionally, until the beet is tender, 5 minutes or so. Remove from the heat and deglaze by adding the vinegar and stirring up any good stuff that is stuck to the bottom of the pan.
- Make the burgers: In a large bowl, combine the cooked chickpeas, quinoa and beet mixture and mash with a potato masher to break up the beans slightly - the mixture should still be fairly chunky. Stir in the parsley, lemon zest and juice, egg, oats, and 1/4 teaspoon salt until combined.
- Cook the burgers: Divide the mixture into 6 equal portions (a large spring-loaded scoop works well) and shape into 1" thick rounds. Coat the bottom of a wide skillet with oil and heat over a medium flame until the oil shimmers. Carefully add the burger patties. Cook until the first side is golden, 2-3 minutes, then flip and cook on the second side until it is golden and the burger is cooked through, 2-3 minutes, reducing the heat if the burger is browning too quickly. Serve the burgers on toasted buns slathered in any toppings you like.

249. Quinoa, Edamame & Cucumber Salad

Serving: Serves 4 | Prep: | Cook: | Ready in:

Ingredients

- Dressing
- 3 tablespoons olive oil
- 2 tablespoons sour cream
- 1 tablespoon lemon juice
- 4 - 6 canned green peppercorns, crushed
- 1 pinch salt
- Salad
- 1 cup quinoa
- 2 cups water
- 1 pinch salt
- 2 tablespoons olive oil
- 1 tablespoon lemon juice
- 1 teaspoon lemon rind
- 1 cup shelled edamame beans
- 1/2 small English cucumber
- 2 radishes
- 2 green onions, chopped
- 2 tablespoons basil, thinly sliced

Direction

- In a medium bowl combine the olive oil, sour cream, lemon juice, peppercorns and salt. Whisk until well combined and set aside.
- Place the quinoa into a fine mesh strainer and rinse in cold water, rubbing the quinoa against the strainer. This will help remove the bitterness from the quinoa. Drain well.
- Place the quinoa in a medium saucepan. Add the water and salt. Bring to a boil over high heat. Cover the pan, reduce the heat to very low and cook for 15 minutes. Remove from the heat and let sit for 5 to 10 minutes longer. Fluff with a fork.
- While the quinoa is cooking place the 2 Tbsp. of olive oil, lemon juice and rind into a medium heat-proof bowl. Add the hot quinoa and toss. Cool to room temperature and then refrigerate.
- Bring a small pot of water to a boil. Add the edamame and cook for 3 minutes. Remove from the heat, drain and let cool to room temperature.
- Using a mandoline slice the cucumber and radishes into paper thin sliced. Add to the dressing in the bowl. Add the green onions and cooled edamame beans and half of the basil. Stir gently. Refrigerate until cold.
- When ready to serve place the quinoa onto a platter or into a shallow serving bowl. Top

with the vegetables. Sprinkle with the remaining basil and serve.

250. Quinoa, Fava Bean, And Chard Veggie Burgers

Serving: Serves 6 | Prep: | Cook: |Ready in:

Ingredients

- 1 cup cooked quinoa
- 2 cups fresh or frozen fava beans (see note)
- 4 ounces chard, center ribs removed
- 1 onion, diced
- 2 garlic cloves, minced
- 1 tablespoon chopped fresh dill (or 1 teaspoon dried)
- 2 large eggs, lightly beaten
- 1/2 cup dry breadcrumbs
- 1/2 teaspoon fine sea salt
- 1/4 teaspoon freshly ground black pepper
- 3 tablespoons olive oil, divided
- 6 ounces Halloumi cheese, cut into 6 slices
- 6 tablespoons olive tapenade (purchased is fine)
- 6 whole grain rolls
- 6 handfuls mixed greens, such as frisee and pea shoots

Direction

- Place the quinoa in a large bowl and set aside for a few minutes.
- Fill a medium pot halfway with water and bring to a boil. Cook the fava beans for two to four minutes, until just tender, and drain thoroughly. If your beans are larger and have tough skins, remove the skins. If they're young and tender, feel free to leave them on. In the bowl of a food processor, pulse the beans until they form a chunky puree. It shouldn't be totally smooth, but it should hold together fairly well. Scrape the bean puree into the bowl with the quinoa.
- Drain and dry the pot you used for the fava beans. Over medium heat, warm one tablespoon of the olive oil. Cook the onion without browning until soft, about five minutes.
- Meanwhile, julienne the chard leaves: stack the leaves on top of one another and roll the stack from tip end to stem end into a cigar shape. Then use a large knife to cut thin crosswise slices of the cigar. When you're done you should have nice long, thin ribbons of chard. Add the chard ribbons to the onions along with the garlic and cook, stirring frequently, until the chard is wilted. Add the contents of the pot to the bowl.
- Add the dill, eggs, breadcrumbs, salt, and pepper to the bowl, and mix everything together thoroughly. Cover the bowl and chill the mixture for 30 minutes.
- When you're ready to make the burgers, heat two tablespoons of the olive oil over medium heat in a cast iron or other heavy pan. Scoop up the mixture by palm-sized amounts and form patties with your hands. (You may have more than enough for six burgers.) Cook burgers, in batches if necessary to avoid crowding, until nice and brown on the underside, about four minutes. Gently flip and cook until the other side browns and the burgers are cooked through, about four minutes more. If cooking in batches, you may need to add more oil. Place each burger into a roll.
- Cook the Halloumi slices in the pan until browned on both sides and place a slice atop each burger. Top with some olive tapenade and a handful of greens and serve immediately. Extra cooked burgers or uncooked mixture will keep in the fridge for two days.

251. Quinoa, Halloumi And Fresh Corn Salad

Serving: Serves 4-6 | Prep: 0hours15mins | Cook: 0hours30mins | Ready in:

Ingredients

- 1 cup quinoa
- 4 Ears of corn, shucked
- 1 cup Cherry tomatoes, halved
- 1/4 cup Mint, roughly chopped (plus some whole leaves to scatter atop the finished dish)
- 1/4 cup Cilantro, roughly chopped (plus some whole leaves to scatter atop the finished dish)
- 2 Scallions, thinly sliced
- 1 Package of helium, cut into 1 inch cubes
- 4 teaspoons Chili powder, divided
- 3 Limes, juiced
- 3 tablespoons Extra virgin olive oil
- 1/4 cup Pepitas

Direction

- Make quinoa: Measure 1 cup quinoa and 1 ¾ cups water into saucepan with a three-finger pinch of salt. Bring water to boil and then lower the heat to simmer. Cover with lid and cook for 10 to 15 minutes, until quinoa has absorbed all of the liquid. Remove from heat and allow to cool for a few minutes, and fluff fork.
- Grill corn: Drizzle corn with olive oil and sprinkle with 2 teaspoons chili powder and a generous pinch of salt. Grill corn on high heat until it begins to develop char marks. Allow corn to cool and then cut the kernels off the cob and into a bowl.
- Toast pepitas: Lightly toast pepitas in a skillet on medium heat with a small drizzle of olive oil, just enough to coat the seeds. Stir frequently and remove the seeds from heat once they have become crunchy and slightly browned.
- Make halloumi croutons: Heat a skillet on high with a glug of olive oil. Fry cheese until golden brown on all sides, flipping with spatula throughout the cooking process. Drain excess oil off croutons by resting on a paper towel lined plate.
- Assemble salad: Combine cooled quinoa, corn, sliced tomatoes, chopped herbs, lime juice, olive oil, remaining two teaspoons of chili powder and half of the halloumi cheese and pepitas. Toss to combine and adjust seasoning as needed. Pile the salad into a bowl and top with the rest of the cheese, peptias and extra herbs.

252. Quinoa, Molasses And Peanuts For Breakfast

Serving: Serves 1 - 2 | Prep: | Cook: | Ready in:

Ingredients

- 1/4 cup quinoa, rinsed
- 1/4 cup barley flakes
- 1/2 tablespoon blackstrap molasses
- 1 tablespoon peanut butter
- 1/2 teaspoon cinnamon
- sea salt
- berries, kiwi or other fruits, cut

Direction

- Put the quinoa, barley flakes and 2 cups of water in a 1 quart pot with a good pinch of sea salt. Bring to a boil, reduce heat to cook at a simmer with the lid slightly ajar (or covered, depending on your pot and your stove). In about 20 minutes, the quinoa should be cooked (showing pits in the top and the little tails unfurled). Most of the water will be absorbed.
- Stir in molasses, peanut butter and cinnamon. Serve with fruit.

253. Quinoa, Oat And Chia Porridge

Serving: Serves 2 | Prep: | Cook: |Ready in:

Ingredients

- 1/2 cup Oats
- 2 tablespoons Quinoa
- 1 tablespoon Chia Seeds
- 1/2 teaspoon Vanilla bean paste
- 1 tablespoon Honey
- 1 1/2 cups Milk (almond, oat, cows)
- 3/4 cup water
- 1 Pear
- 1 tablespoon Almonds

Direction

- In a medium sized saucepan, add all the grains, honey, vanilla, milk, water and salt. Bring to a boil, cover and reduce the heat to a low/medium, and frequently stir.
- After about 12/15mins check if the Quinoa is cooked and the porridge has thickened. Pour into bowls and top with the sliced pear, almonds and a little more milk. Porridge is always best eaten straight away.
- I like to eat this porridge with a brew of rooibos tea. So cozy!

254. Quinoa, Wheat Berry, And Chickpea Salad With Green Beans

Serving: Serves 6-8 | Prep: | Cook: |Ready in:

Ingredients

- 3/4 cup quinoa
- 1 cup dried wheat berries
- 1 cup dried chickpeas
- 2 handfuls fresh green beans
- 1 red bell pepper
- 1 cup whole almonds
- 1 teaspoon smoked paprika
- 6 ounces aged gouda
- 2 tablespoons sherry vinegar
- 1/4 cup olive oil plus 1 Tbsp for the almonds
- 1/2 cup flat leaf parsley leaves
- salt to taste

Direction

- Soak both the chickpeas and the wheat berries separately overnight. For each, rinse and place in 2.5 cups fresh water and simmer on low until they are soft, about 2 hours. Salt generously and reserve. Cook the quinoa on a low simmer in 1.5 cups fresh water with a pinch of salt for about 15 minutes until it releases its halos and the water is absorbed. Strain the chickpeas and wheat berries and combine with the quinoa in a large serving bowl.
- Trim the green beans. Blanch them in boiling salted water until they just lose their firmness (about four minutes). Drain and cool in ice water. Cut into 1.5 inch lengths and mix into the bowl of grains.
- Char the bell pepper directly over a burner until it its black all over. Place in a deep bowl covered with a plate and allow to steam. When it is cool enough to handle, remove the blistered burned skin. Core and seed the pepper. Cut into 1/2 inch wide and 1 inch long strips and mix into the bowl of grains.
- Heat a small skillet over medium heat. Add I Tbsp of olive oil and toss in the almonds to coat them. Add the smoked paprika and a pinch of salt and toss again to coat the almonds with the spice. Cook until the almonds are toasted and fragrant. Mix into the bowl of grains.
- Cut the aged gouda into 1/2 inch chunks and mix into the bowl of grains once they are not too hot.
- Mix together a dressing of lemon juice, sherry vinegar, and olive oil. Pour over the grain salad and mix well. Taste and add more salt, lemon juice, vinegar, or olive oil as needed. Rinse and chop the parsley leaves and toss

into the salad. Serve warm or at room temperature.

255. Quinoa, Cherry Tomato, Tuna And Feta Salad

Serving: Serves 2 | Prep: | Cook: |Ready in:

Ingredients

- Lemon Dressing
- 20 milliliters lemon juice
- 2.5 tablespoons extra virgin olive oil
- 2.5 tablespoons Greek yoghurt
- 1/2 teaspoon lemon zest, finely grated
- 1/2 teaspoon honey, agave syrup or brown rice syrup
- Sea salt & black pepper, to taste
- Salad
- 1/3 cup quinoa, rinsed and drained
- 4.5 ounces can smoked tuna slices in oil, drained and flaked
- 14 ounces coloured cherry tomatoes, halved
- 6 radishes, sliced
- 1 handful Handful Continental parsley, basil, spring onions, chopped
- 2 ounces reduced fat feta cheese, cubed

Direction

- For dressing: Add all ingredients to a glass jar and shake to combine. Set aside.
- Add 1/3 cup of quinoa and 2/3 cup of water to a small saucepan and bring just to the boil on high heat, covered. Once boiling, turn down to low and continue to simmer covered, for around 15 minutes, or until all the water is absorbed. Remove saucepan from the heat and fluff quinoa with a fork then set aside to cool a bit.
- Add the quinoa, tuna, cherry tomatoes, radish and herbs to two plates and crumble over the feta cheese. Drizzle over the dressing and season further if you like.

256. Quinoa Chicken Meatballs With Garlicky Greens

Serving: Serves 4 | Prep: 0hours30mins | Cook: 0hours35mins |Ready in:

Ingredients

- Quinoa-chicken meatballs
- 2/3 cup white quinoa, rinsed
- 1 1/4 pounds boneless, skinless chicken thighs, chopped into 1-inch pieces
- 2 cloves garlic (optional)
- 1 1/4 teaspoons kosher salt
- 2 tablespoons extra-virgin olive oil, plus more as needed
- Garlicky escarole
- 1/4 cup extra-virgin olive oil
- 12 cloves garlic, roughly chopped
- 2 heads escarole, quartered and washed well

Direction

- Add the quinoa to a small pot with 1 ⅓ cups water. Set over medium heat and bring to a boil, then cover and reduce the heat to low-as-possible. Cook for 10 to 15 minutes, until all the water has evaporated, and the quinoa is fluffy and tender. Dump onto a plate and spread out so it cools.
- Pulse the chicken thighs and garlic in a food processor, in small batches, until finely ground (but not pureed!). Transfer to a large bowl and add the salt, 1 tablespoon cold water, and cooled quinoa. Stir gently to combine. Form into small, nugget-size meatballs (figure a heaping tablespoon each—yielding 25 to 30).
- Heat a large cast-iron skillet over medium to medium-high heat and add enough olive oil to create a thin film. When the oil is hot, add about half the meatballs (pan-frying in batches means better browning). Cook for 8 to 10 minutes, turning as needed, until they're crusty and golden-brown all over and cooked through (about 165°F internal temperature); transfer to a plate or wire rack. Repeat with

the remaining meatballs, adding fresh oil if needed.
- While the meatballs are cooking, sauté the escarole. Combine the olive oil and garlic in a super-large sauté pan or pot, then set over medium heat. When the garlic just starts to turn golden, add the escarole and toss. Cover and cook for 5 minutes until the escarole has wilted significantly, then uncover and cook for another 5 minutes or so until it's tender. Season with salt to taste.
- Serve the meatballs with the escarole—or on top of the escarole or whatever you want.

257. Quinoa Lentil Taco Filling

Serving: Serves 4-6 | Prep: | Cook: | Ready in:

Ingredients

- 1/2 cup quinoa
- 1/2 cup red lentils
- 2 tablespoons vegetable oil
- 1 med. onion, diced
- 5 garlic cloves, minced
- 2 teaspoons cumin
- 1-3 teaspoons hot pepper flakes (adjust to your liking)
- 1/2 teaspoon salt
- 1/2 teaspoon black pepper
- 2 teaspoons marjoram (or oregano)
- 1 ounce tequila
- 1 tablespoon soy sauce

Direction

- Rinse quinoa and lentils thoroughly, and drain. Next, place them in a bowl and cover with fresh water. Soak for about 15 minutes and drain.
- While quinoa and lentils are soaking, heat a medium size sauté pan (or wok) over medium heat and add oil, onions and garlic. Sauté until golden, then add in cumin, salt, hot pepper flakes and black pepper (marjoram will be added later) and sauté until fragrant, about 30 seconds. Remove pan from heat and set aside.
- Drain soaked quinoa and lentils, and place in medium sauce pan along with 3 cups water and 1 tsp salt. Bring to a simmer and cover, cooking for 15 minutes (they will be slightly underdone at this point). Pour in to a strainer and rinse briefly Drain well.
- Add cooked quinoa and lentils to pan containing onion, garlic and spice mixture. Add marjoram, tequila, soy sauce and 1/2 c water. Cook and stir over medium high heat until water is absorbed (about 5 minutes)
- To serve: Use as you would any taco filling. Our favorite combo is corn tortillas, sour cream or crema, cheddar cheese, cilantro and lime.

258. Quinoa Oat Chocolate Chip Cookies

Serving: Serves many (or not if you have someone with a sweet tooth) | Prep: | Cook: | Ready in:

Ingredients

- 14 tablespoons butter (at room temperature)
- 3/4 cup brown sugar
- 1/2 cup white sugar
- 2 eggs
- 1/2-1 tablespoons vanilla
- 1 cup white flour
- 1/2 cup white whole wheat flour or quinoa flour
- 1 teaspoon baking soda
- 3/4 teaspoon salt
- 1 cup quinoa flakes
- 1-1/2 cups chocolate chips (I use a mix of semi and bitter sweet)

Direction

- Heat oven to 350 F.

- In a large bowl beat butter, oil and sugars until creamy. Then add eggs and vanilla. Beat well
- Add baking soda and salt and stir to combine. Next add flours. Once they are mixed in, add oats and quinoa flakes. Final addition is chocolate chips.

259.   Quinoa Stuffed Bell Peppers With Basil Sauce

Serving: Serves 4 | Prep: | Cook: | Ready in:

Ingredients

- For the peppers:
- 1 cup uncooked quinoa
- 1 cup vegetable broth
- 2 teaspoons ground cumin
- 1 cup cooked garbanzo beans
- 1/2 cup dried currants
- 1 cup packed chopped baby spinach leaves
- 1/2 cup crumbled feta
- 1/4 cup olive oil, plus more for drizzling
- Salt and pepper
- 4 bell peppers
- For the sauce:
- 1 cup packed chopped basil leaves
- 1/2 cup Greek yogurt
- 3 tablespoons olive oil
- 1 tablespoon water
- 1 garlic clove, coarsely chopped
- salt and pepper to taste

Direction

- Preheat the oven to 400° F.
- Bring quinoa, broth, and cumin to a boil. Cover, lower heat, and cook for 15 minutes, or until the liquid is evaporated. Remove from heat and let sit briefly before dumping into a big bowl.
- To quinoa, add the garbanzos, currants, chopped spinach, feta, olive oil, and salt and pepper to taste. The currants will plump up a little with the heat of the quinoa — this is money.
- Prepare the peppers for stuffing. Lop off the steamy top and run a knife around the inside to remove the ribs and seeds. If the peppers can't stand on their own, carefully level the bottom, being sure not to poke a hole through to the cavernous inside. Stuff peppers with the quinoa mix and then drizzle the tops with olive oil (this well help it get a little golden-brown crust on the top most layer).
- Stick peppers upright in a baking dish (8- by 8-inch works well for this) and pour about 3/4 inch of water into the base around the peppers. Bake for about 1 hour (if things get too brown too fast, cover with foil and continue baking).
- While peppers are baking, throw all sauce ingredients into a food processor or blender and blend until smooth.
- The cooked stuffed peppers are totally attractive and you will be sad to demolish them, but demolish them you must if you are going to make the best use of this crazy addictive creamy pesto-ish magic. I like to grab a big ol' knife and slice the pepper in half longways, from top to bottom, leaving the one pepper in two boat-shaped pieces, each filled with filling. Spoon sauce all over those things, and gobble.

260.   Quinoa Stuffed Mushrooms

Serving: Serves 15-30 people | Prep: | Cook: | Ready in:

Ingredients

- Mushroom Marinade
- 2 pounds crimini mushrooms, stems removed
- 1/2 cup balsamic vinegar
- 1/4 cup extra virgin olive oil
- 3-5 cloves garlic, chopped
- 1 bunch fresh or dried rosemary

- salt to taste
- Quinoa Stuffing
- 1/2 cup quinoa
- 1/2 zuchini, chopped small
- 1/4 red bell pepper, chopped small
- 1/4 green bell pepper, chopped small
- 1/2 white onion, chopped small
- 1 cup feta cheese (optional)
- 1 bunch fresh dill, chopped
- juice from 1/2 lemon
- 1-2 tablespoons extra virgin olive oil OR grape seed oil
- salt to taste

Direction

- Mushroom Marinade
- Wash mushroom caps thoroughly, pat dry, and put into large plastic storage bags which zip closed.
- Add all other ingredients to the bags of mushrooms. Zip bags carefully and shake well to incorporate all ingredients.
- Refrigerate for 30-60 minutes while you work on the filling.
- Quinoa Stuffing
- Cook quinoa according to package instructions. Set aside to cool.
- Preheat oven to 400.
- In an airtight container, combine dill, lemon juice, oil and salt. Shake very well to incorporate. Set aside.
- Lay mushrooms on baking sheet(s) in one layer and cook in the oven for about 20 minutes. They will be ready when they are starting to become soft but still keep their integrity. When they are done, set aside to cool.
- Chop all the veggies very small. Once the quinoa is at room temperature, add all of the veggies in a large mixing bowl. It is very important that the quinoa is not warm, as you do not want the vegetables to cook.
- Add feta cheese and lemon-dill vinaigrette to the quinoa and mix well.
- When the mushrooms are cool, stuff them with the quinoa by using a small spoon. It's can be a little messy, but if you are firm with the spoon, the quinoa will stay put in the cap. Refrigerate until ready to serve.

261. Raddichio Wrapped Quinoa Kale Taco Salad W/ Spicy Avocado Dressing

Serving: Serves 6 | Prep: | Cook: | Ready in:

Ingredients

- Raddichio-wrapped Quinoa Kale Taco Salad
- 1 head of radicchio
- 1 cup red quinoa
- 6 cups kale, de-stemmed and chopped
- 2 cups chickpeas, rinsed and drained
- 1 cup corn, raw or cooked
- 1/4 cup raw pumpkin or sunflower seeds
- 1/2 cup red onion, finely diced
- 1/2 cup cilantro, finely chopped
- Spicy Avocado Dressing
- 1 avocado
- 1 lemon, juiced
- 1/2 cup water
- 1 jalapeno, de-stemmed and seeded
- 2 garlic cloves
- 1/4 cup cilantro
- 1/2 teaspoon salt
- 1/2 teaspoon pepper

Direction

- Cook quinoa according to package directions. When it's done, set it aside to cool.
- Bring a large pot of water to a boil. Blanch the kale leaves in boiling water for 1 min, then remove from heat, drain and let cool.
- To make the dressing, combine all ingredients in a food processor or blender, mixing until smooth. Taste and adjust seasoning as needed.
- In a large bowl, combine quinoa, kale, chickpeas, corn, pumpkin or sunflower seeds, onion and fresh cilantro. Pour dressing on top,

to taste, and toss until everything is well coated.
- Peel a few leaves of radicchio to line your bowl or layer your plate with. Scoop about 1 1/2 cups of the salad into your bowl or onto your plate.

262. Rainbow Quinoa Salad

Serving: Serves 8 | Prep: | Cook: |Ready in:

Ingredients

- Rainbow Quinoa Salad
- 1 cup quinoa
- 2 cups water
- 1 cup cucumber, diced
- 1 cup red, orange and/or yellow pepper, diced
- 1 cup cherry tomatoes, quartered
- 1/4 cup chives, diced
- 1/4 cup mint, chopped
- 1 cup parsley, chopped
- 1/2 cup calamata olives, halved
- 1 cup feta, crumbled
- 1/2 cup pine nuts, toasted
- Dressing
- 1/4 cup extra virgin olive oil
- 1/4-1/3 cups fresh squeezed lemon juice
- salt and pepper to taste

Direction

- Rinse quinoa in fine strainer.
- In a pot bring water and a dash of salt to a boil and add quinoa.
- Reduce heat to low and simmer covered for 20 minutes or until grains are fluffy and water is absorbed.
- Fluff quinoa with a fork; cover and let sit for 10 minutes.
- Transfer the quinoa into a large bowl and combine all ingredients. 6. Whisk dressing ingredients to combine then add to salad and mix gently.

- The inspiration for this recipe was a basic quinoa tabouleh, which I embellished over time to add flavor, color, pizzas and joy!

263. Red & White Meditterranean Quinoa

Serving: Serves 4 | Prep: | Cook: |Ready in:

Ingredients

- 1/2 cup each, red & white quinoa, rinsed with water
- 1 cup each, water and vegetable broth
- 1/4 cup purple onion, minced
- 1/2 cup cucumber, diced
- 1/2 cup red pepper, diced
- 1/4 cup green olives, sliced
- 1/4 cup yellow raisins, plumped in warm water, drained
- 1/8 cup pine nuts, toasted
- 5 ounces feta cheese, crumbled
- 1/4 cup Italian parsley, minced
- 1 tablespoon lemon juice
- 1 tablespoon balsamic vinegar
- 1 tablespoon olives juice
- 4 tablespoons EVOO
- salt & pepper to taste

Direction

- Place rinsed quinoa with water and broth in a lidded pot and bring to a boil. Reduce heat and simmer for 15 minutes. Remove from heat and let sit, covered for 5 minutes.
- In the meantime, chop all vegetables and place everything but the quinoa in a serving bowl.
- Fluff quinoa and add to the serving bowl. Toss well and salt & pepper to taste. Serve warm or at room temperature.

264. Red Quinoa Peach Porridge

Serving: Serves 2 | Prep: | Cook: | Ready in:

Ingredients

- 2 peaches, peeled and sliced
- 1 1/2 cups water
- 1/2 cup milk
- 1/4 cup red quinoa
- 1/4 cup old fashioned rolled oats

Direction

- Place the quinoa, peaches and water in a small saucepan. Cook for 30 minutes.
- Add the oatmeal and milk. Cook until the oats are tender, about 10 minutes, stirring occasionally.

265. Red Quinoa Salad With Citrus And Pistachios

Serving: Serves 8 | Prep: | Cook: | Ready in:

Ingredients

- 1 12-ounce box of red quinoa
- 4 cups low sodium vegetable stock
- 1/4 cup fruity olive oil
- 3 tablespoons Meyer lemon juice - or any fresh lemon juice
- 1 teaspoon ground cumin
- 1 teaspoon orange zest
- 1/4 teaspoon kosher salt
- 1/4 teaspoon ground white pepper
- 3 navel oranges, peeled and cut into sections
- 1 cup shelled pistachio nuts
- 1/4 cup flat-leaved parsley, chopped
- orange and lemon zest curls (optional garnish)

Direction

- Heat the stock in a medium-sized saucepan until it boils. Add the quinoa, cover and reduce heat to low and cook for 20 minutes, until all the stock has been absorbed. Remove from heat and allow the cooked quinoa to "rest", covered, while you prepare the vinaigrette.
- Whisk together in a small bowl the olive oil, lemon juice, cumin, orange zest, salt and pepper.
- Spoon the cooked quinoa into a bowl, add the vinaigrette and toss.
- Add the orange sections, pistachios and parsley. Toss. Add garnish and serve.

266. Red Quinoa Salad With Elephant Garlic And Greens

Serving: Serves 4 | Prep: | Cook: | Ready in:

Ingredients

- 1 cup Red Quinoa, rinsed and drained
- 2 cups Water
- 2 tablespoons Olive Oil
- 1 cup Green Onions, diced
- 1/3 cup Elephant Garlic, sliced
- 1 cup Frozen Peas
- 1 teaspoon Cumin
- 1 teaspoon Coriander
- 1/2 teaspoon Sea Salt
- 1/2 teaspoon Pepper
- 4 cups Kale, chopped small
- 2 cups Broccoli Florets, to garnish

Direction

- In a medium sauce pan, bring water a boil. Add the rinsed quinoa and bring back to a boil. Reduce the heat, cover and simmer for 10 minutes or until liquid is absorbed. Remove from heat and set aside.
- In a large sauté pan over medium heat, add the olive oil, green onions and garlic and sauté for 5 -7 minutes to slightly caramelize onions.

Add peas and stir to combine. Sprinkle in the cumin, coriander, salt and pepper and stir again. Add in the kale, and cook until kale is bright green and wilted. Remove from heat.

- Meanwhile, bring water to a boil in a separate medium sauce pot. Add broccoli and return to a boil. Cook for about 2-3 minutes until bright green
- Add the cooked quinoa to the sauté pan and fold to incorporate and deglaze pan. Plate the quinoa and vegetable sauté and surround the plate with steamed broccoli. Serve and enjoy! Yum!

267. Red Quinoa Tomato Avocado Summer Salad

Serving: Serves 4 as a side | Prep: | Cook: | Ready in:

Ingredients

- .75 cups red quinoa
- 10 ounces water
- 1 large heirloom tomato or 2 medium
- 1 avocado (FIRM)
- 1 handful flat parsley (chopped rough or fine)
- .5 jalapeno diced small, seeds removed (optional)
- 1.5 ounces goat cheese (optional)
- 1 teaspoon salt (more to taste)
- 2 tablespoons extra virgin olive oil
- 2 tablespoons good balsamic (more if desired)

Direction

- Place quinoa in a microwave bowl, add water, and cover with plastic wrap (puncture 1 hole in the plastic wrap) and microwave for 8 minutes. Stir. Microwave for 2 minutes. Let sit for 15 minutes. If quinoa is still a little watery, microwave for 2 more minutes. Let cool to room temp or put in refrigerator.
- Large dice tomatoes. Remove any really seedy/watery parts. Set aside.
- Dice your FIRM avocado. Set aside.
- Chop your parsley. Set Aside.
- Optional: fine dice 1/2 jalapeno. Crumble up goat cheese. Set aside.
- Add salt to quinoa and mix it up. Mix quinoa with tomatoes, avocado, parsley, optional jalapeno (if you use a soft avocado, it will turn to mush). Add olive oil and balsamic. Mix thoroughly. Taste for more salt or balsamic (but NOT to make the salad taste like balsamic. you want to taste the ingredients). Crumble goat cheese on top. Chill for about 30 minutes and serve.

268. Red Quinoa With Honey Glazed Carrots, Thyme Pistou And Pistachios

Serving: Serves 4 | Prep: | Cook: | Ready in:

Ingredients

- 1 pound carrots (young and quite fresh if possible), trimmed, peeled and cut into quarters lengthwise
- 1/4 cup extra virgin olive oil, plus a couple extra tablespoons
- 2 tablespoons orange blossom honey
- Splash of agrodolce (or a similar) vinegar
- 1/2 teaspoon kosher salt, plus a couple pinches later
- 1/4 teaspoon freshly ground white pepper
- zest of 1/2 orange
- 1½ cups vegetable broth
- 3/4 cup red quinoa
- 2 small cloves garlic, peeled
- 4 sprigs fresh thyme, leaves removed from stems
- 1 tablespoon creme fraiche
- Handful shelled, roasted, salted pistachios; gently crushed to small chunks

Direction

- Preheat your oven to 350 F. Place your prepared carrots on a baking sheet large enough to hold them in a single layer. In a measuring cup or small bowl, whisk together the 1/4 cup olive oil, honey and vinegar; pour it evenly over the carrots. Then sprinkle the carrots with the 1/2 teaspoon salt, white pepper and orange zest. Gently toss everything until well combined. Slide the carrots into the oven and bake -stirring occasionally- until they can be pierced with a knife but retain a definite crunch, about 28 minutes.
- Meanwhile, bring the vegetable broth to a boil and then add the quinoa. Cover, turn the heat to medium-low and cook until the quinoa is done to al dente. Remove from heat, keeping the lid on, and let steam until you're ready for it.
- While the quinoa and carrots are cooking, make a quick thyme pistou by crushing into a few tablespoons of olive oil, the garlic, thyme leaves and a small pinch of kosher salt. A mortar and pestle work well for this. Set aside.
- Remove the carrots from the oven and transfer the carrot sticks to a plate; carefully pour the cooking liquid that remains on the pan into a small bowl. You should have just under 1/4 cup. Into that whisk the creme fraiche and a large pinch of kosher salt. Stir this into the quinoa.
- Spoon the quinoa salad into a mound on a serving platter and arrange the glazed carrots around it. Drizzle everything with the thyme pistou and sprinkle crumbled pistachios over top. Serve!

269. Red Quinoa, Red Lentils: A Salad

Serving: Serves 6 - 8 | Prep: | Cook: | Ready in:

Ingredients

- 1 cup red quinoa
- 1/3 cup red lentils
- 4 cups boiling water
- 3 scallions, chopped
- 1/2 - 1 bunches cilantro, chopped
- 1/4 cup walnuts, coarsely chopped
- 1 lemon, juice and pulp
- 2 tablespoons grapeseed oil
- 1/2 tablespoon tamari soy sauce (gluten free)
- 1/4 teaspoon fresh ground pepper
- 2 teaspoons grated fresh ginger
- 3 cloves garlic, pressed

Direction

- Prepare quinoa: Put quinoa in a pot with 2 cups boiling water. Cook covered, at a simmer, about 20 minutes or until water is mostly absorbed.
- Prepare lentils: Pour 2 cups boiling water over lentils, in a heat proof bowl. Let it sit until barely warm, then drain off remaining water.
- In a large bowl, combine remaining ingredients, then gently stir in warm lentils and quinoa. Make sure everything is well distributed, but turn gently so that the quinoa is light and well separated. Check for seasoning.
- Serve at room temperature. You can provide a bed of lettuce, garnish with spears of cucumber, spice it up with Sriracha, and stuff a tomato...

270. Red Quinoa And Garbanzo Bean Salad With Salmon

Serving: Serves 2-3 | Prep: | Cook: | Ready in:

Ingredients

- 2 cups cooked red quinoa
- 1/2 butternut squash
- 3.5 ounces sugar snaps
- 16 ounces garbanzo beans

- 1 small red onion
- 3.5 ounces haricot vert
- 1 bunch arugula
- 2 large salmon filets
- 1 1/2 tablespoons red wine vinegar
- 1 tablespoon olive oil
- 1 teaspoon honey
- 1 garlic clove, smashed
- 1/2 teaspoon cumin
- 1/2 teaspoon paprika

Direction

- Cook the quinoa according to packet instructions. Peel and chop the butternut squash. Thinly slice the onion. Rinse the chickpeas under cold water. Make the dressing by whisking all the ingredients together in a small bowl and season to taste. Boil the haricot verts and sugar snaps in salted water until cooked al dente. Drain and rinse in cold water. Add the cooked and somewhat cooled quinoa to a large bowl. Pour in the dressing and stir to combine. Add the rest of the ingredients to the quinoa. Let it stand to marinate with the dressing until you have cooked the salmon. Season to taste with salt and pepper

271. Red Quinoa And Tofu Miso Bowl.

Serving: Serves 6 | Prep: | Cook: | Ready in:

Ingredients

- 1/2 tablespoon canola oil
- 1 onion
- 1 garlic clove
- 1 carrot
- 1 cup red quinoa
- 1 piece tofu
- 1 packet bok choy
- 1 packet chinese broccoli
- 1 bunch green onions
- 1/4 cup miso paste

Direction

- Sautee chopped onion in the oil at low temperature in a medium sized pan. While it cooks, rinse and drain the quinoa.
- When the onion is transparent add the minced garlic and cook until fragrant. Add the chopped carrots, quinoa, miso paste and cover with 1L [4 cups] of water.
- Leave the pot boiling at medium heat. You might have to add more water while the quinoa is cooking. Since it takes around 15-20 minutes for the quinoa to be cooked; feel free to add the tofu after 10 minutes have passed, so that it absorbs the miso flavor.
- When the quinoa's white germ starts showing, add the chopped veggies reserving the green onions for the end. Taste the broth: if it's too salty, add more water. If it's bland, add more miso or salt. You could even add a dash of soy sauce!
- Cook the veggies for as long as you like [I cook them for 1-2 minutes, I like my veggies to retain their texture] and once you're ready to turn off the heat, add the green onions.
- Enjoy!

272. Red Quinoa Salad With Snow Peas, Spinach, Feta And Poached Egg

Serving: Serves 1 | Prep: | Cook: | Ready in:

Ingredients

- For the salad
- 1/2 cup red quinoa
- 1/2 tablespoon olive oil
- 1 handful of snow peas
- 1 egg
- 1 handful baby spinach leaves
- 50 grams feta cheese
- Sea salt, to taste
- For the sauce

- 1 tablespoon extra virgin olive oil
- 1/4 teaspoon white wine vinegar
- 1/4 teaspoon lemon zest
- 1 small garlic clove, minced
- 1 pinch of cayenne pepper, to taste

Direction

- In a small pot, add the quinoa, a cup of water and a pinch of salt and bring to the boil. Reduce the heat to the minimum and cook, covered, for 15 minutes, or until the quinoa absorbs all water.
- Heat the olive oil in a small frying pan and sauté the snow peas for 2 to 3 minutes on high heat. They should be slightly toasted but still have some texture.
- Put another small saucepan on the stove, add water and a pinch of salt and bring to the boil. Break the egg into a bowl or cup and carefully pour it into the boiling water. Cook for 2 minutes.
- Mix all the ingredients for the sauce.
- On the serving plate, place cooked quinoa, sautéed peas, raw spinach and poached egg. Crumble the feta cheese on top and drizzle with the sauce. Serve right away.

273. Red Quinoa Tabbouleh

Serving: Serves 4 | Prep: | Cook: | Ready in:

Ingredients

- 1 cup red quinoa
- 2 cups water
- 1 bunch parsley
- 1 bunch green onions
- 1/2 bunch cilantro
- 2 sprigs mint
- 1 red onion
- 1 cucumber
- 1/2 cup lemon juice
- Salt
- Olive oil

Direction

- Wash quinoa and strain. Add to a pot of boiling water and let cook for 12-15 mins, until the germ (white curly string) separates from the grain. Turn the heat off and strain. Quinoa should maintain its shape, don't overcook it.
- Chop herbs (the amount of each is up to you); dice the onion (I like to rinse it with cold ice water to remove the strong taste); peel the cucumber and cut it lengthwise, take a spoon and gently scrape the seeds out. Dice it.
- Mix quinoa with the chopped herbs and diced veggies, season with lemon juice and olive oil and sprinkle some sea or kosher salt. Let it rest in the fridge so the flavors blend and meld together. Or if you're in a hurry, eat right away.
- Enjoy!

274. Roast Vegetable Quinoa Salad With Garlic & Parsley Oil

Serving: Serves 4 | Prep: | Cook: | Ready in:

Ingredients

- 1.5 cups Quinoa
- 2 teaspoons Vegetable stock powder
- 2 Eggplant - sliced into 2cm discs
- 8 Dried apricots – chopped
- 1 Garlic clove – finely chopped or crushed
- 2 tablespoons Agave syrup
- Extra Virgin Olive Oil
- Freshly ground black pepper

Direction

- Preheat the oven to 200 C. Toss the sliced red peppers in some olive oil (just enough to coat them), salt and pepper. Place in a baking tray and roast in the oven for about 20 minutes or until they have become limp and soft with a little colour on the edges.

- While they are cooking, bring the quinoa to the boil in just under double its quantity of water with the stock powder. The moment it has come to the boil, reduce the heat to low and place the lid on top. Cook for about 12 minutes until all the water has been absorbed. Turn off the heat, remove the lid and let any remaining water evaporate.
- While the quinoa is cooking, using a pastry brush or even with your fingers, brush or rub both sides of the eggplant discs with olive oil. There is no need to salt them and drain them for this recipe. Heat a pan over a medium flame and once hot add the eggplant discs to the pan. Cook on one side for a few minutes or until golden and then flip over and cook the other side until soft in the centre. Remove from the pan and season with sea salt, pepper and a drizzling of agave syrup.
- Combine the chopped parsley, garlic and enough olive oil to make a lose parsley oil. You don't want it too dry. Then gently stir the eggplant and red peppers through the quinoa, taking care not to mash them so they are unrecognizable. The beauty of this dish, apart from the taste of course, are the gorgeous vegetables vying for attention, so let them shine.
- Drizzle over the garlic and parsley oil and serve immediately with some grilled fish or even just with a light green salad.

275. Roasted Apricot And Quinoa Cakes With Rosemary

Serving: Serves 8 | Prep: | Cook: |Ready in:

Ingredients

- 280 grams Caster Sugar
- 1 Vanilla Bean, split and seeds scraped
- 10 Small apricots, halved
- 1 Orange (juice and thinly peeled rind)
- 125 milliliters Water
- 4 Organic Eggs
- 100 grams Butter, melted
- 80 grams Plain Flour
- 50 grams Almond Meal
- 1 teaspoon Baking Powder
- 1 Rosemary stalk, leaves finely chopped

Direction

- Preheat Oven to 180 degrees (Celsius) and lightly flour 8 muffin holes.
- In a baking tray scatter 110g of the caster sugar. Add the vanilla seeds and mix to combine. Place the apricots cut side down in the sugar and press into the sugar before turning over. Drizzle with the orange juice and scatter the rind over. Roast for 25 minutes until golden and tender.
- Transfer half the apricots to a food processor and purée.
- Meanwhile, place the quinoa in a small saucepan along with the vanilla bean and water. Bring to the boil over a medium-high heat and reduce to a low simmer. Simmer for 12-15 minutes, until the quinoa is tender and all the liquid has evaporated.
- Add the apricot purée and quinoa and mix to combine.
- Pour into the muffin holes and bake for approximately 25 minutes or until golden and springy to the touch.
- Cool in the tin for 10 minutes before turning out onto a rack.
- Serve warm with the remaining apricots and their syrup, orange zest and rosemary.
- To store in an airtight container in a cool dry place for up to three days.

276. Roasted Beet & Quinoa Salad.

Serving: Serves 4 | Prep: | Cook: |Ready in:

Ingredients

- For the salad
- 1 cup quinoa, cooked & cooled (cooking the quinoa in broth gives it a little more flavor)
- 6 beets (small to medium sized)
- 1 leek, chopped
- 1 avocado, chopped
- a handful of spinach, roughly chopped
- a handful of cilantro, roughly chopped
- a small handful of roasted, salted almonds, roughly chopped
- for the dressing
- 2 TBL extra virgin olive oil
- 1 TBL agave syrup
- 2 tsp apple cider vinegar
- a super healthy pinch of sea salt & cracked pepper

Direction

- For the salad
- Preheat the oven to 450 degrees. Rub olive oil over the beets & place them in a tinfoil packet. Put on the bottom rack for about 40 minutes. Remove from the oven & let cool. When they are cool enough to handle, peel them (the skin comes right off) & dice them.
- Meanwhile in a serving bowl add the rest of the ingredients & toss. You can add the beets in, or if you don't want everything to turn pink, you can add the beets right before serving (sprinkled on top of the salad). But either way, feel free to let it sit for a while & let the flavors develop before eating. Serve with agave dressing.
- For the dressing
- Whisk together in a small bowl.

277. Roasted Butternut Squash Salad With Quinoa

Serving: Serves 4 | Prep: | Cook: | Ready in:

Ingredients

- Salad
- 1 Pomegranate (Large)
- 2.2 pounds Butternut Squash
- 1 cup Quinoa, rinsed
- 2 Avocados (Medium)
- 1 teaspoon Salt
- 1 tablespoon Extra Virgin Olive Oil
- 1/2 Lemon
- For the Dressing
- 4 teaspoons Honey
- 4 teaspoons Freshly Squeezed Lemon Juice
- 4 teaspoons Extra Virgin Olive Oil

Direction

- Rinse and cut the squash into bite size cubes. Get rid of the skin by trimming off each cube or peel it beforehand.
- Transfer the squash onto a baking tray lined with baking paper. Season with salt and pepper. Drizzle some olive oil over (about a tablespoon).
- Bake in a preheated oven @ 200C/400F for 30-35 minutes or until soft throughout. 15 minutes into baking, open the oven and toss the squash pieces around (use a fork or spatula).
- Meanwhile: Rinse quinoa and transfer it in a small/medium sauce pan. Cook according to the package information (I use 1 part quinoa, 3 parts water).
- Deseed the pomegranate and dice avocados (first cut in half, remove the stone, scoop out the flesh and dice).
- Prepare the honey dressing (optional) by mixing 4 teaspoons of honey with 4 teaspoons of freshly squeezed lemon juice and 3-4 teaspoons extra virgin olive oil.
- Once the squash is cooked throughout and has nice brown color, take it out from the oven.
- Transfer onto a serving plate/bowl or serve on a baking tray (this way the salad stays warm for longer). Throw in pomegranate seeds, quinoa & diced avocado.
- Squeeze half a lemon over (optional) or drizzle with honey dressing (optional).
- Serve as a starter, main or a side dish.

278. Roasted Fig And Hazelnut Quinoa Salad

Serving: Serves 2 | Prep: | Cook: | Ready in:

Ingredients

- For the salad:
- 1 cup arugula, washed
- 1/2 cup red quinoa, uncooked
- 1 cup water
- 1/2 cup blue cheese, crumbled
- 12 Mission figs, stems removed, and quartered
- 1/3 cup roasted hazelnuts, coarsely chopped
- 1/2 cup fresh flat leaf parsley, coarsely chopped
- For the dressing:
- 1 tablespoon balsamic vinegar
- 1 tablespoon sherry vinegar
- 1/2 tablespoon Maple syrup
- 4 tablespoons olive oil, plus a bit more for the figs
- Pinch salt
- Pinch coarse ground black pepper

Direction

- Preheat oven to 350F
- Line a baking sheet with the figs and coat them with about 1 tsp olive oil, salt and pepper. Place in the oven and roast for no longer than 20 minutes.
- In a small saucepan, add the quinoa and water and cook until the liquid is absorbed and the quinoa has cooked.
- In a small bowl, whisk together the vinegars, syrup and olive oil. Set aside.
- In a large bowl, add the arugula, cooked figs, cooked quinoa, blue cheese, hazelnuts, and parsley. Add the dressing, season with salt and pepper, and toss thoroughly to coat.

279. Roasted Kale, Squash And Quinoa Salad

Serving: Serves 2 | Prep: | Cook: | Ready in:

Ingredients

- For the veg and dressing
- 1 tablespoon coconut oil, melted
- 350 grams butternut squash
- salt, pepper, to taste
- 150 grams kale
- 1 tablespoon coconut oil
- salt, pepper, to taste
- 2 garlic cloves
- ½ teaspoons chili powder
- 1 handful basil
- 1 handful olives
- 1 handful sun-dried tomatoes
- 2 tablespoons lemon juice
- 2 tablespoons EVOO
- water/milk, to thin
- To assemble
- 140 grams quinoa
- 1 handful olives, chopped
- 1 handful sun-dried tomatoes, chopped
- 1 handful dried mulberries/raisins
- 1 handful salt, pepper, to taste
- 2 poached eggs
- hummus, to serve

Direction

- Preheat the oven to 220C. Toss the squash in the coconut oil, salt and pepper, then spread on a baking tray then roast for around 40 minutes, or until tender and beginning to char.
- Meanwhile, Bring a pan of salted water to the boil, then drop the kale in it. Cook for a few minutes, then drain and dry. Toss with the coconut oil, transfer to a baking tray and roast for 10-20 minutes, until beginning to crisp.
- Now for the dressing: using a mortar and pestle, grind each ingredient to a paste one by one, starting with the garlic and working your way down to the EVOO. Thin with milk or water to taste.

- Spread each plate with a thick layer of hummus. Cook your quinoa the way you like it, then toss it with the squash, kale, dressing and remaining ingredients. Pile on top of the hummus, and crown with a creamy poached egg.

280. Roasted Quinoa With Potatoes And Cheese

Serving: Makes 4-6 servings | Prep: | Cook: | Ready in:

Ingredients

- 1/4 cup Extra virgin olive oil
- 1 pound Small waxy potatoes, like new red or Peruvian purple, cut into wedges
- 3-4 Cloves garlic, peeled
- Salt
- 3/4 cup Quinoa
- Freshly ground black pepper
- 1/2 cup Sliced scallion
- 1 Medium red bell pepper, cored, seeded, and chopped
- 1-2 tablespoons Minced fresh chile, or to taste, or hot red pepper flakes
- 6 ounces Cheese, preferably smoked, like cheddar or Gouda, grated
- 1/4 cup Minced parsley for garnish

Direction

- Preheat the oven to 400F. Grease an 8x10 inch roasting pan with a tablespoon or so of the olive oil.
- Put the potato wedges and garlic in a large pot with water to cover, salt it, and turn the heat to high. When the water begins to boil, stir in the quinoa. Adjust the heat so that the water boils assertively and cook, stirring once or twice, for about 5 minutes.
- Drain the quinoa, garlic, and potatoes in a strainer, but leave them fairly wet. Spread them into the prepared pan, sprinkle with salt and pepper, drizzle with the remaining olive oil, and gently toss with a spatula. Spread them out again. Roast, undisturbed, for 15 minutes. Gently toss again, scraping up any browned bits from the bottom of the pan, and return the pan to the oven for another 10 minutes or so, until the potatoes are tender on the inside and golden on the outside.
- Add the scallion, bell pepper, chile and toss everything one last time. Taste and adjust the seasoning, keeping in mind. That the cheeses will add some saltiness. Spread the cheese over all and return to the oven for another 5-8 minutes, until the cheese is melted and bubbling. Sprinkle with parsley and serve.

281. Roasted Sweet Potato, Quinoa And Arugula Salad

Serving: Serves four | Prep: | Cook: | Ready in:

Ingredients

- 1 large sweet potato, peeled and diced (about 2 cups)
- 2 tablespoons melted coconut oil
- 1/2 teaspoon ground cinnamon
- 1 1/2 cups cooked quinoa
- 3 cups baby arugula leaves, roughly chopped
- 3 tablespoons extra virgin olive oil
- 1 tablespoon freshly squeezed lemon juice

Direction

- Preheat the oven to 425°F.
- Toss the sweet potatoes, coconut oil and cinnamon together on a parchment-lined baking sheet with a pinch of salt.
- Roast the sweet potatoes until softened and a little bit browned, about 20 minutes.
- Transfer the sweet potatoes to a large bowl and combine them with the quinoa and arugula. Drizzle over the olive oil and lemon juice and stir the ingredients together to combine. Season to taste with salt and a bit

more lemon juice if you'd like it. Serve warm or at room temperature.

282. Roasted Vegetables & Quinoa Tartlets

Serving: Serves 4 | Prep: | Cook: | Ready in:

Ingredients

- 1/2 large shallot diced
- 1 tablespoon extra-virgin olive oil
- 1 cup quinoa
- 2 cups water
- salt & pepper to taste
- 2 tablespoons basil pesto
- 1 tablespoon parmesan cheese
- 10.5 ounces grape tomatoes
- 1 bunch baby carrots
- 12 asparagus spears
- 4 handfuls mache rosette - one for each tartlet (or arugula)
- 1 tablespoon fresh lemon juice
- 2 tablespoons extra-virgin olive oil
- 1 teaspoon honey
- 1 teaspoon Dijon mustard or to taste

Direction

- Quinoa: Place 1 tablespoon olive oil in a non-stick skillet with diced shallots and sauté for 1-2 minutes. Add quinoa. Stir to combine, continue cooking on medium heat until quinoa becomes fragrant, about 2 minutes. Add water and bring to a simmer. Cook for approximately 15 minutes or until liquid is absorbed. Remove from heat. Add pesto, parmesan, salt and pepper. Stir to combine. Set aside and allow to cool.
- Preparing Tartlets: In the meantime, prepare 4 (4 3/4 -inch) tartlet pans. Spray with non-stick spray. Take 1/2 cup of quinoa mixture and add to each tartlet pan. Using your fingertips, gently press quinoa mixture into bottom and up sides of the tartlet pan. Be sure to create at least a 1/8-inch border of quinoa around the edges for stabilization. Place quinoa filled tartlet pans into a 350F degree oven for 20 minutes or until golden brown.
- Roasted Vegetables: Wash tomatoes, carrots, and asparagus and place on a sheet tray lined with heavy-duty foil. Drizzle lightly with olive oil and salt. Place veggies in a 425F degree oven for 20 minutes.
- Remove tartlets from oven and allow to cool briefly before removing them from their container, onto a plate. Top with greens, veggies, and drizzle with a touch of lemon vinaigrette.
- Lemon Vinaigrette: Combine lemon juice, 2 tablespoons olive oil, honey, Dijon, salt & pepper to taste. Whisk and drizzle over roasted veggies and greens.

283. Roasted Vegetables With Bright & Crunchy Herbed Topping

Serving: Serves 4, as a side | Prep: 0hours4mins | Cook: 1hours0mins | Ready in:

Ingredients

- root vegetables for roasting (such as carrots, parsnips, potatoes, beets, squash), scrubbed
- 1/2 teaspoon salt
- 1/4 teaspoon pepper
- 2 tablespoons extra-virgin olive oil, plus more as needed
- 2 tablespoons finely chopped shallot (about 1/2 shallot)
- 2 tablespoons lemon zest (from about 1 lemon)
- 1/4 teaspoon MSG
- 1/4 cup pepitas
- 2 tablespoons red quinoa (or millet or sesame seeds)
- 1/2 cup finely chopped parsley

Direction

- Preheat the oven to 425° F and prepare the vegetables for roasting. Depending on the vegetable, cut them as you wish: For small carrots, perhaps leave them whole; for squash, cut down into bite-size pieces.
- Toss the vegetables with the salt, pepper, and enough olive oil to coat. Spread out on a baking sheet and roast until fork-tender, about 20 to 60 minutes, depending on the vegetable. (If you're roasting red beets, roast them on their own section of the pan or on a separate pan as they will bleed into their neighbors.)
- Meanwhile, stir together the shallot, lemon zest, and MSG, which will allow the shallot to lightly pickle. While the shallots are sitting, toast the pepitas in a dry pan, then add to the shallots. Toast the quinoa in the same dry pan until they start to pop, then stir into the shallots, as well. Add the parsley, followed by 1/2 teaspoon olive oil, and stir to combine. Season to taste with the MSG, olive oil, pepper, and lemon juice.
- To serve, put the vegetables on a large platter then sprinkle with the crunchy topping. Serve warm or at room temperature.

284. Roasted Veggie Quinoa Medley

Serving: Serves 4-6 | Prep: | Cook: | Ready in:

Ingredients

- 2 cups quinoa
- 2 white or yellow onion, chopped
- 3 cloves garlic, chopped
- 1 green zucchini, chopped
- 1 yellow squash, chopped
- 1 large eggplant, chopped
- 1 red bell pepper, chopped
- 2 large tomatoes, chopped
- 1/4 cup pumpkin seeds or walnuts
- 1 lemon
- 1 1/2 tablespoons dried oregano
- 1-2 teaspoons red chili flakes
- olive oil
- salt + pepper

Direction

- Preheat oven to 375 degrees F.
- Chop veggies in cube like pieces.
- Place in baking sheet and drizzle with olive oil.
- Sprinkle veggies with oregano, red chili flakes, salt + pepper.
- Bake for 25-30 minutes until golden.
- While the veggies roast, cook the 2 cups of quinoa in 4 cups of water.
- It will cook in approximately 20 minutes.
- Stir occasionally and fluff with a fork when done and all the water has evaporated.
- In a separate bowl, combine quinoa with veggies.
- Add your favorite nut. I especially like sunflower seeds or walnuts in this recipe.
- Give the mixture a squeeze of lemon and more salt + pepper to taste.
- Voila you're done! This dish is great on its own as a vegetarian option or can be served as side.

285. Roasted Zucchini And Scallion Quinoa Bowl

Serving: Serves 4 | Prep: | Cook: | Ready in:

Ingredients

- 3 cups cooked quinoa (from 1 cup uncooked)
- 3 medium zucchini
- 1 bunch scallions
- 1 cup fresh feta cheese, crumbled
- 2-3 tablespoons fresh basil, chiffonaded
- 1 lemon
- olive oil
- kosher salt

- freshly ground black pepper

Direction

- Preheat the oven to 425F. Slice the zucchini into batons, about two inches long, and place on a foil-lined baking sheet. Slice the scallions into 2-inch lengths, and add to the sheet. Drizzle liberally with olive oil and season well with salt and pepper. Roast in the oven until caramelized, about 25 minutes total, tossing the vegetables every so often to ensure even cooking.
- To assemble, layer the bottom of your bowl with quinoa, top with the roasted vegetables, sprinkle with feta and basil, and finish with a squeeze of lemon juice and a drizzle of olive oil.

286. Sautéed Kale & Sun Dried Tomatoes With Mixed Red & White Quinoa

Serving: Serves 4 | Prep: | Cook: |Ready in:

Ingredients

- mixed red & white quinoa, water, coarse sea salt
- 1 cup Mixed red & white quinoa
- 1 3/4 cups Water
- 1/2 teaspoon Coarse Sea Salt
- extra virgin olive oil, 1-2 cloves of garlic, water, kale leaves chopped fine (spine discarded), sun dried tomatoes, cooked mixed quinoa, coarse sea salt, ground black pepper, grilled chicken.
- 3 tablespoons Extra virgin olive oil
- 1-2 Cloves of garlic finely chopped (depending on your taste)
- 6-8 large kale leaves (spine discarded) finely chopped
- 1/4 cup water
- 4 sun dried tomatoes finely chopped
- 2 cups cooked mixed red & white quinoa
- 1 grilled chicken breast
- 1 pinch coarse salt
- 1 ground pepper (to taste)

Direction

- Mixed red & white quinoa, water, coarse sea salt
- Rinse quinoa well. Place in quinoa in the salted water. Bring to a boil, reduce to a simmer and cover the pot. Let cook until there is no more liquid, about 13-15 minutes. Remove from heat, put a dry paper towel between the pot and lid, let quinoa sit for 5 minutes, then fluff with fork.
- Place quinoa aside until you prepare second part of recipe.
- extra virgin olive oil, 1-2 cloves of garlic, water, kale leaves chopped fine (spine discarded), sun dried tomatoes, cooked mixed quinoa, coarse sea salt, ground black pepper, grilled chicken.
- Heat olive oil in a large saucepan over medium-high heat. Add the garlic and cook until soft, but not colored. Raise heat to high, add the water and kale and toss to combine. Cover and cook for 5 minutes. Remove cover and continue to cook, stirring until all the liquid has evaporated. Add sun dried tomatoes, and toss for about 3 minutes. Add 2 cups of the already prepared quinoa along with grilled chicken. Toss to heat through. Serve immediately.

287. Seared Scallops Over Pesto And Quinoa Paste

Serving: Serves 4 | Prep: | Cook: |Ready in:

Ingredients

- For Pesto and Quinoa
- ½ cups Rinsed quinoa
- 1 cup Vegetable stock
- 1/2 packet Basil leaves

- 1 tablespoon Extra virgin olive oil
- 1/2 tablespoon Parmesan cheese
- 2 1/2 tablespoons Vegetable stock
- 2 Cloves minced garlic
- Salt and Pepper to taste
- 1/4 cup Walnuts
- Red pepper flakes (optional)
- 1 pound Fresh scallops

Direction

- For Pesto and Quinoa
- Make the Quinoa: Add quinoa and water/vegetable stock to a small pot. Bring mixture to a boil, then reduce to a simmer and allow to cook for 15-20 minutes, or until quinoa is tender and the liquid is absorbed. Remove from heat, fluff with a fork, and then set aside.
- Make the Pesto: While the quinoa is cooking, add basil, olive oil, nutritional yeast/cheese, stock, and garlic to a small blender or food processor and blend until smooth. Taste, season with salt + pepper if needed, then blend again to combine. Add walnuts and pulse until small bits remain (I like a little crunch in my pesto, but you can blend until smooth, too).
- Assemble the Pesto & Quinoa: Pour pesto into the quinoa pot and mix until combined. Season with additional salt + pepper if needed. Top with red pepper flakes, walnuts, and/or cheese if desired.
- Season scallops with salt and pepper. Pan-fry the scallops for one and a half minutes on each side, depending on thickness – they should feel slightly springy when pressed. Make sure you turn them in the same order you put them into the pan to ensure even cooking.
- Remove ready scallops and plate the dish as you like, but scallops over the Pesto and Quinoa paste.

288. Sesame, Quinoa & All The Greens Power Wrap

Serving: Serves 4-6 | Prep: | Cook: |Ready in:

Ingredients

- sesame seeds, ground flax, hemp seeds, kale, nori, sesame oil, tamari, maple syrup, rice syrup, sea salt
- 1/2 cup sesame seeds
- 2 tablespoons ground flax
- 1 tablespoon hemp seeds
- 1 kale leaf (large)
- 1 sheet of nori
- 1 tablespoon tamari
- 2 tablespoons maple syrup
- 1 tablespoon rice syrup
- 1/4 teaspoon sea salt
- quinoa, garlic, fresh ginger, tamari, oil (sesame or olive), fresh ground pepper, whole leaves of napa cabbage or collards plus a variety of leafy greens (I used: green kale, tuscan kale, red kale, rapini but I'm sure the addition of collards, watercress,
- 1 cup quinoa
- 2 cups curly kale (chopped)
- 2 cups tuscan kale (chopped)
- 2 cups red kale (chopped)
- 2 cups rapini (chopped)
- 2 tablespoons garlic (about 3 cloves, crushed)
- 2 teaspoons ginger (about 2 inches, pealed and minced)
- 1 tablespoon tamari
- 2 tablespoons oil (olive or sesame)
- 8-10   large and whole leaves of napa cabbage or collard greens
- 1 carrot
- 1 beet

Direction

- Sesame seeds, ground flax, hemp seeds, kale, nori, sesame oil, tamari, maple syrup, rice syrup, sea salt
- Preheat oven to 350ºF

- Chop kale into very fine pieces and place in a small mixing bowl.
- Cut nori into slivers and add to mixing bowl (I recommend using clean kitchen scissors for cutting).
- Add sesame seeds, flax and hemp and stir a few times so ingredients are combined.
- Mix all wet ingredients (plus sea salt) in a small jar. Shake until combined, then pour over sesame mixture and mix until coated.
- Using a spatula, transfer sesame mixture onto a cookie sheet lined with parchment paper and spread out (don't worry too much about it being even, the clumping is the best part!)
- Cook for 10 minutes, then flip seeds and cook 5 minutes. Remove from the oven and place somewhere cool.
- To make a quick dipping sauce that goes amazing with these wraps combine 1T maple syrup, 1T tamari, 1/4 c. water, 2 T cilantro (finely chopped), 1/4 t. red pepper flakes, 1/4 t. wasabi powder (optional).
- quinoa, garlic, fresh ginger, tamari, oil (sesame or olive), fresh ground pepper, whole leaves of napa cabbage or collards plus a variety of leafy greens (I used: green kale, Tuscan kale, red kale, rapini but I'm sure the addition of collards, watercress,
- It's always important to wash grains and fresh vegetables before cooking! And it actually does make a difference the flavour of the food we make so, wash the quinoa in a strainer then put in a pot with 2 c. water and a pinch of sea salt. Wash all the greens and set aside.
- Bring quinoa to a gentle boil for 5 minutes and then reduce heat to low and cover for 15 minutes, or until grain is cooked and fluffy (but not mushy).
- As the quinoa is cooking proceed with the sautéed mixed greens.
- Chop the greens, and peel and mince garlic and ginger.
- Place ginger and garlic in a large frying pan (cast iron works well) with oil, and sauté on high until fragrant.
- Add the chopped greens and stir. Cover pan with lid, reduce heat to medium/low and let cook for one minute.
- Remove lid and stir. Add tamari and fresh ground pepper to taste.
- Sauté until greens are bright green (about another minute, making sure not to overcook — 'cause there's nothing worse than overcooked greens!) then remove from heat and transfer to a bowl.
- Add the cooked quinoa to the greens mixture and set aside. Make sure to poor out any additional liquid that may be in the pan after sautéing so the quinoa and greens mixture isn't wet and saucy.
- Bring 2 inches of water to a simmer in your pan and place up to 3 leaves at a time in the simmering water. Blanch leaves until bright green (about 1 minute), then remove and place on a plate to cool (or submerge briefly in cold water if you want to be fancy and fast).
- Pat leaves dry with paper towel.
- Flatten one leaf on a cutting board. Add two heaping spoonfuls of quinoa and greens to the centre of the leaf (lengthwise).
- Cut the beet and carrot into thin matchsticks.
- Add matchstick carrots and beets if you'd like to add some colour, crunch and other flavour to the wraps.
- Add a few clusters of the now cooled and crunchy sesame mix.
- Roll the bottom of the leaf up and over the vegetables and quinoa greens you've just places in the centre. Fold over the left side of the leaf and then the right side as you roll, making sure to keep the roll as tight as you can as you complete.
- Place the roll on a plate with the leaf-fold face down to ensure all your hard work doesn't unravel!
- Cut in half and sprinkle with additional sesame crunchies.
- Mix. Dip. Eat. Repeat.

289. Shaved Fennel & Asparagus Quinoa Salad

Serving: Serves 6 | Prep: | Cook: | Ready in:

Ingredients

- 1/2 cup quinoa, uncooked
- 1 bunch asparagus
- 1 bulb fennel, thinly sliced
- 1/2 red onion
- 1.8 ounces Manchego, thinly sliced
- 2 tablespoons freshly squeezed lemon juice
- 1 tablespoon olive oil
- zest of one lemon
- 1 teaspoon salt
- 1/2 teaspoon pepper

Direction

- Combine the quinoa with 1 cup of water in a small saucepan. Bring to a boil, cover, reduce heat and let simmer for 15 minutes. Remove from heat and let sit for 15 minutes, covered. Fluff with a fork.
- Combine asparagus, fennel, onion, and Manchego on a large plate.
- Sprinkle quinoa across the salad.
- Combine ingredients for dressing (lemon juice, zest, olive oil, salt, and pepper) and dress salad. Serve immediately.

290. Shrimp Quinoa Salad With Feta And Tomatoes

Serving: Serves 2-3 | Prep: | Cook: | Ready in:

Ingredients

- 4 cups fresh salad greens
- 1 cup cooked quinoa (or rice)
- kosher salt, fresh ground pepper
- 2 tomatoes, chopped
- 3/4 cup feta, cubed
- 8 ounces cooked shrimp
- 2 tablespoons Each: red and green bell peppers, minced
- 1 tablespoon dried oregano
- 1 lemon (use juice of half and rest sliced for garnish)
- 1/3 cup kalamata olives, chopped (optional)

Direction

- Line the edges of a large platter with salad greens and mound the quinoa at center. Sprinkle the quinoa with a bit of salt, pepper, crushed red pepper, and drizzle with olive oil. Add the tomatoes in an even layer over quinoa and then layer feta and shrimp on top of the tomatoes. Top shrimp with minced peppers. Sprinkle entire salad with dried oregano and squeeze half of the lemon over all. Sprinkle salad with salt and pepper and garnish with olives, if using. Drizzle with other 2 tablespoons olive oil. Garnish with lemon slices and serve cold.

291. Smoky Coconut Broth With Quinoa

Serving: Serves 2 | Prep: | Cook: | Ready in:

Ingredients

- 1 cup quinoa
- 1-1/4 cups water
- 1 red onion chopped
- Large pinch sea salt
- 2 cloves garlic minced
- 1 teaspoon smoked paprika
- 1/4 teaspoon turmeric powder
- 3/4 teaspoon cumin powder
- 1 can coconut milk, full fat or light
- 1 cup vegetable broth
- small pinch cayenne powder
- 2 teaspoons fresh lime juice
- 1 teaspoon pure maple syrup
- parsley or cilantro to finish
- 1 cubed avocado

Direction

- For the Quinoa: Rinse quinoa until there is no foam, add it to a medium pot along with the water, bring to a boil then simmer covered 15-18 minutes. Water should be all absorbed. Remove from heat and keep covered another 10 minutes, the quinoa will fluff even more.
- For the Broth: Sauté onion in oil with large pinch of sea salt until tender about 4 minutes, add the garlic, paprika, cumin and sauté another minute, add the coconut milk and stir followed by pinch of cayenne, add the veggie broth and cook until hot and bubbly, turn down the heat add the lime juice, maple syrup and simmer for 2 minutes. Taste for seasoning add more salt if needed. Steam cauliflower (broccoli is good too) four minutes covered until fork tender.

292. Soupa De Quinoa Con Pollo (Peruvian Quinoa Soup With Chicken)

Serving: Serves 4 | Prep: | Cook: | Ready in:

Ingredients

- 3 large boneless, skinless chicken breasts
- 1 cup quinoa (organic is best)
- 1 onion, sliced thin
- 2 carrots, skinned and sliced into chunks
- 2 russet potatoes, peeled and cubed
- 1 sweet potato, peeled and cubed
- 1 stalk celery, cubed
- 1 can white (navy) beans, drained
- 1 teaspoon cumin
- 1 teaspoon oregano
- 1 tablespoon minced garlic
- 1 dried red pasilla pepper, sliced (or any smoked red pepper)
- 3 bay leaves
- Salt and pepper to taste
- Cilantro or parsley to garnish

Direction

- Wash the chicken breasts in cold water, then place in a pot with 4 to 5 quarts of water, 3 bay leaves, salt, and a dried, smoked red pepper (sliced). Cover, bring to a boil, and cook for half hour or so, until tender. Take out chicken, cut into large cubes, and return to the pot.
- Peel and cube the potatoes, slice the onions, cut the celery and carrots in pieces, and add them all to the broth with the chicken. Add the garlic and spices.
- Bring the soup back to a boil and let it simmer uncovered for 10 minutes, then add the quinoa, cover, and cook over medium heat for another 30 minutes. Serve with chopped cilantro as a garnish (or parsley, if you prefer) and steamed rice on the side.

293. Southwest Quinoa Salad With Sweet & Spicy Honey Lime Dressing

Serving: Serves 6 | Prep: | Cook: | Ready in:

Ingredients

- 3 cups quinoa, cooked
- 14 ounces black beans, drained and rinsed
- 1 cup frozen corn, thawed
- 1 Jalapeno pepper, seeded and diced
- 1 roma tomato, chopped
- 1/2 small red onion, chopped
- 2 green onions, chopped
- 1 avocado, seeded and chopped
- 1/4 cup cilantro, roughly chopped
- 4 ounces crumbled queso fresco or feta cheese
- Dressing
- 1/2 cup freshly squeezed lime juice
- 1/4 cup extra virgin olive oil
- 2 tablespoons honey
- 1 teaspoon cumin
- 1/2 teaspoon black pepper
- 1/2 tablespoon salt

Direction

- Prepare quinoa according to package instructions. Set aside to cool. Remember to rinse quinoa in cold water prior to cooking.
- While quinoa is cooking, drain and rinse beans and thaw corn. Chop and prepare red pepper, jalapeno, tomato, red onion, green onion, avocado, and cilantro.
- Once quinoa is cool, combine with beans, corn, veggies, and cheese in a large mixing bowl. Toss to combine.
- Prepare dressing by combining lime juice, olive oil, honey, cumin, cayenne pepper, black pepper, and salt in a small bowl. Whisk until well combined.
- Pour dressing over quinoa and veggie mixture and stir to combine.
- Spoon into serving bowl. 1 serving equals roughly 1 cup.

294. Southwestern Quinoa

Serving: Serves 2 as entree, 4 as side dish | Prep: | Cook: | Ready in:

Ingredients

- 1 cup red quinoa
- 2 cups low sodium chicken stock
- 2 ears of corn
- 1 cup canned black beans, rinsed and drained
- 1 lime, juiced
- 1/2 cup cilantro, finely chopped
- 1 tablespoon extra virgin olive oil, plus more for drizzle
- 2 teaspoons ground cumin
- 1/2 cup sour cream
- 1 tablespoon liquid from canned chipotle peppers in adobo sauce
- 1/2 cup shredded cheese
- salt and pepper
- cilantro sprig, for garnish

Direction

- Heat your grill or grill pan on high heat for at least 10 minutes.
- Shuck the ears of corn and wrap in aluminum foil. Place on the grill and cook, turning every few minutes, until the corn is cooked through and the kernels begin to brown. Remove from foil and grill an additional 2 minutes to char the corn. Let corn cool, then cut off kernels and reserve.
- Pour the chicken stock into a medium size saucepan and stir in quinoa. Bring to a boil, reduce to a simmer, and cover. Cook for approximately 10-15 minutes, or until all the liquid has been absorbed and the quinoa is fluffy. Season with salt and pepper and drizzle with extra virgin olive oil, stir and cover to keep warm.
- Add the charred corn, black beans, lime juice, cilantro, oil, and cumin into a bowl and mix well. Season with salt and pepper to taste. Let sit out at room temperature while the quinoa cooks.
- Mix the sour cream, 1 tablespoon lime juice, and chipotle liquid in a small bowl until incorporated. Taste and adjust seasoning based on level of heat desired.
- Fluff the quinoa with a fork and spoon into a serving bowl. Sprinkle shredded cheese on top of warm quinoa. Spoon on the corn and black bean mixture and a scoop of the chipotle sour cream. Garnish with cilantro sprig. Serve additional chipotle sour cream on the side.

295. Southwestern Quinoa Salad

Serving: Serves 2 | Prep: | Cook: | Ready in:

Ingredients

- 1 cup quinoa
- 1 tablespoon butter
- 2 cups chicken broth
- ½ cup diced green bell pepper

- ½ cup diced red onion
- 1 cup corn
- 1 (15 ounce) can black beans, drained
- ¼ cup chopped cilantro
- 1 large tomato, diced
- ½ cup fresh lime juice, or to taste
- 2 tablespoons red wine vinegar
- 2 tablespoons olive oil
- 1 tablespoon adobo seasoning
- ½ cup feta cheese
- salt and black pepper to taste

Direction

- Rinse the quinoa thoroughly under cold water, and drain. Melt butter in a large saucepan over medium heat, and cook and stir the quinoa until the water has evaporated and the quinoa is lightly toasted, about 3 minutes. Pour in the chicken broth, bring to a boil, reduce heat to low, and simmer until the quinoa has absorbed all the broth, about 10 minutes. Cool quinoa in refrigerator at least 10 minutes.
- Mix together green pepper, red onion, corn, black beans, cilantro, tomato, lime juice, red wine vinegar, olive oil, adobo seasoning, and feta cheese in a large salad bowl. Lightly stir in the quinoa, and season with salt, pepper, and additional lime juice to taste, if desired. Chill the salad at least 30 minutes before serving; serve cold.
- Nutrition Facts
- Per Serving:
- 195 calories; protein 6.3g 13% DV; carbohydrates 22.1g 7% DV; fat 9.8g 15% DV; cholesterol 17.8mg 6% DV; sodium 196.7mg 8% DV. Full Nutrition-----
- #700434f3-52e9-40a7-b86d-9826b8eea5a3
- To prepare coconut cream: Refrigerate an unopened 14oz cans of coconut milk (look for an organic brand with minimal preservatives) overnight or for at least 6 hours. Remove chilled coconut milk can from fridge. Flip upside down and open both cans, pour separated liquid into a two cup measure. Scoop coconut cream into a mixing bowl and, using either a hand mixer or a whisk (this will require a bit more elbow grease), adding 2-3 teaspoons of unrefined sugar (maple syrup or agave will work as well) and 1/2tsp of vanilla while mixing. Whip until light and fluffy, cover and chill until serving.
- Add lukewarm water to a large mixing bowl and sprinkle yeast over top. Let stand for 5 minutes. Take reserved coconut milk liquid, you should have somewhere around 1.5 cups and add enough water to fill the two cup measure.
- Gently warm coconut milk, either in a microwave or on the stovetop. Pour milk and oil mix into yeast bowl, stirring until combined.
- Add flours, sugar, salt and vanilla and mix thoroughly. Cover mixing bowl with plastic wrap or a well-fitting lid and place in a warm spot to rise for at least an hour. A slightly warm oven with the light left on works perfectly. Dough will be roughly doubled and bubbly when ready.
- Once dough has risen combine ground flax seed and boiled water. Whisk together and allow to sit until thickened and gelatinous, about 5 minutes. Preheat waffle maker.
- Add thickened flax and baking soda to risen waffle batter, stir well to combine. Pour batter by the half cup into your waffle maker. Waffles are done when lightly golden brown and crisp on the outside.
- Remove coconut whip from the fridge and rewhip until fluffy. Serve waffles with a healthy sprinkle of blueberries (or other fresh fruit) and a spoon of coconut whip.

296. Southwestern Quinoa Salad, By Way Of The Pantry

Serving: Serves 4 | Prep: | Cook: | Ready in:

Ingredients

- 1 1/2 cups quinoa

- 1 cup corn (or two ears of corn, with the kernels sliced off)
- 1 teaspoon cumin seeds
- 1 1/2 cups black beans, cooked
- 1 pint cherry tomatoes, halved
- 1 cup feta, crumbled
- 3 green onions, sliced (the whites and the greens)
- 1/2 teaspoon smoked paprika
- 2 poblano chiles
- 2 tablespoons olive oil
- 2 tablespoons lime juice
- 1/4 cup orange juice

Direction

- Bring three cups of salted water to boil in a large saucepan. While it warms, rinse the quinoa well under cold water. When the water boils, add the quinoa and stir. Cover the pot, reduce to a simmer, and cook for about 15 minutes -- the quinoa should still have a slight bite. (You want it well before mushy.) Then drain it well and add to a large salad bowl.
- While the quinoa cooks, heat a cast-iron skillet or wok on high, without adding oil. When the pan is hot, toss in the corn, stirring occasionally, until the kernels are singed. It should take at least five minutes, possibly as much as ten. When they are almost done, add the cumin seeds to the skillet and toast briefly. Then add both to the large salad bowl.
- To the same salad bowl, add the halved cherry tomatoes, the cooked beans (drained and rinsed, if using canned), the feta, the sliced green onions, and the smoked paprika.
- Roast the poblano peppers until blackened. (I use the open flame on the stove.) Let cool, then peel, seed, and chop roughly. Add these to the bowl too.
- Toss the salad together and add salt to taste. Then whisk together the oil, lime juice, and orange juice. Toss the salad with the dressing. Taste. You may want more oil or more lime juice. Adjust as desired. Taste again. Serve.

297. Soy Sauce Quinoa Bowl

Serving: Serves 2 | Prep: | Cook: | Ready in:

Ingredients

- For the quinoa
- 1 teaspoon vegetable oil
- 1/2 teaspoon sesame oil
- 1/2 cup quinoa
- 2 teaspoons soy sauce
- 1 cup chicken stock or vegetable stock
- 1/2 inch knob ginger, peeled
- 4 stalks cilantro, leaves removed and set aside
- For the veggies:
- 1 teaspoon sesame oil
- 1 teaspoon vegetable oil
- 1/4 teaspoon salt
- 7 ounces firm tofu, cut into 1 inch cubes
- 1/2 red bell pepper, sliced
- 8 heads baby bok choy
- 1/2 tablespoon toasted sesame seeds
- Leaves of 4 stalks cilantro, finely chopped

Direction

- For the quinoa
- In a small Dutch oven, heat vegetable oil and sesame oil. Toast quinoa until covered with oil.
- Add soy sauce, chicken broth, ginger, and cilantro stalks. Cook on low heat until liquid is absorbed and quinoa is fluffy, about 30min. Discard ginger and cilantro stalks.
- For the veggies:
- In a bowl, coat the tofu, bell pepper, and bok choy with sesame oil, vegetable oil, and salt. Stir gently to prevent breaking up the tofu.
- Grill everything until bok choy is cooked through and bell peppers are slightly charred.
- Serve on a bed of quinoa and garnished with sesame seeds and chopped cilantro.

298. Spicy BLAQ (Bean, Leek, Avocado And Quinoa) Salad Tacos

Serving: Serves 4 | Prep: | Cook: | Ready in:

Ingredients

- 1/2 cup Bob's Red Mill quinoa
- 1 cup fat free, low-sodium chicken stock
- 1 teaspoon canned Chipotle chiles in adobo sauce, seeded and minced plus 2 teaspoons adobo sauce from can
- 2 tablespoons extra virgin olive oil, divided
- 2 cloves garlic, minced
- 1 leek, washed, exterior thick leaves discarded and finely chopped
- 15 ounces can organic black beans, drained and rinsed
- 2 large sage leaves, minced
- 2 avocados, halved, pits removed, flesh spooned out and chopped, divided
- 1 tablespoon mayonnaise
- 1 tablespoon lime flavored or plain Greek yogurt
- 1 tablespoon minced cilantro
- juice of 2 limes
- zest of 1 lime
- 2 Roma tomatoes, quartered and chopped
- 8 whole wheat tortillas
- 16 ounces bag shredded cheddar cheese

Direction

- Bring quinoa, stock (in place of water), chiles and sauce to a boil in a saucepan. Reduce heat to low, cover and simmer until quinoa is tender, and stock has been absorbed; about 10 to 20 minutes (depending upon package instructions). Stir and set aside uncovered to cool.
- While quinoa cooks, saute garlic and chopped leek with 1 tablespoon oil in a skillet on medium-high heat for 3 minutes. Add beans. Cook for 3 minutes; stirring occasionally. Mix in sage and remove skillet from heat and set aside to cool.
- Place half avocado chunks in a small bowl and mash. Add mayonnaise, yogurt, cilantro, lime juice, zest and remaining oil; mix to combine. In a large bowl, add black bean mixture, quinoa, avocado mixture and tomato. Toss to combine. Fold in remaining avocado. Spoon into warm tortillas and sprinkle with shredded cheese. Serve.

299. Spicy Black Bean And Quinoa Salad

Serving: Serves 4-6 | Prep: | Cook: | Ready in:

Ingredients

- 1/2 cup red quinoa (or sprouted quinoa)
- 1 cup water
- Juice and zest of one lime, about 1.5-2 oz. juice, and 1-2 teaspoons zest
- Kosher or sea salt
- 1/2 teaspoon ground cumin
- 1/2 teaspoon chili powder
- 1/2 teaspoon chipotle powder
- 1/4 cup extra virgin olive oil
- 3 scallions, thinly sliced (white and green parts)
- 1 cup roasted red/yellow bell peppers, chopped
- 1.5 to 2 cups cups cooked black beans
- 1/4 cup picked fresh cilantro, roughly chopped

Direction

- Bring the quinoa and water to a boil in a small saucepan. Cover, reduce the heat to low, and simmer for about 15 minutes. Fluff with a fork and set aside.
- In a large serving bowl, whisk the lime juice with the zest, a pinch or two of salt, the chili powder, chipotle powder, and the cumin. Add the olive oil and whisk until the dressing comes together.

- Add the quinoa to the dressing and toss. Add the scallions, red peppers, black beans, and cilantro and toss well to combine. Garnish with additional cilantro and lime zest, if desired.

300. Spicy Delicata Squash Boats With Fruity Quinoa Pilaf

Serving: Serves 8 side dishes | Prep: | Cook: |Ready in:

Ingredients

- Squash and Roasting Glaze
- 2 tablespoons minced chipotles in adobo sauce
- 2 teaspoons hoisin sauce
- 2 tablespoons maple syrup
- 1 tablespoon apple cider
- 1/8 teaspoon kosher salt
- 4 Delicata squash, halved lengthwise with seeds and pulp removed
- 2 teaspoons chocolate nibs
- 2 teaspoons coconut palm sugar
- Fruity Quinoa Pilaf
- 1 cup quinoa
- 2 cups water or vegetable broth
- 1 cup apple cider
- 1 tablespoon Calvados Apple Brandy
- 1 apple
- 1 tablespoon minced dried apricots
- 2 tablespoon dried cranberries
- 1 tablespoon chocolate nibs

Direction

- Preheat the oven to 425 degrees F. Line a baking sheet with parchment paper.
- In a small bowl, whisk together all of the Roasting Sauce ingredients except the squash. Lay each Delicata half, cut side facing up, on the lined baking sheet and brush the Roasting Sauce on all cut surfaces. Coat the squash well, and roast for 15 minutes. Remove the squash and baste a second coat of the Roasting Sauce on the surfaces. Roast for another 15 minutes, or until tender.
- Remove from the oven and sprinkle the bowl of each Delicata half with Mocha Sprinkles while still hot.
- Rinse the quinoa very well, rubbing it between your hands as you rinse it. In a small pot over medium heat, bring the water (or vegetable broth, if preferred) to a simmer. Add the quinoa and simmer for 20 minutes or until tender.
- While the quinoa is cooking, bring the apple cider and Calvados to a simmer in a second small pot. Peel the apple, core and seed it, and chop it into very small chunks. Add to the simmering cider along with the remaining Fruity Pilaf ingredients. Simmer until the cider is reduced by half, about 15 minutes. Strain, retaining the reduced apple cider.
- Combine 2 cups cooked quinoa with the fruit and toss. Add a couple of tablespoons of the reduced apple cider, to taste. Spoon it over the Delicata boats.
- Serve warm.

301. Spicy Quinoa Pilaf With Warm Beet Greens

Serving: Makes 1 pot meal | Prep: | Cook: |Ready in:

Ingredients

- 3 cups quinoa washed
- 2 large onions julienned
- 2 carrots sliced
- 1 large parsnip sliced
- 4 celery sticks chopped
- 1 red bell pepper chopped
- 1 bunch fresh basil
- dry spices: anise seed, thyme, paprika, curry, cumin powder, cayenne pepper,
- salt adjusted to taste
- 1/2 cup oil
- 1/2 cup water

- 1 can coconut milk

Direction

- 1. Turn the heat on medium. In a large cast iron pot pour the oil and the water, then add the carrots, onions, and parsnips. Sauté for 5-6 minutes.
- 2. Add the peppers and celery along with all the dry spices and salt. Sauté for 5 minutes.
- 3. Add the coconut milk and let everything simmer until the vegetables are tender, about 15 minutes (the quinoa boils fast that is why you want your vegetables tender). If you feel the vegetables mixture is too thick add some more water.
- 4. Add the quinoa. Stir. Turn the heat down at low. Let it simmer for about 10- 15 minutes.
- 5. Add the garlic and fresh basil, check if it needs more salt and turn the heat off. Let it sit for half an hour before serving.
- While the quinoa is simmering prepare the beet greens: 1. Give them a rough chop. 2. In a separate pot (preferably a wok) pour some oil (3-4 tablespoons), some soy sauce (1-2 spoons) and add the greens. 3. Sauté for 3-4 minutes

302. Spicy Quinoa Tabouli

Serving: Serves 4 | Prep: | Cook: | Ready in:

Ingredients

- 1 cup quinoa
- 4 finely diced roma tomatoes
- 1 diced English cucumber
- 1/2 bunch cilantro leaves, chopped
- 1/2 small red onion, finely minced
- 2 jalapeno peppers, seeded and minced
- 1 tablespoon lime juice
- 2 tablespoons sherry vinegar
- 1 avocado, chopped
- 1/4 cup olive oil, good quality
- 1 teaspoon kosher salt

Direction

- Cover the quinoa with cold water and let it sit for 5-10 minutes. Put it in a fine mesh colander and rinse until the water runs clear. Transfer to a medium saucepan. Cover with 3 cups water and salt and bring to a boil. Reduce heat to low, and simmer 15 minutes. Drain excess water, cover the pot with a dish towel, replace the lid, and let it sit for 10 minutes.
- Combine the cucumber, tomato, cilantro, onion, olive oil, lime juice, and vinegar.
- Stir the quinoa into the veggies. Serve with chopped avocado on top.

303. Spicy Tempeh Quinoa Tacos

Serving: Serves 6 | Prep: | Cook: | Ready in:

Ingredients

- Tempeh Quinoa Filling
- 8 ounces tempeh, crumbled
- 1 1/2 cups vegetable broth
- 3 cloves of garlic, minced or pressed
- 1/2 small red onion, chopped
- 1 cup cooked quinoa
- 2 tablespoons chili powder
- 1 teaspoon cumin powder
- 1 teaspoon smoked paprika
- 1/4 teaspoon cayenne pepper, add more or less depending on desired amount of heat
- 1 pint cherry tomatoes
- 1 red pepper, seeded and chopped
- 1/2 teaspoon salt
- 1/2 teaspoon your favorite hot sauce, such as Sriracha or Cholula
- 1/4 cup cilantro, washed and chopped
- Tofu Cheese and Salsa
- 7 ounces firm tofu, crumbled.
- 10 ounces jar of pimento stuffed green olives, drained and rinsed well
- 3 tablespoons fresh lemon juice

- 2 tomatillos, husked, washed, and chopped
- 2 small tomatoes, washed and chopped
- 1/2 small red onion, chopped
- 2 scallions, washed and chopped
- 1 lime, juiced

Direction

- Place crumbled tempeh, garlic, and onion in a large sauté pan. Add 1 cup of broth to cover and simmer until almost all the liquid is gone.
- Add quinoa, chili powder, cumin, paprika, and cayenne. Stir to coat.
- Place cherry tomatoes and red pepper in a food processor and pulse until finely chopped.
- Add additional ½ cup of broth and tomato mixture to tempeh mixture in pan and sauté until liquid has evaporated. You want the mixture pretty dry or the tortillas will get soggy very quickly.
- Season with salt to taste.
- Place tofu, olives and lemon juice in food processor and pulse until chopped. Set aside.
- Place tomatillos, tomatoes, onion, scallions and lime juice in a bowl. Stir to coat and set aside.
- Warm soft corn tortillas in a hot cast iron skillet or griddle. If using taco shells gently warm in oven. Fill just before serving. Start with tempeh mixture in tortilla then top with cheese and salsa. Finish with hot sauce, cilantro and a squeeze of lime.
- If using soft tortillas, skewer tacos with a piece of lime on either side to keep together [or you can just wrap it up – depends on the pliability of your tortilla].
- Note: Tacos tonight, taco salad tomorrow – layer tempeh, cheese, and salsa over a bed of shredded lettuce or massaged kale.
- Nutrition Facts: Calories per serving, 250; Carbohydrates, 33g; Fat, 7g; Protein, 15g; Fiber, 8g; Vit A, 21%; Vit C, 30%; Calcium, 13%; Iron, 19%.

304. Spicy Quinoa Pilaf With Beet Greens

Serving: Makes 1 pot | Prep: | Cook: | Ready in:

Ingredients

- 3 cups quinoua washed
- 2 large onions julienned
- 2 large carrots sliced
- 1 large parsnip sliced
- 4 celery sticks chopped
- 1 red bell pepper julienned
- 7 cloves garlic crushed
- 13. 66 ounces coconut milk (1 can)
- 1 bunch fresh basil chopped
- dry spices: paprika, anise seed, curry powder, cumin powder, thyme, cayenne pepper, salt
- 3/4 cup grapeseed oil
- some water
- 1 bunch beet greens chopped

Direction

- 1. Prepare a large iron cast pot. Turn the heat on medium and pour the oil and 1/2 cup water. Then add the carrots, onions, and parsnips. Sauté for 5-6 minutes.
- 2. Add the peppers and celery along with all the dry spices and salt. Sauté for 5 minutes.
- 3. Add the coconut milk and let everything simmer until the vegetables are tender, about 15 minutes (the quinoa boils fast that is why you want your vegetables tender). If you feel the vegetables mixture is too thick add some more water.
- 4. Add the quinoa. Stir. Turn the heat down at low. Let it simmer for about 10- 15 minutes.
- 5. Add the garlic and fresh basil, check if it needs more salt and turn the heat off. Let it sit for half an hour before serving.
- 6. In a different pot (wok preferably) sauté the greens with a bit of oil, salt, soy sauce for about 3 minutes.

305. Spinach Potato Quinoa Croquettes With A Spinach Sorrel Pesto

Serving: Serves 8 croquettes (or 24 small croquette appetizers) | Prep: | Cook: | Ready in:

Ingredients

- Spinach Croquettes
- 1 large russet potato
- 2 cups chicken broth
- 1/2 cup quinoa, well rinsed (I use a mixture of red and white quinoa)
- 1 1/2 cups yellow onion, finely diced (about 1/2 of a large onion)
- 5 cloves of garlic, 2 that are smashed and 3 that are minced
- 1 large bunch of spinach or 2 small bunches (leaves only)
- 1 tablespoon lemon juice
- lemon zest from 1 lemon
- 1/2 cup parmesan cheese, grated
- 4 teaspoons Dijon mustard
- 1/2 teaspoon yellow mustard seeds
- 3/4 teaspoon salt
- 1/4 teaspoon pepper
- 1/4 teaspoon cayenne pepper
- 1 large egg
- 1 cup panko bread crumbs (or toasted bread crumbs)
- Spinach - Sorrel Pesto
- 2 little bunches of sorrel leaves, coarsely chopped (about 15 leaves per bunch)
- 20 small baby spinach leaves, coarsely chopped
- 1 clove of garlic, coarsely chopped
- 1 tablespoon toasted pine nuts
- 1/4 cup parmesan cheese, grated
- 1/4 teaspoon salt, to taste
- 1 teaspoon lemon juice
- 1 cup olive oil

Direction

- Spinach Croquettes
- Peel the potato and boil in a mixture of water and chicken broth until tender (I used 2 cups of my Chicken Broth with a Mexican Twist but any will work fine, and then filled the pot with enough water to cover the potato.) Let cool and then grate using a coarse grater.
- Cook the quinoa by bringing 3/4 cup of water with the 2 smashed garlic cloves, along with a healthy pinch of salt and pepper to a rapid boil. Add the quinoa, cover the pot and simmer for about 12 minutes or until the liquid is completely absorbed. Turn off the heat and let the quinoa sit covered for another 10 minutes.
- Wash the spinach and spin in a salad spinner to remove as much water as possible from the leaves. In a large Sautee pan, Sautee the onion until soft and translucent. Add the garlic and Sautee another minute. Add the spinach and lemon juice and Sautee until the spinach is tender and completely wilted, but still defined leaves. Remove from the pan and coarsely chop the spinach. Place in a large mixing bowl.
- Add the grated potato, 1 cup of cooked quinoa and all the rest of the ingredients except the bread crumbs to the spinach mixture and mix well with your hands or a large spatula.
- Form little croquettes that are about 3" across, or about 3 ounces in weight. I weigh everything so that the cooking time won't vary between the different croquettes. Cover in bread crumbs.
- Sauté in olive oil over medium heat until lightly browned on each side. Try to flip the croquettes only once to avoid breaking any.
- Spinach - Sorrel Pesto
- Put all the ingredients except the olive oil in a food processor and pulse 10-12 times. Then process fine while slowly pouring in the olive oil.

306. Sprouted Quinoa Salad With Peanut Ginger Dressing

Serving: Serves 4 | Prep: | Cook: | Ready in:

Ingredients

- Sprouted quinoa(rinse in cold water then put in a bowl overnight covered with water, then strain in a sieve and put in a plate one layer thick/ rinse in sieve 2 or 3 times a day and it will sprout a tail
- one cup quinoa sprouted the red on is best
- one yellow pepper diced
- 1 cup green onion thinly sliced diagonal
- 1 cup shredded carrot
- 3/4 cup cilantro
- 3 cups shredded cabbage
- 1 tablespoon toasted sesame seeds
- peanut ginger dressing(if peanut allergy replace with cashew butter)
- 1/2 cup peanut butter(preferably one that is fresh ground in grocery store)
- 1 teaspoon sesame oil
- 2 tablespoons peanut oil
- 3 tablespoons tamari
- 1 lime juiced
- 2 teaspoons red chili paste
- 3 cloves of garlic minced
- 2 teaspoons of grated ginger

Direction

- You can boil quinoa for 2 min in a little water and allow to cool or you can mix it in raw with the other salad ingredients
- Dressing, put all in food processor and mix till smooth after mixing dressing and salad, sprinkle on 1 tbsp. of toasted sesame seeds

307. Steak Quinoa Salad With Avocado Lime Ranch Dressing

Serving: Serves 4 | Prep: | Cook: | Ready in:

Ingredients

- 2 garlic cloves, minced
- 1/4 cup olive oil
- 3 tablespoons Worcestershire sauce
- 2 tablespoons fresh lemon juice
- 2 tablespoons light brown sugar
- 1/2 teaspoon ground cumin
- 1/4 teaspoon cayenne pepper
- 1 pound flank steak
- 1 avocado, pitted and peeled
- 1/3 cup prepare ranch dressing (homemade, or a good store brand)
- 1-1/2 tablespoons fresh lime juice
- 8 ounces salad greens (whatever you want - I used 1/2 spring mix, 1/2 spinach)
- 1 cup cooked quinoa
- 3/4 cup grape tomatoes, halved
- 1/2 cup crumbled feta cheese
- 1/4 cup thinly sliced red onion
- 2 tablespoons chopped fresh basil

Direction

- In a small bowl, whisk together garlic, oil, Worcestershire, lemon juice, brown sugar, cumin and cayenne. Place steak in large Ziploc bag; pour marinade over steak. Seal bag and refrigerate at least 1 hour or up to 8 hours.
- Meanwhile, in a small bowl, mash together avocado, ranch dressing and lime juice until everything is nicely combined - you can leave the avocado chunky, or keep mashing until the mixture is smooth.
- Preheat an outdoor grill for direct grilling over medium-high heat. Remove steak from marinade; discard marinade. Grill steak 8 to 10 minutes or until internal temperature reaches 135° for medium-rare, flipping once halfway through cooking. Transfer to plate; let rest at least 5 minutes.
- To serve, divide salad greens, quinoa, tomatoes, feta, onion and basil between 4 plates. Thinly slice steak across the grain, and divide between plates. Serve with dressing.

308. Strawberry And Quinoa Salad With Tarragon, Soft Goat's Cheese And Poached Egg

Serving: Serves 4 | Prep: 0hours0mins | Cook: 0hours0mins | Ready in:

Ingredients

- 150 grams (5½ oz) quinoa
- 500 grams (1 lb 2 oz) strawberries
- 3 to 4 mint sprigs
- 3 to 4 tarragon sprigs
- 2 tablespoons olive oil
- 60 milliliters (2 fl oz/ 1/4 cup) white-wine vinegar
- Pinch of finely grated orange zest
- 1 orange, juice of
- 4 small eggs
- 1 handful rocket (arugula), red sorrel, or mizuna
- 1 pinch salt and freshly ground black pepper, to taste
- 100 grams (3½ oz) soft goat's cheese

Direction

- Rinse the quinoa under cold water, to wash away any bitterness. Combine 300 ml (10 fl oz.) water and ½ teaspoon salt in a saucepan, then cover and bring to the boil. Rain in the quinoa and simmer gently over very low heat for 5 minutes. Remove from the heat and leave, covered, for about 15 minutes to swell up.
- Meanwhile, slice the strawberries or chop into wedges. Pick the mint and tarragon leaves and roughly chop. In a bowl, combine the quinoa, olive oil, 1 tablespoon of the white-wine vinegar, and the orange zest and juice.
- Fill a saucepan with 2 liters (68 fl oz./8 cups) water and add the remaining vinegar. Bring to the boil. Break the eggs, one at a time, into a cup, taking care not to break the yolk. Carefully slide the eggs, one at a time, into the bubbling water and spoon the white over the yolk. Reduce the heat – the water should be just under boiling. Cook the eggs for 3–4 minutes then, using a skimmer or slotted spoon, remove the poached eggs from the water and drain on paper towel.
- Toss the herbs, salad leaves and strawberries with the quinoa and transfer to a serving plate. Season with salt and pepper, crumble over the goat's cheese and top with the poached eggs.

309. Strawberry Basil Skillet Quinoa Cornbread

Serving: Serves 8-10 | Prep: | Cook: | Ready in:

Ingredients

- 1 tablespoon butter, for skillet
- 1 cup all-purpose flour
- 3/4 cup coarse yellow cornmeal
- 1 teaspoon baking powder
- 1/2 teaspoon baking soda
- 1/4 cup fresh basil, finely chopped
- 2 large eggs
- 1.5 cups quinoa, cooked
- 3 tablespoons butter, melted and cooled slightly
- 1/4 cup light brown sugar (honey works here, too)
- 1 teaspoon kosher salt
- 2 cups milk
- 1.5 tablespoons lemon juice
- 1 teaspoon vanilla
- 2 cups strawberries, hulled and sliced
- 1 cup heavy whipping cream
- 1 teaspoon vanilla

Direction

- Preheat the oven to 350 F and place a rack in the top third. Butter a 10-inch oven-proof skillet or equivalent baking dish. Once the

oven has preheated, place buttered skillet on oven rack and heat for about 10 minutes.
- Meanwhile, in a large bowl, stir together the flour, cornmeal, baking powder, baking soda, and fresh basil.
- In a separate bowl, beat the eggs, quinoa, and melted butter until well-mixed. Add the sugar, salt, milk, lemon juice, and vanilla and stir again. Fold the dry ingredients into the wet ingredients until the batter comes together. It will be very thin. No need to fear.
- Take skillet from oven and layer sliced strawberries in the bottom. You'll want to work quickly so the skillet will stay hot when it's time for the batter to be poured in.
- Next, pour the batter over the strawberries.
- In a spouted measuring cup, mix cream and vanilla. Pour the heavy cream into the center of the batter. Do not stir. Carefully (you don't want to spill because the batter's really loose) place skillet in the oven and check after 45 minutes.
- The skillet bread is done when the top becomes lightly browned and the center just set. If it's not set after 45 minutes, cook for 5-10 minutes more, checking occasionally.

310. Stuffed Tomatoes With Quinoa

Serving: Serves 4 | Prep: | Cook: | Ready in:

Ingredients

- 4 large field tomatoes
- 1/2 cup Quinoa
- 1/2 cup Parmesan cheese grated

Direction

- Spoon out 4 large field tomatoes so that all pulp is removed and shell is wide open
- Turn upside down on paper towels for a few minutes to drain any excess moisture
- Cook quinoa according to directions.
- When quinoa is done sprinkle in 1/4 cup grated parmesan cheese and mix throughout
- Add a sprinkle of parmesan to the inside bottom of the tomatoes and fill with quinoa pressing down to make a dense filling.
- Sprinkle tops with remaining parmesan cheese and pop in the oven at 350 degrees for about 20 minutes. Tomatoes should be slightly soft to touch.

311. Summer Chili With Quinoa And Black Chick Peas

Serving: Serves 8 | Prep: | Cook: | Ready in:

Ingredients

- 1 pound Organic Ground Bison
- 2 cups Black Chick Peas
- 1 cup Red Quinoa
- 1 Medium Size Yellow Onion
- 3 pounds Organic Tomatoes or 2 Large Cans of Organic Stewed Whole Tomatoes
- 1 Sweet Red Pepper
- 1/2 cup Raisins
- 1/4 teaspoon Cinnamon
- 1/4 teaspoon Mixed Chile and Peppercorns
- 1/4 teaspoon Freshly Ground Black Pepper
- 1/2 teaspoon Oregano
- 1 teaspoon Smoked Paprika
- 3 tablespoons Agave Syrup
- 1-2 tablespoons Ground Cumin
- 1 tablespoon Olive Oil

Direction

- In a large bowl soak the chick peas in water for at least 3 hours and then discard the water.
- Dice the onion and red pepper.
- In a large sauce pot, sauté the onion and pepper in the olive oil until softened.
- Add the bison to the onions and sauté until browned.
- If you are using fresh tomatoes, dice them and add them to the already cooking vegetables

and meat. Let the mixture cook down for at least 20 minutes before proceeding to the next step. If you are using canned tomatoes, add them to the meat and vegetables. Fill the can with water and add it to the tomatoes, meat and vegetables. There should be enough water to cook the quinoa and chick peas.

- Once the tomatoes have reduced add the quinoa and continue to cook on a low to medium flame for at least 20 minutes.
- After the quinoa has fully cooked, add the black chick peas. These are smaller than regular chick peas and don't cook down as much. This will result in a thinner chili but the flavor and texture they add make a beautiful contrast to traditional chile.
- Once the chick peas have been added to the chile, you may now add all of the remaining ingredients.
- Turn the flame down to low and allow the chile to simmer for 30 minutes to an hour.
- Season to taste. Dish out and enjoy this sweeter variation on a winter classic.
- P.S. This dish freezes and thaws beautifully, so don't worry if you have leftovers!

312. Summer Fresh Quinoa And Kale Salad

Serving: Serves 3 | Prep: | Cook: | Ready in:

Ingredients

- 1/2 cup Quinoa
- 1 bunch Kale
- 2 teaspoons Argan Oil
- 15-20 pieces Cherry Tomatoes
- 1/3 piece Red Onion
- 1 piece Corn on the Cob
- 1 pinch Salt

Direction

- Start by boiling the Quinoa. Bring water to a boil in a saucepan. Stir quinoa into the boiling water, reduce heat to medium-low, place cover on the saucepan, and cook until water absorbs into the quinoa, about 12 minutes. Remove the saucepan from heat and let rest covered for 5 minutes. Remove the cover and let the quinoa to cool completely.
- Then, either oven roast the corn still on the cob, or grill it on charcoal to add a smoky flavor. You could also just boil it before slicing the kernels off the cob.
- Finally chop the kale, dice the red onion, and cut the cherry tomatoes in half.
- Toss the whole with some salt, and of course drizzle it with Argan Oil. Simple and deliciously health!

313. Summer Herb Salad With Fresh Crab, Quinoa Tabouleh, And Harissa Vinaigrette

Serving: Serves 4-6 | Prep: | Cook: | Ready in:

Ingredients

- 2 tablespoons harissa
- 3 tablespoons champagne vinegar
- 1/4 cup canola oil
- 1/4 cup extra-virgin olive oil
- kosher salt and freshly ground black pepper to taste
- 1 pound backfin crabmeat, picked over
- 2 tablespoons shallot, minced
- 1 tablespoon fresh lemon juice
- 1 tablespoon extra-virgin olive oil
- 3 heads little gem or bibb lettuce, rinsed
- 3/4 cup quinoa tabouleh
- 1/2 cup each of fresh mint and basil leaves
- 1/2 cup each of chopped dill and snipped chives

Direction

- For vinaigrette: Whisk harissa and sherry vinegar together. Gradually add canola oil a

few drops at a time, whisking constantly. Add olive oil a drizzle at a time, continuing to whisk and emulsify. Season with salt and pepper.
- To assemble, combine crabmeat with shallot, lemon juice, and olive oil. Season with salt and pepper and carefully toss to combine.
- In a large serving bowl, toss lettuce with fresh herbs and enough vinaigrette to delicately coat the greens (about ½ cup).
- Carefully fold in crab mixture and serve with fresh lemon wedges and extra vinaigrette on the side.
- Enjoy!

314. Summer Quinoa Salad, Mexican Style

Serving: Serves 4 as a side dish | Prep: | Cook: | Ready in:

Ingredients

- 1/2 tablespoon olive oil
- 3 ears fresh corn, kernels cut from cob
- 1/2 tablespoon chipotle powder (or another smoky chili powder)
- 1 ripe avocado
- 1/2 cup fresh cilantro, divided
- 1/4 cup sliced green onions, divided
- 1 serrano pepper, seeded and minced
- juice of 2 limes, divided
- 2 cups cooked quinoa (from 1/2 cup uncooked)
- 1 cup cherry tomatoes, halved
- salt and pepper, to taste

Direction

- Heat the olive oil in a large skillet until shimmering. Add the corn kernels and cook on medium-high heat for 3 minutes, letting them brown (do not touch or stir them). After one side is charred, toss the kernels and let another side cook, undisturbed, for 2-3 minutes, repeating until the kernels are evenly charred on all sides. Toss with the chipotle or chili powder, then set aside to cool.
- In a large bowl, make a basic guacamole: mash the avocado, half of the cilantro, half of the green onions, serrano pepper and juice of one lime.
- Stir in the cooled corn, quinoa and cherry tomatoes into the guacamole. Toss with the remaining cilantro, green onions and lime juice, then add salt and pepper, to taste. Serve at room temperature or chilled.

315. Sunshine Quinoa Salad

Serving: Serves 4 | Prep: | Cook: | Ready in:

Ingredients

- For the Quinoa:
- 2 cups quinoa
- 4 cups water
- 1/4 teaspoon fine sea salt
- 1 teaspoon turmeric
- For the Salad:
- 1 large lemon, juiced
- 1/4 cup extra virgin olive oil
- 3 tablespoons apple cider vinegar
- 1 tablespoon honey
- 3/4 teaspoon fine sea salt
- fresh ground pepper
- 1/2 cup pine nuts
- 1/2 cup craisins
- 1/3 cup chopped mint
- 1/3 cup chopped flat leaf parsley
- 2 cups finely shredded green cabbage
- 10 radishes, thinly sliced

Direction

- For the Quinoa:
- To prepare the quinoa: Place quinoa, water, turmeric, and sea salt in a 2-quart saucepan and cover with lid. Bring to a boil, stir, and immediately turn off heat, leaving the pan on the hot burner. Keep covered and allow to sit

for at least 30 minutes. Uncover and fluff with fork.
- For the Salad:
- To prepare the citrus vinaigrette: Meanwhile, using a citrus juicer juice the lemon and pour into a large serving bowl. Add extra virgin olive oil, apple cider vinegar, honey, and sea salt. Stir until honey and sea salt are dissolved. Add fresh ground pepper to taste.
- To prepare the salad: In a skillet over medium heat, toast pine nuts until golden. Stir frequently to avoid burning. Set aside and allow to cool. Add the mint, parsley, cabbage, radishes, and cooled pine nuts to the vinaigrette. Mix well. Slowly fold the cooled quinoa into the vinaigrette mixture making sure to break up any quinoa clumps. Mix well.

316. Sweet Onion & Corn Quinoa Fritters With Fresh Corn & Basil Salad

Serving: Serves 4 to 6 | Prep: | Cook: |Ready in:

Ingredients

- Fresh Corn and Basil Salad.
- 1 ear of fresh corn, shucked
- 1/2 cup loosely packed torn basil
- 1/4 cup finely minced sweet onion
- 1 teaspoon apple cider vinegar
- 1 teaspoon freshly squeezed lime juice
- 2 teaspoons olive oil
- Salt, black pepper, and crushed red pepper, to taste.
- Quinoa Fritters with Sweet Onion, Fresh Corn and Basil
- 1 ear of fresh corn, shucked
- 1 cup uncooked quinoa, rinsed and well drained
- 1/2 cup all purpose flour
- 1/3 cup minced sweet onion
- 1/2 cup loosely packed minced fresh basil
- 2 tablespoons ground flax seeds
- 6 tablespoons boiling water
- 2 teaspoons sea salt
- 1 teaspoon black pepper
- 1 teaspoon crushed red pepper
- 1 teaspoon paprika
- 2 tablespoons nutritional yeast (optional but strongly encouraged)
- Oil for frying: 2 to 3 tablespoons to start, plus more as needed.

Direction

- Fresh Corn and Basil Salad.
- Carefully shave kernels from the ear of corn with a kitchen knife into a medium mixing bowl.
- Add basil and sweet onion.
- In a small bowl, whisk together apple cider vinegar, lime juice, and olive oil.
- Pour dressing over corn mixture and toss to combine.
- Season with salt, black pepper, and crushed red pepper to taste.
- Quinoa Fritters with Sweet Onion, Fresh Corn and Basil
- In a medium saucepan over medium-high heat, toast rinsed quinoa for 4 to 5 minutes, stirring constantly, until lightly browned and fragrant.
- Add two cups of water and bring to a boil. Reduce to a simmer, cover, and let cook for 12 to 15 minutes until all liquid is absorbed.
- Allow cooked quinoa to cool completely before continuing with the recipe. The quinoa can easily be made a day ahead of time.
- In a small bowl, whisk together ground flax seeds and 6 tablespoons of boiling water. Set aside and allow to cool completely and thicken.
- Place a box grater over a bowl or dish and grate the ear of corn until all kernels are removed. You will wind up with about 1/3 cup of pulpy corn mash.
- In a large mixing bowl combine the cooled quinoa, grated corn, minced onion, basil, flour, nutritional yeast, salt, peppers, and paprika. Stir to combine, being careful not to over-mix.

- Add cooled flax mixture, then stir gently until combined. Season to taste.
- Using a tablespoon, scoop out dough and gently form it into balls using your hands. Roll in a little bit of flour, flatten into a patty and set in a single layer on a plate or baking sheet.
- Heat 2 tablespoons of oil in a heavy skillet over medium-high heat. In batches, add fritters and cook for 3 to 4 minutes on each side, until golden brown and crispy. Add more oil as needed.
- Drain cooked fritters on paper towels. Serve with Corn and Basil Salad.

317. Sweet Potato & Mushroom Quinoa Burgers

Serving: Serves 6 | Prep: | Cook: |Ready in:

Ingredients

- 1/2 cup quinoa
- kosher salt and pepper to taste
- 1 tablespoon olive oil or grapeseed oil, plus more for frying
- 1 shallot or small red onion, minced to yield about 1/3 cup
- pinch red pepper flakes
- 5 to 6 ounces cremini mushrooms, about 8, or 1 portobello
- 1 medium sweet potatoes, about 11 oz, scrubbed but not peeled, cut into wedges, see notes above
- 1/2 cup panko bread crumbs
- 1/2 cup finely minced parsley or cilantro
- 1/2 cup grated Parmigiano Reggiano
- 3 eggs, beaten
- buns, mashed avocado, quick-pickled onions, optional, for serving, see notes above

Direction

- In a medium pot, combine the quinoa with 1 cup of water. Add a pinch of salt. Bring to a boil, turn heat to low, cover, and cook until tender, about 20 minutes. Remove from heat, and let stand covered. You should have about 1 1/2 cups.
- Meanwhile, place a large sauté pan over medium-high heat. Add a tablespoon of oil. When it shimmers, add the shallots or onion and a pinch of red pepper flakes. Turn the heat down to medium, and cook until the shallots soften, about 2 minutes.
- Meanwhile, run the mushrooms down the chute of a food processor fitted with the shredder attachment. Run the sweet potato wedges down the chute next. (If you don't have a food processor, shred the sweet potato using a cheese grater and finely mince the mushrooms.) Dump the mushrooms and sweet potatoes into the pan with the shallots. Turn the heat up to medium-high and cook until the vegetables are just soft, about 2 minutes more. Season with salt to taste. Transfer to a large bowl. Add the cooked quinoa, panko, parsley, and Parmigiano Reggiano. Stir to combine. Taste. This is your chance to get the seasoning right. If it needs more salt and pepper, and them now. Add the eggs, and stir to combine.
- Make a test patty: Place a large skillet over high heat. Add oil to coat the bottom in a thin layer. Scoop out some of the quinoa mix with your and cup it to form a ball. Gently flatten to form a patty. When the oil shimmers, carefully lower the patty, season with salt and pepper, cook 2 minutes, or until underside is deeply golden brown, flip, cook 2 minutes more. Remove from skillet. Let cool briefly. Taste, make adjustments to your vegetable mix accordingly — if the patty fell apart, add another egg. If it feels too wet, add more panko. Adjust seasoning with more salt and pepper if necessary.
- When ready to cook, form patties using a 1/3 cup measuring cup. Scoop out the mix, squeeze with your hands, form into a ball, then pat to form into a patty — mixture will be delicate/wet. Portion out all of the mixture. Return the skillet to medium-high heat. Add more oil if necessary — there should be a thin

layer. Carefully lower patties into the oil and cook two to three minutes a side or until each side has formed a nice, golden-brown crust. It's best to let the patties cook undisturbed for a minute or two before peeking to check for doneness—you want to give them a chance to develop a crust.
- Serve with buns, mashed avocados, lettuce, and pickled onions if you wish.

318. Sweet Potato Quinoa Salad

Serving: Serves 4 | Prep: 0hours20mins | Cook: 0hours20mins | Ready in:

Ingredients

- 2 tablespoons butter
- 1 tablespoon olive oil
- 1 pound sweet potato, peeled and cut into 1/2" dice
- 2 teaspoons maple syrup
- 2 cups cooked quinoa, warm or room temp
- grated zest of navel orange
- juice of 1/2 navel orange
- 1/4 cup dried cranberries
- pistachios, or peanuts, or both, lightly crushed (about a small handful)
- 1 jalapeno, ribs and seeds removed, cut into small dice
- 1/3 cup diced red onion
- 1 tablespoon chopped cilantro
- 1 tablespoon chopped mint
- salt and pepper

Direction

- Heat butter and oil in a large saute pan over medium heat. When butter begins to foam, add the diced potatoes. Cook, stirring occasionally, for about 10 or so minutes, until potatoes just begin to brown. Stir in the maple syrup. Season with salt to taste. Turn off heat.
- In the saute pan, combine the remaining ingredients with the potatoes. Season with salt and pepper. Serve warm or room temperature.

319. Sweet Quinoa

Serving: Serves 2 | Prep: | Cook: | Ready in:

Ingredients

- 1 cup quinoa
- 1.5 cups water
- 1 cup coconut milk
- 1 tablespoon cinnamon
- 1 tablespoon nutmeg
- 1 tablespoon honey

Direction

- (Always soak your grains for hours before cooking and consuming. This removes Phytic Acid from the grain, which prevents calcium absorption.) Place water and quinoa in small saucepan and bring to a boil. Reduce to simmer and cover for 12-15 minutes, until water is boiled out.
- Leave quinoa in saucepan and add coconut milk. Keep on simmer, cover and allow quinoa to soak up coconut milk. After about 15 minutes, add cinnamon and nutmeg. Once the quinoa is at a consistency of your liking, (depending on if you would rather it a bit more soupy or grainy) remove from saucepan and place in bowl. Let sit for 20 minutes to cool, then add honey. (Waiting is crucial so that the enzymes are not sacrificed in honey!)
- Serve and enjoy!

320. Sweet And Crunchy Quinoa Salad

Serving: Serves 6 | Prep: | Cook: | Ready in:

Ingredients

- Recipe Ingredients
- 1 cup quinoa
- 2 cups low-sodium chicken or vegetable broth
- ? cups sliced almonds, toasted
- 1 cup thinly sliced green onions (about one bunch)
- ½ cups dried cherries*, chopped / * May substitute chopped apricots, cranberries or raisins
- ½ cups chopped parsley
- For the dressing
- ¼ cups orange juice
- 1 tablespoon olive oil
- 2 tablespoons buttermilk
- 2 tablespoons honey
- ¼ teaspoons salt, optional
- ½ teaspoons freshly ground black pepper, or to taste

Direction

- Place quinoa and broth in a large saucepan and bring to a boil. Cover and reduce heat; simmer 15-20 minutes or until liquid is absorbed. Remove from heat.
- Meanwhile, place almonds in a small pan over medium heat and toss until lightly browned and fragrant.
- Whisk together the dressing ingredients in a small bowl until well blended.
- While the quinoa is still warm, stir in the green onions, cherries, parsley, and almonds, then toss with the dressing and serve.
- Per serving: 262 calories, 8g protein, 39g carbohydrate, 9g fat, 1g sat fat, 5g mono fat, 0mg cholesterol, 3g fiber, 44mg sodium (with optional salt: 141mg sodium)

321. Taco Tuna Quinoa Sliders

Serving: Makes 12 | Prep: | Cook: | Ready in:

Ingredients

- 5 ounces drained solid white tuna
- 1 cup cooked quinoa
- 2 eggs
- 2 laughing cow swiss wedges
- 1 tablespoon taco seasoning

Direction

- Preheat oven to 350F & spray/oil muffin tin.
- Combine all ingredients in large bowl, mix till well combined.
- Divide mixture into 12 cakes and bake for 30 minutes. Let cool 10 minutes before removing from muffin tin.

322. Tandoori Quinoa Cakes With Garden Herbs

Serving: Makes 12 | Prep: | Cook: | Ready in:

Ingredients

- Quinoa, vegetable stock, eggs, onion, sweet red pepper, garlic chives, thyme, oregano, basil, cheese, masala tandoori, breadcrumbs, ghee or coconut oil
- 1 cup Quinoa
- 2 cups vegetable stock
- 1 medium onion
- 1 sweet red pepper
- 8 sprigs garlic chives
- 3 sprigs fresh thyme
- 6 oregano leaves
- 6 basil leaves
- 1 tablespoon masala tandoori powder
- 2 cups shredded cheese (I use a nacho blend)
- 1 cup fine breadcrumbs
- 2 tablespoons ghee, coconut oil or your preferred oil
- 4 large eggs
- Mayonnaise, masala tandoori powder, agave syrup

- 1/2 cup mayonnaise, preferably olive oil based
- 2 teaspoons masala tandoori powder
- 1 tablespoon agave syrup

Direction

- Cook the quinoa in the vegetable stock as you normally would. Set aside to cool. Finely dice the onion and red pepper and gently saute for a few minutes, just to soften. Set aside to cool.
- In a large mixing bowl, beat 4 whole eggs. Wash and finely chop the herbs and add to the eggs. Add the onions & peppers, the cheese, the masala tandoori and the breadcrumbs. You may need more breadcrumbs as needed. Form 12 even patties, approximately 4 inches in circumference.
- Heat the oil in a frying pan on medium. Fry each patty for approximately 4 minutes on each side until heated through and nicely browned.
- Make a garnishing sauce by mixing the mayonnaise, tandoori masala and agave syrup together.
- For a meal, serve 2 alongside a crisp garden salad. These are also fantastic on a bun....quinoa burgers!

323. Thai Inspired Peanut Quinoa Salad

Serving: Serves 4 | Prep: | Cook: | Ready in:

Ingredients

- Salad
- 1.5 cups uncooked quinoa
- 10-12 ounces chicken breast
- 1 red bell pepper, cut into strips
- 1 cup snow peas, ends trimmed
- 2 cups broccoli florets
- 2 tablespoons vegetable oil, divided
- 1/4 cup chopped or crushed peanuts
- 1/4 cup chopped cilantro
- 2-3 tablespoons chopped green onions
- 1 tablespoon sesame seeds
- Peanut sauce
- 1/3 cup creamy peanut butter
- 3 tablespoons sesame oil
- 1/4 cup soy sauce
- 1 tablespoon rice vinegar
- 3 tablespoons brown sugar
- 1 teaspoon grated fresh ginger
- 1 clove garlic, minced
- 2-3 tablespoons water

Direction

- Cook the quinoa according to the directions on the package. This will most likely call for 1 part quinoa to two parts water.
- Heat 1 tablespoon vegetable oil in a skillet over medium heat for 1-2 minutes. Place the chicken in the skillet and cook until no pink remains, flipping at least once partway through the cooking time. Set aside to cool.
- In a small saucepan, combine all the ingredients for the sauce, except the water. Heat over medium-low, stirring periodically, until smooth and slightly thickened, about 5-7 minutes. Be careful not to turn the heat too high, or the sauce will begin to sputter! After removing the sauce from the stove, stir in up to 3 tablespoons of water to thin it to the consistency of a salad dressing.
- Once the chicken is cool enough to touch, chop or shred it into bite-sized pieces. Pour half of the peanut sauce over the chicken and stir until all surfaces are coated.
- Cook the vegetables. You may do this however you prefer: steaming, stir-frying, parboiling, etc. I sautéed the bell pepper strips and snow peas with 1 tablespoon of vegetable oil for about 2-3 minutes, until just slightly softened, and steamed the broccoli in the microwave. To do this, put the broccoli in a microwave-safe bowl, place 1/3-1/2 cup water in the bowl, and microwave, covered, for about 2 minutes (the time will vary, depending on the power of your microwave).

- Pour the other half of the peanut sauce over the quinoa and toss to combine. Add in the chicken and cooked vegetables. Garnish with peanuts, cilantro, green onions, and sesame seeds as desired.

324. The Best Quinoa Salad Ever

Serving: Serves 6-8 | Prep: | Cook: |Ready in:

Ingredients

- 1 cup Quinoa
- 1 tablespoon Butter
- 2 tablespoons Basil, roughly chopped
- 1 tablespoon Mint, roughly chopped
- 1 Apple, cored, diced
- 1/2 cup Dried cranberries
- 1/2 cup Sunflower seeds
- 2 Cloves garlic, minced
- 1/2 Jalapeno, grated (remove seeds and rind if you don't like heat!)
- 2 Lemons, juiced
- 1 Lime, juiced
- 2 tablespoons Agave nectar
- 1/2 cup Olive oil
- Salt and pepper

Direction

- Prepare quinoa according to directions on package. Once cooked, add in butter and stir until melted.
- In a large bowl combine the rest of the ingredients through the jalapeno.
- Add quinoa and vinaigrette to the large bowl with herbs and stir together. Season with salt and pepper and serve cold or hot.

325. The Family Waffle

Serving: Makes 4 belgian waffles | Prep: 0hours10mins | Cook: 0hours30mins |Ready in:

Ingredients

- 1 1/2 cups (235 g) gluten-free flour blend or (210 g) all-purpose flour
- 3 tablespoons cooked quinoa, cooled
- 2 tablespoons chia seeds
- 2 teaspoons unrefined cane sugar
- 1 1/2 teaspoons baking powder
- 1/2 teaspoon fine sea salt
- 1 1/2 cups (360 ml) real milk
- 1/2 cup (120 ml) vegetable oil, plus more for the waffle iron
- 2 large eggs, lightly beaten
- 1 teaspoon pure vanilla extract
- Plain yogurt (optional) and fresh berries (or any fruit), for serving
- 4 eggs, fried, for serving (optional)
- Pure maple syrup, for serving

Direction

- Preheat a waffle iron (we like a Belgian waffle maker, but any will work). Whisk together the flour, quinoa, chia seeds, sugar, baking powder, and salt. In a separate bowl, whisk together the milk, oil, eggs, and vanilla. When your waffle iron is hot and ready to use, stir the milk mixture into the flour mixture until just combined; the batter will be loose, the consistency of heavy cream.
- Spray or brush the waffle iron very lightly with oil. (If your waffle iron is seasoned or nonstick, you should only need to do this once before you begin, not between every waffle, which makes them taste greasy.) Ladle 1 heaping cup (240 ml) of the batter into the waffle iron and cook until golden brown, 12 to 14 minutes. Set aside on a rack while you cook the remaining waffles to keep them crispy (stacking will make them steam and get soggy). Serve the waffles warm with berries, a dollop of yogurt or a fried egg (if desired), and

a drizzle of maple syrup, or anything else you desire.
- Keep prepared batter in the refrigerator, covered, up to overnight. Or bake the waffles, cool, and freeze them in batches of two in large resealable freezer bags. To eat, bring to room temperature for 5 to 10 minutes, and toast to warm through. If you are making them fresh to order, you should know—as my kids and guests do—that waffle cooking is a one-by-one affair; everyone is allowed to eat their waffle hot and fresh off the press, when they're best, while the rest cook.

326. The Leigh Anne (Farro, Sausage And Brussel Sprouts)

Serving: Serves 4 | Prep: 0hours30mins | Cook: 0hours30mins |Ready in:

Ingredients

- 1 cup Farro
- 1 pound sausage (we like Dartagnan rabbit, pork & ginger sausage)
- 1/2 pound brussel sprouts, halved and cleaned
- freshly grated parmesan to finish

Direction

- Follow the instructions to make your faro. We like to use chicken stock instead of water.
- If sausage has a casing, take the sausage out of its casing and crumble into a hot skillet. Otherwise, crumble into hot skillet. Cook until nice and browned
- Toss the Brussels sprouts in olive oil, salt & pepper. Roast at 400 degrees for about 20min or until nice and crispy (Roasted broccoli is also sublime with this recipe)
- Once all of the ingredients are prepped, toss together in a bowl and top with grated parmesan

327. The Red And The Black. Roasted Red Peppers, Black Quinoa And Allioli (with Apologies To Stendhal)

Serving: Serves 4 | Prep: | Cook: |Ready in:

Ingredients

- stuffed peppers
- 4 red bell peppers
- 1 cup black quinoa
- 2 cups water or chicken stock
- 1/4 cup pine nuts, toasted
- 1 scallion
- Olive oil
- Allioli
- 5 (or more cloves of garlic)
- 2 egg yolks
- ½ teaspoon fleur de del (or other sea salt)
- 1 cup arbequina olive oil* (or other light Spanish olive oil)

Direction

- Stuffed peppers
- Grab your tongs and light your burners. Grill the peppers directly on your flaming range top or else outside over a wood grill. Either method works. Turn the peppers constantly while they are over the hot flames. When black all around drop them into a paper sack and seal up, or else into a large bowl which you can cover with plastic wrap.
- Toast the pine nuts in a dry skillet and set aside.
- Chop the scallion.
- When the peppers are cool enough to handle rub off the burnt black skin (it's okay if a little is left on---it looks sexy), stem and seed them.
- Cook the quinoa as usual using the 1 to 2 ratio, quinoa to liquid for about 15 minutes until cooked through.

- In a bowl mix cooked quinoa, pine nuts and scallions along with a drizzle of olive oil and salt and pepper to taste.
- To plate up scoop the black quinoa mixture in to the pepper shells (it should be spilling out). Add a big smear of allioi to each plate.
- Allioli
- Being a lazy sod I use a blender or food processor for this job.
- Begin by chopping the garlic and then mash it into a paste along with the salt in a mortar. Add that to the bottom of your blender along with the egg yolks.
- With the motor running drizzle in the arbequina oil until it becomes a mayonnaise you would recognize.
- *Note to cook, arbequinas are olives native to Catalonia and it's fairly easy to find imported oil made from them but I must add that arbequina oils are being produced in California now and I really like the intensity of flavor you get from them.

328.   The Red And The Black: The Sequel. Black Quinoa, Pearl Couscous ,Tomato Coulis

Serving: Serves 4 | Prep: | Cook: |Ready in:

Ingredients

- 1 pound ripe tomatoes
- 2 Hatch chilis roasted*
- 2 cloves garlic chopped
- Extra virgin olive oil, as needed up to ½ cup
- 1/2 of 1 bunch cilantro washed and torn up by hand
- 1 cup black quinoa
- 1 cup pearl couscous (aka Israeli couscous), Bob's Red Mill™ preferred
- 4 cups water
- salt

Direction

- Begin by roasting your chilies over an open gas flame or on an outside grill. Once the skin has blackened place them in either a paper bag or a bowl covered with cling wrap to steam. After they are cool enough to handle peel off as much black skin as you can. Don't worry if there are some residual streaks. Cut off the tops and yank out the seeds. A few strays aren't going to hurt. Give the peppers a rough chop.
- Core and then cut your tomatoes into chunks.
- Heat up the olive oil in a sauce pan over medium-low heat. Add the garlic and allow it to color a bit. Then add the peppers and the tomatoes. Season with salt. Allow this mixture to simmer until soft and gooey. You are going to mill it anyway so don't worry about texture right now.
- Meanwhile prepare your quinoa and couscous. In one pot get water boiling (for pearl/Israeli couscous follow the package directions as cooking time can vary). Add the couscous and cook until al dente. This might take 10-15 minutes or more.
- In another pot heat up two more cups of water just to where it's beginning to boil. Add salt and then your black quinoa. Cover and hold at a simmer for about 15 minutes. You will know it is done when that little ring (the germ) begins to appear and the texture is soft. Turn off the heat and hold covered.
- Now that the tomatoes and peppers have simmered down place a food mill over a large bowl and work the mixture through. This will remove the skins and most of the residual seeds. You can use a blender or food processor for this but the results will be somewhat less elegant. I'll leave that up to you.
- Wipe out the pan you used for the tomatoes and return the mixture and re-warm. It doesn't need to be very hot.
- In another large bowl combine the cooked quinoa and couscous along with the chopped cilantro, more olive oil and salt. Taste it!
- To the plate! Ladle out the tomato and chili mixture and top with the quinoa/couscous.

- *Few things smell better than fresh roasted Hatch chili when it's in progress. As noted you can substitute the canned variety in the off season. You can also substitute long Anaheim chilies which are available most of the year but the flavor is weak in comparison

329. Toasted Almond And Coconut Quinoa Porridge

Serving: Serves 4 | Prep: 0hours5mins | Cook: 0hours35mins | Ready in:

Ingredients

- 1/2 cup Slivered almonds
- 1 cup Dried quinoa
- 1 cup Water
- 1 1/2 cups Full fat coconut milk, divided
- 2 tablespoons Maple syrup
- 1/4 teaspoon Sea salt
- 1 Cinnamon stick (or 1 tsp cinnamon)
- 1/3 cup Pitted dates, chopped into small pieces (optional)

Direction

- Heat a shallow pan or a dry skillet over medium heat. Toast almonds till they're golden. Quickly remove from heat and transfer to a cool plate to stop them from burning.
- Rinse quinoa using a sieve until the rinse water runs clear. Bring the quinoa, maple syrup, sea salt, cinnamon, 1 cup coconut milk and 1 cup water to boil. Reduce heat to a simmer. Let simmer until quinoa is fluffy and all liquid has absorbed (about 15-20 minutes). Turn off heat and fluff quinoa gently with a fork. Remove cinnamon stick.
- Quickly, before it gets cold, divide quinoa into four bowls. Top each with about 2 tablespoons of coconut milk, along with 2 tablespoons of toasted almond slivers and a sprinkle of dates, if desired. Serve.

330. Tomato Peanut Butter Quinoa Soup

Serving: Serves 6 | Prep: | Cook: | Ready in:

Ingredients

- 1 tablespoon peanut oil
- 1 tablespoon minced garlic
- 4 cups low sodium, gluten free vegetable broth
- 1 tablespoon balsamic vinegar
- 1 28 ounce can chopped tomatoes in juice
- 1 6 ounce can tomato paste
- 1/2 cup creamy, unsalted peanut butter
- 1/4 teaspoon cayenne pepper
- salt to taste
- 1 cup cooked quinoa
- 6 scallions, chopped
- slivered almonds or peanuts for sprinkling

Direction

- In a medium saucepan, heat oil over medium heat.
- Add garlic & cook until fragrant then add tomatoes with their juices, tomato paste, broth, vinegar, peanut butter, cayenne & salt
- Whisk to combine and bring to a boil
- Once it has boiled, allow to simmer on medium low 15 to 20 minutes
- Add cooked quinoa to the pot
- Ladle soup into bowls, garnish with the scallions & nuts

331. Tomato Quinoa With Zucchini Red Pepper And Corn

Serving: Serves 3 | Prep: | Cook: | Ready in:

Ingredients

- 1 cup quinoa
- 3 tablespoons olive oil
- 1 medium sized red onion, chopped
- 1 red bell pepper, chopped
- 1 zucchini, chopped
- 1 cup frozen corn kernels, or 1 ear of corn (kernels shaved)
- 1/4 cup chopped parsley
- 4 tablespoons tomato paste
- 1 lemon

Direction

- Rinse quinoa and add to a pot with 1½ cups water.
- Cover, bring to a simmer, then turn heat down to low and cook for 15 minutes with the cover on the pot.
- Check to make sure all the water has absorbed into the quinoa (and there is none at the bottom of the pot). Then remove from heat.
- Meanwhile, heat a large skillet over medium high heat.
- Add the oil, onion, pepper, and zucchini and sauté for 10 minutes.
- Add the corn and sauté another minute.
- Add the parsley and tomato paste, and cook for 30 seconds, stirring.
- Remove from heat and add the cooked quinoa and the juice from 1 lemon. Season with salt and pepper to taste.

332. Tomato And Chard Quinoa Bake

Serving: Serves 4 | Prep: | Cook: | Ready in:

Ingredients

- 2 cups Cooked quinoa
- 1 cup Chopped Swiss chard, about 4 stalks with leaves cut into ribbons
- 3 Green Onions, finely chopped
- 3/4 cup Feta cheese, crumbled
- 1 Egg
- 1/2 teaspoon Cumin
- 1/2 teaspoon Smoked Paprika
- 1/2 teaspoon Salt
- 1 1/2 cups Sliced Roma tomatoes

Direction

- Preheat oven to 350 degrees.
- In a medium sized bowl, add egg and spices and whisk together. Add quinoa and 1/2 c of the crumbled feta cheese and stir together.
- Then, fold in the chard, tomatoes and onions.
- Place in a greased 1 1/2 quart casserole dish and top with remaining feta cheese.
- Bake in oven 20 to 25 minutes until warmed through.

333. Tomato And Fresh Herbs Quinoa Salad

Serving: Serves 4-6 | Prep: | Cook: | Ready in:

Ingredients

- 1 cup uncooked quinoa (rinsed)
- 2 cups water
- 1 large tomato
- 1 handful fresh parsley
- 1 handful fresh dill
- 1/2 small red onion
- juice from 1/2 lemon
- 2-3 tablespoons extra virgin olive oil
- salt (to taste)
- fresh ground pepper (to taste)

Direction

- Put the quinoa and 2 cups of water into a medium-sized pot with a cover and bring to a boil. Once the water begins to boil, turn the heat down to low and cook for 15-20 minutes (still covered) until there is only a small amount of water left. Turn off the burner and keep the quinoa covered for another 10 or so

minutes to allow the rest of the water to be absorbed then fluff quinoa with a fork.
- While the quinoa cooks, dice the tomato (~1cm cubes), chop the parsley and dill, and finely dice the 1/2 small red onion, and add them to a large mixing bowl. Add the lemon juice and extra virgin olive oil and gently mix everything together.
- When the quinoa has cooled down, but is still pretty warm, add a little (~1/2 cup) at a time to the mixing bowl with the tomato herb mixture and gently mix together until all is incorporated. The key is to get the tomato and herb mixture to release some of its flavors without causing the herbs to wilt. Add salt and pepper, to taste.
- Allow to cool to room temperature if eating immediately, or store in an airtight container in the refrigerator.

334. Tomatoes Stuffed With Quinoa, Spinach And Feta

Serving: Serves 4 | Prep: | Cook: | Ready in:

Ingredients

- 4 large Roma tomatoes, halved lengthwise, seeded and cored
- 3/4 cup rinsed and drained quinoa simmered for about 15 minutes in 1 1/2 cups water and then cooled
- 2 tablespoons butter
- 2 green onions, thinly sliced
- 1 clove garlic, minced
- 1 tablespoon dried dillweed
- 4 ounces fresh baby spinach leaves (a great big handful)
- 1/2 cup crumbled feta cheese plus a little more for topping
- Salt and pepper to taste
- 2 tablespoons extra virgin olive oil for drizzling

Direction

- Place the cut sides of the tomatoes on paper toweling to drain while you prepare the filling.
- In a medium sauté pan sauté the green onion and garlic in the butter for about one minute. Stir in the dried dill weed.
- With the heat still on, add the spinach a little at a time, stirring all the while until it wilts. Stir in the cooked quinoa and 1/2 cup of the crumbled feta. Taste and season with a little salt and pepper if needed.
- Generously fill the tomato halves with the spinach-quinoa mixture and place in a medium baking dish. Sprinkle with a little more feta and then drizzle the tomatoes with the olive oil and bake in a 325F oven for 40 to 45 minutes.

335. Top Shelf Trek Mix

Serving: Makes 5 cups | Prep: 0hours10mins | Cook: 0hours15mins | Ready in:

Ingredients

- 1 cup Macadamia nuts
- 1 cup Marcona almonds
- 1 cup puffed quinoa
- 1 cup dried Strawberries
- 1 cup cacao nibs

Direction

- Toast nuts on a parchment paper-lined baking sheet in a 350°F oven for 8 to 15 minutes, tossing at least once, or in a skillet over medium heat for 3 to 5 minutes, tossing frequently, until fragrant and one shade darker.
- Mix to combine.

336. Tropical Quinoa And Fruit Pudding

Serving: Serves 3 | Prep: | Cook: |Ready in:

Ingredients

- 1 cup quinoa, rinsed
- 1 can (14 ounces) light coconut milk
- 1 tablespoon finely chopped gingerroot
- 1/4 cup water
- 1 tablespoon brown sugar or honey
- 1 container (6 ounces) Yoplait® Greek Fat Free honey vanilla yogurt
- 1 cup medium mango, seed removed, peeled and chopped (1 cup)
- 2 tablespoons chopped slivered almonds
- 1/4 cup cup pomegranate seeds, dried cranberries or cherries

Direction

- In 2-quart saucepan, stir together quinoa, coconut milk, gingerroot and water. Heat to boiling; reduce heat to medium-low. Cover and simmer 10 to 15 minutes or until most of the liquid is absorbed. Turn off heat; let stand covered 5 minutes. Stir in brown sugar or honey. Divide pudding among 3 bowls, top with yogurt, mango, almonds and pomegranate seeds.

337. Turkey Quinoa Burger

Serving: Serves 5 | Prep: | Cook: |Ready in:

Ingredients

- 1 pound ground Turkey
- 1 cup cooked quinoa
- 1/2 cup chopped parsley
- 2 small shallots, minced
- salt and pepper

Direction

- Mix everything together, without squishing it. Make 1-2 inches balls and flatten to shape as mini burgers. Cook for 3-4 minutes on each side
- I baked potato slices in the oven at F400 for 10-12 minutes and used them as buns....I served it with a siracha aioli, mixing vegenaise (or mayonnaise) and siracha sauce.
- Et Voila, Bon Appetit!

338. Vegan Quinoa Lentil Curry Burger

Serving: Serves 2 | Prep: 10hours10mins | Cook: 0hours45mins |Ready in:

Ingredients

- 4 cups Vegetable Stock
- 1/2 cup quinoa
- 1/4 cup lentils
- 1/8 cup oats
- 1/2 white onion, finely chopped
- 4 sun dried tomatoes, chopped
- 1/4 teaspoon turmeric
- 1/4 teaspoon coriander powder
- 2 teaspoons curry powder
- 1 pinch red chili powder
- Salt & pepper, to taste
- 2 stalks mint
- 1 handful coriander
- 1 lime, quartered
- 1 cup yogurt (skip if vegan)

Direction

- In a heated pot, cook the quinoa, lentils, oats and onions in chicken stock.
- Add in the remaining veggie patty ingredients and cook on medium heat for 20-30 minutes, till quinoa is cooked through. If required, add extra water to continue cooking. Then let cool.
- Meanwhile, preheat your oven to 180C, and prepare your patties. Use a shaper/mold for consistency.

- Bake on a lined baking tray for 25 minutes. Remove from heat and let cool for a few minutes before serving.
- Serve the veggie patty with a squeeze of lime topped with mint leaves, with a side of yogurt.

339. Vegan Rosh Hashanah Recipe: Pomegranate Glazed Tofu & Quinoa

Serving: Serves 6-8 | Prep: | Cook: | Ready in:

Ingredients

- Quinoa & Veggies
- 1 cup tri-colored quinoa
- 2 carrots, diced
- 1/3 cup yellow onion, diced
- 1/2 cup diced crimini, shitake and oyster mushrooms
- 1 tablespoon chopped rosemary
- 1/2 eggplant
- 1 cup cherry tomatoes, cut lengthwise
- 2 tablespoons extra-virgin olive oil
- 2 tablespoons concentrated pomegranate juice
- Tofu & Glaze
- 15 ounces extra-firm tofu (1 package)
- 1 tablespoon soy sauce
- 1 teaspoon Dijon mustard
- 1 tablespoon extra-virgin olive oil
- 1/4 cup concentrated pomegranate juice

Direction

- Preheat the oven to 400 F, and prepare the grill.
- Cook the quinoa on the stovetop according to the package directions.
- While the quinoa is cooking, roast the carrots at 400 F for 20-30 minutes, and test for doneness. They should be tender and sweet.
- Grill the sliced eggplant and then dice.
- Fry the onion in a skillet until brown, and add in the mushrooms.
- Now add the cherry tomatoes and rosemary to the mixture, then toss with olive oil and pomegranate juice.
- Prepare the tofu marinade sauce and place horizontally cut tofu in sauce.
- Grill both sides of the tofu for 3-4 minutes each.
- When done, place the grilled tofu on top of the quinoa mixture, and garnish with rosemary. Enjoy!

340. Vegetable Quinoa Pilaf

Serving: Serves 4 | Prep: | Cook: | Ready in:

Ingredients

- 1 cup quinoa
- 3 cups water
- 1 large zucchini, shredded
- 1 mdium carrot, shredded
- 2 large radishes, shredded
- 2 small beets, shredded
- 5 garlic scapes, chopped
- salt
- oil

Direction

- Rinse the quinoa and drain. Place the quinoa in a sauce pan and toast over medium high heat. Add the water and cook until the water is absorbed (about 30 minutes).
- Combine the vegetables on a large platter or shallow bowl. Sprinkle generously with salt and let it sit for 30 minutes to draw out excess liquid. Place the mixture in a strainer or colander and squeeze out the liquid
- Heat up pan and coat the bottom with oil. Add the vegetable mixture and cook until it starts to crisp. Fold in the cooked quinoa to combine, and cook the mixture for a few minutes.

341. Vegetable Quinoa Salad

Serving: Serves 5+ | Prep: | Cook: | Ready in:

Ingredients

- 1 cup quinoa
- 1 1/2 cups meat or vegetable stock or broth
- 1 teaspoon sea salt
- 1/2 cup chopped broccoli
- 1 chopped carrot
- 1/2 cup chopped zucchini
- 2 tablespoons grass-fed butter

Direction

- Add the quinoa, stock, and sea salt to a medium-sized pot and bring to a rolling boil.
- Bring the heat down to a simmer and add the broccoli and carrot.
- After 7 minutes, add the zucchini and butter.
- Cook for 5 more minutes (or until the liquid has been absorbed).

342. Vegetarian Summer Rolls With Quinoa

Serving: Makes 6 rolls | Prep: | Cook: | Ready in:

Ingredients

- Summer Rolls
- 1/2 cup red quinoa
- 1/2 cup water
- 1/2 teaspoon seasoned rice vinegar
- 1/2 teaspoon sesame oil
- 1 packet banh trang - rice paper spring roll wrappers
- 1 large carrot (or 2 small), peeled and julienned
- 1/2 English cucumber, peeled, seeded and julienned
- 1 small red bell pepper, seeded and julienned
- 6-8 leaves red leaf lettuce
- 2-3 mint sprigs (12-18 leaves)
- 7 ounces (1/2 a brick), extra firm tofu, julienned
- soy sauce
- black sesame seeds
- Nuoc Cham (dipping sauce)
- 1-2 cloves garlic, crushed
- 1 Thai chile, minced
- 1 tablespoon fresh lime juice
- 1 teaspoon seasoned rice vinegar
- 1/2 cup fish sauce
- 1/2 cup water

Direction

- Combine quinoa and water in a medium sauce pan and bring to a boil. Reduce heat to low and simmer for 15-20 minutes until water is fully absorbed and the quinoa is completely cooked. Transfer to a bowl to cool and dress it with rice wine vinegar and sesame oil. Set aside.
- Make sure you have all vegetables, herbs and tofu cut and ready to go. Drizzle the tofu with soy sauce and sprinkle with sesame seeds, if using. Fill a plate or pie pan with water and make sure it's large enough to submerge the rice paper wrappers.
- Soak each rice paper wrapper as you go, turning it over in the water 5 times. It'll still feel a little bit stiff, but resist the urge to oversoak. The water will continue to hydrate the wrapper as you're adding your filling.
- Lay the lettuce and mint down first, followed by 2 T. quinoa, 2-3 slices of each vegetable and tofu. Carefully wrap the bottom edge over the filling and pull it back slightly to create a tight roll. Fold the right side of the wrapper to the center, fold the left side of the wrapper to the center and roll upwards to complete the roll. Set on a plate and continue rolling with the remaining ingredients.
- To make the sauce, stir together all ingredients in a medium bowl. Use less chile if you're heat sensitive.

343. Veggie Fried Quinoa

Serving: Serves 4 | Prep: | Cook: | Ready in:

Ingredients

- 1 cup quinoa
- 1 1/3 cups water
- 1 tablespoon coconut oil
- 8 ounces sliced mixed mushrooms
- 1 tablespoon fresh ginger, peeled and finely chopped
- 2 garlic cloves, thinly sliced
- 1 packet broccoli slaw or stir fry mix
- 1/2 cup shelled edamame
- 3 handfuls fresh spinach
- 2 eggs, beaten
- 4 scallions, sliced diagonally in half inches
- 1-2 tablespoons tamari or soy sauce
- 1-3 teaspoons sriracha
- 1 teaspoon sesame oil
- 1 tablespoon toasted sesame seeds
- Olive oil
- Kosher salt

Direction

- In a medium saucepan over medium high heat, add about a tablespoon of olive oil and swirl to coat the pan. Add the quinoa and stir occasionally until lightly toasted, about 3 minutes. Add the water and a pinch of salt, bring to a boil, cover and reduce the heat to low. Cook for 20-25 minutes, until water is absorbed, then fluff with a fork and set aside until ready to use.
- In a wok or large pan, heat the coconut oil over medium high heat. Add the garlic and ginger and stir fry for 1 minute. Add the mushrooms and cook, stirring often, until they have released their juices and are slightly browned. Next, add the broccoli slaw and continue to stir fry for 1-2 minutes. Add the tamari (or soy), sesame oil and sriracha to taste and fry for another minute. Add the edamame then the cooked quinoa and stir to mix well. Next, add the handfuls of spinach, one at a time, mixing in as they wilt, followed by the scallions. Lastly, make a well in the middle of the stir fry and pour in the eggs, stirring in circles as you scramble. Mix all ingredients well, adjust seasoning as necessary, and serve sprinkled with sesame seeds.

344. Veggie Quinoa Stuffed Chiles

Serving: Serves 4-6 | Prep: | Cook: | Ready in:

Ingredients

- 8 Poblano peppers-roasted peeled and seeded
- 1 cup Quinoa
- 1 cup Orange Juice
- 1 cup Chicken or vegetable stock
- 1/2 teaspoon salt
- 6 Shitake Mushrooms Finely Diced
- 1 /2 Butternut squash
- 1/2 cup Dried Currants
- 1/2 cup Toasted Pecans -chopped
- 1/2 teaspoon Ground Coriander
- 1/2 teaspoon Ground Cumin
- 1/2 cup Feta -diced into small dice

Direction

- HEAT THE OVEN TO 450*
- PLACE THE QUINOA, ORANGE JUICE AND STOCK INTO A SAUCEPAN. COOK UNTIL ALL THE LIQUID IS ABSORBED. ADD THE SALT TO TASTE.
- N A SMALL SKILLET, SAUTE THE MUSHROOMS UNTIL LIGHTLY BROWNED. REMOVE FROM HEAT AND ADD THE SPINACH. STIR TO COMBINE AND SET ASIDE.
- PLACE THE 1/2 SQUASH IN A GLASS PIE PAN WITH ABOUT A 1/4 INCH OF WATER. COVER WITH PLASTIC WRAP AND MICROWAVE FOR 8-10 MINUTES UNTIL JUST SOFT BUT NOT MUSHY. REMOVE FROM THE WATER AND DICE THE

SQUASH INTO 1/4"CUBES AND SET ASIDE TO COOL SLIGHTLY.
- ADD THE CURRANTS, CUMIN AND CORIANDER TO THE QUINOA, STIR TO COMBINE. ADD THE MUSHROOMS & SPINACH, FETA AND THE SQUASH. TOSS LIGHTLY.
- FILL THE PEELED & SEEDED POBLANOS WITH THE QUINOA MIXTURE AND PLACE ON A COOKIE SHEET. BAKE FOR 10-15 MINUTES UNTIL THE MIXTURE IS HOT AND THE CHEESE IS SOFT.
- YOU CAN SERVE THESE ON A POOL OF ROASTED TOMATO SAUCE, WITH A MANGO SALSA OR TANGY TOMATO VINAIGRETTE.

345. WHEAT BERRIES, RED QUINOA, AND WILD RICE WITH SUN DRIED TOMATOES

Serving: Serves 2 as a main course | Prep: | Cook: | Ready in:

Ingredients

- 1 cup cooked red quinoa
- 1/2 cup cooked wild rice
- 1/2 cup cooked wheat berries
- 2 tablespoons pine nuts
- 2 large cloves garlic, minced
- 3 tablespoons sun-dried tomatoes, packed in oil, slivered
- 2 tablespoons extra-virgin olive oil
- 2 tablespoons minced fresh herbs (basil and/or oregano)
- Salt and pepper to taste

Direction

- Sauté pine nuts, sun-dried tomatoes, and garlic until pine nuts become toasted.
- Add cooked grains, stir well, and heat until hot.
- Season with salt, pepper, and herbs.

346. Walnut & Sage Smothered Lentil Quinoa Pilaf

Serving: Serves 3-4 | Prep: | Cook: | Ready in:

Ingredients

- 1/2 cup organic white Quinoa
- 1/2 cup Beluga lentils
- 1 cup Walnuts, toasted
- 20-22 Sage leaves
- 1/2 teaspoon Kosher Salt
- 2 cups water
- 2 tablespoons unsalted butter
- 1/2 cup Crumbled Feta Cheese
- 1-1 1/2 tablespoons orange zest
- 1-2 tablespoons Extra Virgin Olive Oil (EVOO)
- Juice of 1/2 a lemon

Direction

- In a large saucepan, combine the water & salt & bring to a boil. Add the beluga lentils, cover & cook for 5 minutes. Add the Quinoa and lower the heat to medium. Cover & allow to cook till all the water is absorbed (~ 15 minutes). Once cooked, fluff the lentil quinoa mix with a fork.
- Combine 1/2 a cup of toasted walnuts and about 15 torn sage leaves & coarsely mince in a food processor till they resemble coarse bread crumbs (albeit with a tantalizing aroma)
- Add 1 tablespoon of butter in a small skillet and add the minced walnut/sage mixture. Sauté till the bits of sage begin to wilt.
- In a large mixing bowl, combine the remaining walnuts (broken into small bits), Lemon juice & orange zest. Add the feta cheese, quinoa/lentil mix, the sautéed walnut/sage blend and fold to combine all the ingredients.

Drizzle with the EVOO, taste and adjust for seasonings as per your preference.
- Heat the remaining butter and add the remaining sage to it, sauté till the leaves crisp up and add the mix to the lentil quinoa pilaf as a garnish.

347. Walnut And Quinoa Salad With Goat Cheese, Dried Cherries And Arugula

Serving: Serves 5 | Prep: | Cook: |Ready in:

Ingredients

- .5 cups Balsamic Vinegar
- 1 pinch Salt
- 1.5 cups Cooked and chilled quinoa
- 1 cup Arugula, coarsely chopped
- 1/4 cup Walnuts, chopped
- 1/4 cup Dried cherries, coarsely chopped
- 1 tablespoon Extra virgin olive oil
- 1 Lemon, juiced
- 1 teaspoon Salt
- 2 ounces Goat cheese

Direction

- In a small saucepan, bring balsamic vinegar and pinch of salt to boil. Reduce to low and simmer for @15 minutes or until thickened. Remove balsamic glaze from heat and allow to cool.
- In large bowl mix together quinoa, arugula, walnuts, dried cherries, evoo, lemon juice and salt until well combined. Add goat cheese and mix until fully distributed. Serve with a drizzle of the balsamic glaze.

348. Warm Red Quinoa & Squash Salad

Serving: Serves 2 | Prep: | Cook: |Ready in:

Ingredients

- 1/4 cup red quinoa
- 1/2 cup water
- 1/4 teaspoon Kosher salt
- 1 1/2 cups chopped, peeled butternut squash (3/4" chunks)
- 1 teaspoon extra virgin olive oil
- 8 grape tomatoes, halved lengthwise
- 1/4 cup crumbled feta cheese
- 1/4 cup chopped fresh basil (loosely packed)
- Freshly ground pepper

Direction

- Combine the quinoa, water, and salt in a small saucepan. Bring to a simmer over high heat. Reduce heat to low, stir in squash, cover, and cook for 10 to 15 minutes, or until the quinoa has popped and the squash is soft. (You may need to add another tablespoon or two of water, depending on how juicy your squash is.)
- Remove from heat and fold in the olive oil, tomatoes, feta, and basil. Season to taste with freshly ground pepper.

349. Watermelon Pizza Salad With Curried Quinoa

Serving: Serves 8 | Prep: | Cook: |Ready in:

Ingredients

- For the curried quinoa -
- 1 teaspoon oil
- 1/2 teaspoon ghee
- 1/2 teaspoon mustard seeds
- 1/2 teaspoon cumin seeds
- 1/8 teaspoon asafetida powder

- 1/4 serrano pepper
- 1/4 teaspoon turmeric powder
- 1/4 cup quinoa
- 1/2 cup hot water
- sea salt to taste
- 2 cups baby kale leaves, julienned
- 1/4 cup diced red onion
- 1 cup grated carrots
- 1/4 cup feta cheese
- For the dressing and base
- 1/4 cup balsamic vinegar
- 1/2 teaspoon brown sugar
- 1/2 teaspoon curry powder
- 1/2 teaspoon ghee
- sea salt to taste
- 8 watermelon triangle shaped slices
- tajin seasoning to taste

Direction

- Heat the oil and ghee over medium heat. Add the mustard and cumin seeds. When they start to splutter, add the asafetida and chili pepper.
- Lower the heat, add the turmeric powder and the washed and drained quinoa. Roast the quinoa well with the spices for about 2 minutes. It will start to make a crackling sound.
- Add the half cup of hot water and sea salt to taste. Stir and let the quinoa cook, covered, on low heat, until cooked, about 25 minutes.
- Let it cool. Remove the green chili pepper slices and discard. Fluff with a fork and add the kale, onion, carrots and feta cheese.
- In a saucepan, reduce the balsamic vinegar for about 2 minutes on low heat. Add the brown sugar, curry powder, ghee and the sea salt and whisk to combine. Remove from heat.
- Sprinkle the tajin seasoning over the watermelon slice base. Top with the quinoa salad and drizzle the dressing over the top!

350. White Bean And Quinoa Chili

Serving: Makes about 6 to 8 servings | Prep: | Cook: | Ready in:

Ingredients

- 1 1/2 cups diced onion
- 2 tablespoons olive oil
- 1 cup diced green bell pepper
- 5 cloves minced garlic
- 2 tablespoons ground cumin
- 3 tablespoons ancho chili powder
- 2 teaspoons salt
- 1 teaspoon black pepper
- 1/4 teaspoon crushed red pepper flakes
- 2 14 to 15 ounce cans tomatoes, chopped
- 1 to 2 12 ounce cans V8 or tomato juice
- 12 ounces beer, preferably a brown ale
- 1 to 2 teaspoons brown sugar
- 3 cups cooked white beans (or two 14 to 15 ounce cans drained and rinsed)
- 3/4 cup quinoa simmered in 1 1/2 cups water for 10 to 15 minutes

Direction

- In a soup pot or Dutch oven saute the onions and bell pepper in the olive oil until the onions begin to soften. Add the garlic and saute another minute or two.
- Stir in the cumin, chili powder, crushed red pepper flakes, salt and pepper and saute another minute or two.
- Add the tomatoes, beer and one can of the tomato juice, bring up to the boil and gently simmer for about 15 minutes. Taste at this point and if the mixture seems to acidic, stir in some of the brown sugar.
- Stir in the cooked beans and cooked quinoa and if the chili seems too thick, add some or all of that second can of tomato juice. Bring up to the boil and serve. You can certainly garnish with your favorite toppings - green onion, avocado, grated cheese, sour cream, etc.

- Note: Make this early in the day or the day before serving for better flavor.

351. Wintry Mushroom, Kale, And Quinoa Enchiladas

Serving: Serves 6 | Prep: | Cook: | Ready in:

Ingredients

- Homemade Enchilada Sauce
- 1 tablespoon olive oil
- 1 cup onion, diced
- 2 cloves garlic, minced
- 1/2 tablespoon chili powder
- 1 teaspoon ground cumin
- 1 teaspoon fresh oregano (or 1/2 tsp dried)
- 1 14 oz can diced tomatoes (I like the Fire Roasted diced tomatoes from Muir Glen)
- 1 teaspoon maple syrup
- 1/3 cup water (or as needed)
- sea salt to taste
- Kale, Mushroom, and Quinoa Enchiladas
- 2 cloves garlic, minced
- 1 small yellow onion, chopped
- 3/4 pound baby bella or button mushrooms, chopped
- 1/2 cup diced green chilis
- 3 cups kale, chopped
- 1/2 teaspoon ground cumin
- 1/4 teaspoon sea salt (or to taste)
- 1 1/2 cups cooked black beans
- 1 1/2 cups cooked quinoa
- 10 6-inch whole wheat or corn tortillas
- 1/2 cup chopped cilantro

Direction

- To make the enchilada sauce, heat olive oil in a medium skillet or pot. Sautee onion for three minutes. Add garlic and continue cooking for another five minutes, or until onions are translucent.
- Add the chili powder, cumin, oregano, tomatoes, and maple syrup. Add sea salt to taste.
- Transfer sauce to a blender or food processor, and blend till it's smooth. Add water to adjust the consistency as you wish. Set sauce aside till you're ready to use.
- Preheat oven to 350 degrees.
- In a large pot over medium heat, heat 1 tbsp. olive oil. Sautee onion and garlic till onion is translucent. Add mushrooms and cook until liquid has been released and evaporated.
- Add the chilis to the pot and give them a stir. Add the kale and allow it to wilt slightly. Add the cumin, sea salt, black beans and quinoa, and continue heating the mixture until it's completely warm and well mixed.
- In the bottom of a casserole dish, spread a thin layer of the enchilada sauce. Place about a quarter cup mushroom and quinoa mixture in the center of a tortilla. Roll the tortilla up and place it into the dish. Repeat with the remaining tortillas. Cover them all with a layer of enchilada sauce and bake for 25 minutes. Top the enchiladas with chopped cilantro.

352. Yogurt With Toasted Quinoa, Dates, And Almonds

Serving: Serves 1 (can easily be doubled, tripled, etc.) | Prep: | Cook: | Ready in:

Ingredients

- 1/2 tablespoon red quinoa
- 5 shelled pistachios (raw or salted, either will work), chopped
- 5 almonds, chopped
- 6 ounces whole milk Greek yogurt
- 2 medjool dates, pitted and chopped
- Pinch of freshly grated lemon zest
- Flaky sea salt or other coarse salt -- or olive salt if you can get hold of some
- 1 to 2 teaspoons best quality olive oil

Direction

- Heat the oven to 350 degrees F. Pour the quinoa into a small sauté pan and place over medium heat. Toast the quinoa -- it will begin popping when it's toasted, and as soon as it is pour it into a bowl to cool. Spread the pistachios and almonds in a small baking dish and toast in the oven for 5 minutes. Remove and let cool.
- Spread the yogurt on a small plate or shallow bowl. Sprinkle on the quinoa, pistachios, almonds, and dates. Fleck with lemon zest and sea salt, and finish with a sprinkling of olive oil.

353. Zesty Red Quinoa Salad

Serving: Serves 4 to 6 | Prep: | Cook: |Ready in:

Ingredients

- 1 cup red quinoa
- 1½ cups water
- 1/2 sweet potato, diced and parboiled
- 1/2 red pepper, diced
- 3 kumquats finely chopped, plus a few slices for garnish
- 1 tablespoon olive oil
- 1 tablespoon good quality maple syrup
- 1 tablespoon chopped cilantro, plus a little for garnish

Direction

- Soak the quinoa in hot water for 5 minutes. Strain and rinse. Put in a pot with the 1½ cups water and bring to a boil. Lower the heat, cover, and cook until water is absorbed and quinoa is tender, about 20 minutes.
- Transfer the cooked quinoa to a large bowl. Add the sweet potato, red pepper, kumquats, olive oil, and maple syrup and mix to combine. Add the cilantro and lightly toss. Serve hot, at room temp, or cold. Garnish with chopped cilantro and sliced kumquat.

354. Beet, Quinoa, Tahini Bowl

Serving: Serves 4 | Prep: | Cook: |Ready in:

Ingredients

- for the beets and quinoa
- 1 cup uncooked quinoa, rinsed
- 1 1/2 cups water
- 2 pounds red and yellow beets
- 2 tablespoons olive oil
- 1/4 cup fresh mint leaves
- for the yogurt tahini dressing
- 1/2 cup greek yogurt
- 2 tablespoons tahini
- 1 clove garlic, finely minced
- 1 tablespoon extra-virgin olive oil
- 2 tablespoons fresh mint, chopped
- 2 tablespoons lemon juice

Direction

- Pre-heat the oven to 375 degrees. Remove the stems and leaves from the beets. Place the beets on a large piece of tinfoil and toss with a tablespoon of olive oil and season with salt and pepper. Tightly wrap the foil packet and place on a rimmed baking sheet. Bake the beets for 1 hour and 15 minutes or until they are easily pierced with the tip of a knife. Let cool slightly and then peel the skins off and slice into quarters.
- Meanwhile, cook the quinoa. Rinse it well and then add it along with the 1 1/2 cups of water in a medium saucepan with a pinch of salt. Bring to a boil, reduce the heat to medium and cook for 15 minutes or until all the water is absorbed. Take off the heat, cover and let steam for 5 minutes.
- Pour the remaining tablespoon of olive oil into a skillet over medium heat. Cut the beet stems

into small pieces and add to the oil, cook for 3-4 minutes until they begin to soften. Slice the beet greens into ribbons and then add them to the pan along with the stems and season with salt and pepper. Cook for 3-5 minutes until the greens are wilted.

- In a blender place all the ingredients for the dressing and process to combine, taste and add more salt or pepper if desired.
- Divide the quinoa, beet greens and beets among four bowls. Top with a tablespoon or two of the tahini sauce and top with the fresh mint.

355. Crunchy Quinoa & Veggie Roaster

Serving: Serves 6 as a side | Prep: | Cook: | Ready in:

Ingredients

- 3 cups cooked quinoa (leftover is ideal)
- 3 tablespoons olive oil
- 2 tablespoons lemon juice
- 1 teaspoon dried basil
- 1 teaspoon fennel seeds
- 1 teaspoon dried oregano
- 1 teaspoon garlic, minced
- 10 mushrooms, quartered
- 1/2 red onion, diced
- 1/2 red pepper, diced
- 12-15 cherry tomatoes, halves
- 1/2 cup pomegranate seeds
- 1/4 cup kalamata olives, quartered
- 1/2 cup fresh parsley, rough chopped
- 1/2 cup crumbled goat or feta cheese (optional if you want it vegan)
- salt and pepper
- olive oil sprayer, or 1-2 additional tablespoons olive oil if you don't have a sprayer

Direction

- Place large (full) sheet pan in oven (if you don't have a large/full then you might be best to use two regular sized sheets) and preheat oven to 415 degrees Fahrenheit. Allow baking sheet to heat up while you prep all other ingredients.
- In a small bowl, mix together olive oil, lemon juice, oregano, basil, fennel and garlic. Pour over quinoa and stir to incorporate very well. Set aside.
- bring hot baking sheet out of oven and spray with olive oil spray (if you don't have olive oil spray, just pour a little glug on the sheet pan and spread around using a pastry brush, or paper towel if you're absolutely in a bind). Pour quinoa onto oiled sheet pan, and spread evenly over entire pan. The thinner the layer of quinoa, the faster it will crunch up. Place in oven for about 10 minutes.
- While the quinoa is taking its first go in the oven, on another sheet pan, add mushrooms, red onion, bell pepper, and cherry tomatoes, and drizzle with about 1 tablespoon olive oil. Toss to coat all vegetables very well.
- Bring quinoa out of the oven and turn it very well using a spatula. Return to oven on the bottom rack, and place the sheet pan of vegetables on the top rack. Allow both to roast for another 15 minutes. Make sure to keep an eye on your quinoa through the oven window to ensure that the quinoa around the edges doesn't burn (if it is starting to brown too much, you will just need to toss the quinoa more often)
- Once the 15 minutes is up, turn the quinoa and the vegetables again, and season both with salt and pepper to taste (I use about 1 teaspoon of each) if the quinoa is still more moist than crunchy, it needs another go around in the oven. Ultimately, you want about 70% crunchy quinoas and 30% moist quinoas. In my opinion, the more you roast the vegetables, the sweeter and better they will be. There is no right or wrong "doneness" for roasted veg.
- Once quinoa and veg have reached your desired roasted-ness (I make up words apparently), pour both into a large bowl and toss to incorporate. Season again with salt and pepper if required. Add pomegranate seeds,

parley and olives and any additional optional toppings and serve immediately. Note: if you are using the cheese, I don't add it until the quinoa is served up on plates or in bowls as I prefer it as a garnish. If you add it into the bowl, it will inevitably melt and disappear. Which isn't necessarily a bad thing!
- Notes:
- 1. If you prefer, you can grill the veggies as it adds nice smokiness, however since the oven is on already, and if you're sort of lazy like me....enough said.
- 2. As the quinoa is a good protein, this can be a main dish for 3-4 people
- 3. This dish is excellent served cold the next day. An excellent lunchbox item!

356. Goat Cheese & Quinoa Stuffed Artichoke Heart Bottoms

Serving: Makes 4 to 6 pieces | Prep: | Cook: | Ready in:

Ingredients

- 4-6 fresh OR canned artichoke bottoms, drained and dried
- resh plain goat cheese (1 package to taste)
- 1 packet plain quinoa (cooked until tender in vegetable stock) cooled to room temperature
- 1/2 bunch fresh italian flat leaf parsley, chopped finely
- 1 cup chopped frozen, thawed & drained spinac
- good quality olive oil
- 2 fresh ripe plum tomatoes finely chopped
- homemade vegetable stock (or store bought)
- grated parmigiano cheese (for topping)
- sea salt and black peeper to taste
- (i.e. you can add in other favorite items, like sauteed mushrooms, black olives, etc. all chopped finely and mixed in to the goat cheese base... have fun and enjoy!)

Direction

- if using fresh artichoke bottoms: Once your artichoke heart bottoms are prepped and ready, drop them in a bowl of ice water with lemon to keep them from turning color. In a medium sauce pan bring the vegetable stock to a boil, add the artichoke heart bottoms to the stock and cook on medium heat until cooked through (carefully test with a fork for doneness.) Remove from the stock and set aside to cool.
- Using additional vegetable stock, cook your quinoa until tender and done (store leftover quinoa for serving as a side dish for other meals, etc.)
- In a small bowl, add the cooked quinoa and chopped tomato and parsley leaf and chopped spinach and blend well. Add in the small package of goat cheese and begin to blend with your fork until mixed well. Add some cracked black pepper to taste and blend well.
- Take the cooled artichoke bottoms, season lightly with sea salt and black pepper. Using a small spoon, add the goat cheese filling to the bottoms and form evenly in a rounded shape. Continue until all the bottoms are filled and set inside an oven baking dish right side up. Sprinkle a healthy amount of grated Parmigianino cheese on the top of the filling for each one, this will create a savory crunchy crust.
- Place in a preheated 350-375 degree oven on the middle rack. Bake for about 15 minutes or so depending on how fast your oven cooks, etc. Check them and when you see the tops begin to brown lightly, turn to broil for 2 minutes or so until the tops are golden and crispy.
- Remove from oven and serve immediately or allow to come to room temperature and serve, delicious both ways! Serve along with a crisp white wine and other small plates of your desire. P.S. For extra crunch & flavor, top with a small amount of crumbled oven roasted bacon… wonderful indeed.

357. Mandarin Quinoa And Kale Bowl

Serving: Serves 4 | Prep: | Cook: | Ready in:

Ingredients

- for the salad:
- 1 cup quinoa
- 5 cups kale
- 1/2 cup dried cranberries
- 1 cup mandarin orange segments from a 15 ounce can
- 1/4 cup toasted sliced almonds
- 1/2 cup feta cheese, crumbled
- for the vinaigrette:
- zest of one orange
- 2 large cloves garlic, minced
- 1/4 teaspoon fresh ground black pepper
- 1/2 teaspoon salt
- 1 1/2 teaspoons teaspoons dijon mustard
- 1 1/2 teaspoons whole grain mustard
- 2 tablespoons orange juice (from the zested orange)
- 2 tablespoons rice wine vinegar
- 4 tablespoons olive oil

Direction

- Prepare the quinoa as instructed on the package. When quinoa has absorbed the water, stir in the dried cranberries and remove from heat. Cover and let rest for 10 minutes. Remove the lid and cool to room temperature.
- Meanwhile, rinse and dry the kale. (I used my salad spinner). Remove the tough stems and massage the kale with your hands to break down the fibers a little. Bunch the kale into a tight ball with one hand and slice the kale very thinly with a sharp knife. Set aside.
- Drain the can of mandarin oranges and pat dry. Set aside.
- In a small bowl combine the orange zest, garlic, pepper, salt, Dijon, whole grain Dijon, orange juice, vinegar and olive oil. Whisk until emulsified.
- Combine the cooled quinoa and cranberries, kale and oranges in a bowl. Toss with a few tablespoons of the vinaigrette, until well coated, but not soupy (you may not use all the vinaigrette in this salad, but keep it to serve with other vegetables or over chicken or fish.)
- Lightly toss the salad with the feta cheese and almonds. Serve.

358. Quinoa Salad With Vegetables & Poached Egg

Serving: Makes 1 serving | Prep: | Cook: | Ready in:

Ingredients

- 1 tablespoon olive oil
- 1/4 cup quinoa
- 1/2 cup water
- 1/2 onion, chopped
- 1 clove garlic, chopped
- 1/4 cup soaked & cooked chickpeas
- 1/4 cup corn
- 2 small roasted beets
- salt + pepper to taste
- 1 egg
- chopped mint, rosemary, mint

Direction

- Heat the oil in a small saucepan. Add the garlic and onion and cook until soft, about 5-6 minutes. Add the chickpeas and corn, cook for another few minutes.
- Add the quinoa and water. Bring to a boil, then reduce heat and cover. Cook for about 15 minutes, or until all the liquid is absorbed. Note: you can also use vegetable stock instead of water for even more flavor.
- Meanwhile, in another small saucepan, bring water to a boil. Crack an egg into a small bowl. Once the water is boiling, turn off the heat, carefully slide the egg into the water, and

cover for 5 minutes. If you like your eggs a little more runny, reduce that time a little.
- While all of this is going on, cut some herbs, or use what you have on hand. The more the better! I chopped up a lot of mint, oregano, and rosemary.
- Once the quinoa is done, add the salt and pepper, give it a quick stir. Transfer to a bowl and top with chopped herbs. Add the quartered beets. With a slotted spoon, carefully lift the poached egg out of the water and lay on top of the dish.

359. Quinoa With Roasted Vegetables & Wine Glazed Chicken

Serving: Serves 4 | Prep: | Cook: | Ready in:

Ingredients

- 2 uncooked chicken breasts, trimmed of fat
- Sea salt
- Juice of one lemon
- Olive oil for drizzling
- Dry red or white wine
- 1 cup raw quinoa (I used tri-color here, but white works well, too)
- 1 tablespoon unsalted butter
- 1 teaspoon sea salt
- 3 red bell peppers, stems removed, cut in half, inner veins and seeds removed
- 1 large sweet potato (around 1 pound), cut into roughly 1/2-inch square pieces
- 1 full head of garlic, left in one piece, but with the papery outer skin removed
- 1/4 cup minced red onion
- 2 tablespoons fresh garlic chives, minced
- 1/4 cup extra-virgin olive oil
- 2 tablespoons sherry vinegar

Direction

- Place the chicken breasts on a designated cutting board, cover with plastic wrap, and pound with a meat tenderizer so the meat becomes thinner and slightly larger. Remove the plastic wrap and place the chicken in a shallow flat glass container, sprinkle both sides of each breast liberally with sea salt, and drizzle with the fresh lemon juice and olive oil. Cover and let marinate in a refrigerator until ready to cook.
- Prep the red bell peppers and place the halves on a large baking sheet. (This makes more than you'll need for the recipe, but roasting several red bell peppers this way is more efficient). Turn the oven broiler on high, place baking sheet about eight to ten inches from the heat (generally on the second-highest rack from the top), and roast until the skins are well-blackened. Remove and tent with aluminum foil for several minutes until cool to loosen blackened skins.
- Remove skins by lightly rubbing and peeling them off with your fingers. Discard skins. Dice one whole (two roasted halves) of roasted red bell pepper. Place the remaining roasted bell peppers in a glass storage container with a little bit of olive oil drizzled over them. Refrigerate for future use.
- Rinse the raw quinoa well in a fine strainer to remove any of the bitter coating. Drain. To cook the quinoa, place it in a medium saucepan with two cups of water, the butter, and the salt. Bring to a boil, then reduce the heat to a gentle simmer, cover, and cook until the quinoa has absorbed all the water, about fifteen to twenty minutes. Remove from the heat.
- Once the quinoa is cooked, let it cool for a few minutes, and then dump it on a separate large baking sheet, spreading it out evenly over the entire sheet. I do this to let some of the moisture evaporate so the quinoa doesn't become soggy when mixed with all the other ingredients. Once the quinoa has cooled to room temperature, fluff it up using a fork before placing it into a larger bowl for mixing in the other ingredients.

- Preheat the oven to 400°F. Cut the sweet potato into 1/2-inch pieces, place in a bowl, drizzle with about a tablespoon of olive oil, and sprinkle with a little sea salt and freshly ground black pepper. Dump the sweet potato on a large baking sheet and spread the pieces out over the sheet. Prep the garlic as directed by removing all the loose papery skin, leaving the head in one piece, and trim the very tip of the cloves off with a sharp knife. Place the head of garlic, stem side down, on a piece of aluminum foil that is big enough to completely wrap around the head of garlic. Create a cup shape underneath the garlic with the foil, and drizzle the garlic with a little olive oil. Fold the sides of the foil upwards and pinch together to seal. Place the foil package in the middle of the same baking sheet with the sweet potato pieces. Place in the oven on the middle rack and roast for thirty minutes until the potato is tender and slightly caramelized.
- While the sweet potato and garlic are roasting, mince the onion and the chives. After thirty minutes, remove the sweet potatoes and garlic from the oven. Carefully remove the foil package with the garlic inside from the baking sheet and place back in the oven for an additional five minutes, then remove and let cool slightly.
- Once the garlic has cooled slightly, remove the foil. Let sit a little longer until cool enough to handle, then gently remove the cloves from their skins by squeezing from the bottom. Some of the outside cloves may be a little softer then the inside ones, which should be softened but whole. Chop the roasted garlic into smaller pieces as well as you can manage; the cloves will be very soft and mushy.
- Once the garlic has cooled slightly, remove the foil. Let sit a little longer until cool enough to handle, then gently remove the cloves from their skins by squeezing from the bottom. Some of the outside cloves may be a little softer then the inside ones, which should be softened but whole. Chop the roasted garlic into smaller pieces as well as you can manage; the cloves will be very soft and mushy.
- Scoop the fluffed quinoa into a large bowl. Stir in the roasted sweet potato, red onion, diced roasted red bell pepper and chives. Place the chopped roasted garlic on top, pour the olive oil/sherry vinegar mixture over, and fold into the quinoa.
- Remove the chicken from the refrigerator. Heat a skillet over medium high heat, and sauté the chicken on both sides until it is no longer pink and gives very slightly when pressed. Remove to a separate plate. With the skillet still hot, add about a 1/4 cup of wine to deglaze the pan, and reduce until slightly thickened. Pour sauce over the chicken. Let chicken rest for several minutes, then slice diagonally into thick strips.
- Divide quinoa among four plates. Divide sliced chicken breasts evenly among each plate, placed on top. Garnish with extra minced chives if desired.

360. Quinoa With Sauteed Vegetables & Soft Cooked Egg

Serving: Serves 1 | Prep: | Cook: |Ready in:

Ingredients

- 1 organic medium to large raw egg (soft cooked)
- 3 to 5 fresh thin asparagus spears (trimmed and chopped)
- small bunch of fresh baby spinach leaves
- leftover sauteed, grilled or baked mushrooms (any variety: button, baby bella, portobella, etc.)
- leftover red & white quinoa (cooked in beef, chicken or vegetable stock)
- 1 large very ripe tomato (washed & chopped)
- 1 small garlic clove (peeled and chopped)
- olive oil
- salt and pepper to taste (red chili flake, if desired)

Direction

- In a medium skillet, drizzle olive oil and add the chopped garlic, asparagus and spinach leaves. Sauté gently for 2 to 3 minutes; add the chopped tomato and sauté slowly for another 3 to 4 minutes; add in the leftover mushrooms until warmed through and season with salt and pepper; remove from heat and set aside.
- In a small stockpot, place water to boil; add the raw egg right before the water comes to a full boil; cook for 4 1/2 to 5 minutes maximum. Remove immediately from the heat; place in cool water and set aside.
- On a serving plate, spoon the leftover reheated quinoa (quantity to individual preference); add the sautéed vegetable mixture on the side.
- Remove the egg from the cool water and peel gently; place on top of the quinoa and carefully cut in half allowing the soft yolk to run out (I love my egg yolk runny so I cook it for about 4 1/2 minutes; any more will harden the yolk.)
- Season the egg with salt and pepper and serve immediately. If desired, you can add some grated Parmigiano or asiago cheese.

361. Quinoa With Wild Mushrooms, Black Eyed Peas And Dandies

Serving: Serves so many | Prep: | Cook: | Ready in:

Ingredients

- 2 handfuls of wild mushrooms
- a cup of quinoa, soaked overnight
- a cup of black eyed peas, soaked overnight
- a bundle of dandelion greens
- your choice of herbs, a few sprigs of whatever you decide
- a shallot, diced
- 2 fatty cloves of garlic, minced

Direction

- First order of business, get your black-eyed peas going. In enough water to cover, bring to a boil, skimming the foam that arises, then reduce the fire to low, and simmer. Thank goodness it's a quick cooking legume. They should take about 20 minutes or so. (When tender, drain and set aside).
- Slice your mushrooms into lovely bite-size pieces. And now that you're into this project knee-deep, you're probably facing a fungal horror show with your porcini. A word on these lovelies: they usually come with teeny white worms. Flick the squirmy things into the trash, what you see anyway. The ones that you will inevitably miss... think of them as extra protein. I'm sorry friends, this is the price you pay for eating some of the most expensive mushrooms around. Oh, by the way, I'm using porcini, chanterelle, oyster and cinnamon enoki.
- Speaking of diamonds of the woods, or, mushrooms. You never want to wash them. Unless you've got a stash of black trumpet or morel which can be caked with dirt and pine needles. In which case, give 'em a dunk or two, but quickly. They should never sit in water, because mushrooms are like sponges, and a sodden fungus is a gross one. So, don't rinse. Instead, brush them clean with one of a mushroom brush.
- Dice your shallot. Chop your garlic. Tear the leaves from the stems of your herbs. I'm using thyme, marjoram and sage.
- Sauté the mushrooms and shallot in olive oil using your favorite cast iron pan; do this until the mushrooms are browned. Add the garlic, sauté for another minute. Be sure to season all this with salt.
- Drain and rinse the quinoa, then add it to the pan with two cups of water and another pinch of salt. Pop a lid atop, and steam till the grains are tender. Should take about 15 minutes or so.
- When the quinoa is tender, gingerly fluff with a fork and sprinkle with your herbs. Avoid

vigorous stirring. Aggression makes this grain gluey.
- Add your dandies, a fatty handful or three, which you've given a rough chop, with a pinch of salt. Fluff them into the quinoa. They should wilt in less than a minute.
- Add your black-eyed peas with a pinch of salt.
- And drizzle with a little olive oil. Fluff all of this with a fork. Taste. Adjust seasoning as needed. Et voila! Quinoa with wild mushrooms and dandelion greens!

- Toss the cherry tomatoes and shallots in 1 tbsp of olive oil and place on a baking sheet or pan.
- Roast the tomatoes + shallot for 10-12 minutes, right when the juices of the tomatoes begin to pop their skin.
- Put the cooked quinoa on a dish. Place the roasted tomato + shallot mixture on top of the quinoa. Garnish with cilantro. Drizzle the pomegranate molasses over the entire dish. Enjoy!

362. Roasted Cherry Tomatoes + Pomegranate Molasses Over Quinoa

Serving: Serves 4 | Prep: | Cook: |Ready in:

Ingredients

- 1 pint cherry tomatoes, heirloom medley
- 2 shallots, sliced
- 1 tablespoon extra virgin olive oil
- 2 tablespoons pomegranate molasses
- 1 pinch salt
- 1/2 pinch ground black pepper
- 1 cup dry uncooked quinoa
- 1 tablespoon fresh cilantro, chiffoned
- 2 cups water
- 1 dash extra virgin olive oil

Direction

- Preheat the oven to 400 degrees.
- First, cook the quinoa according to the package. Typically you will rinse off one cup in a mesh strainer, dry, and then place in a pot with a dash of olive oil. Mix it around in the pot. Then, add 2 cups of water. Bring contents to a boil, reduce to simmer, and cover. Let the quinoa cook for 15 minutes before removing from heat. Let it sit for 5 minutes before you fluff it with a fork.
- Slice the roasted cherry tomatoes in half. Slice the shallots in thin pieces.

363. Tomates Farcies: Vegetarian & Beef Stuffed Tomatoes, Bonus QUINOA Salad

Serving: Serves 6-8 | Prep: | Cook: |Ready in:

Ingredients

- vegetarian stuffed tomatoes
- 1 cup cooked quinoa
- 1 fennel bulb, finely minced
- 2-3 scallions, finely sliced (or chopped chives)
- 1 small bunch flat leaf parsley, finely chopped
- 1 small bunch chopped fresh dill
- 6-8 ripe roma tomatoes, emptied (inside juices and softer pulp set aside)
- sea salt & freshly ground pepper to taste
- 1-2 tablespoons extra virgin olive oil
- french style tomatoes farcies with grass fed beef
- 1 pound grass fed lean ground beef
- 1 yellow onion, finely minced
- 1-2 garlic cloves, finely minced
- 8 large ripe tomatoes (heirlooms are good)
- 1 large bunch flat leaf parsley, finely chopped
- Handful thyme sprigs (leaves)
- 1 small bunch fresh basil leaves
- 3 tablespoons good quality bread crumbs
- 2 tablespoons extra virgin olive oil
- sea salt & fresh ground pepper to taste

Direction

- Vegetarian stuffed tomatoes
- 1. Combine the cooked quinoa with all of the chopped herbs, green onions, very finely chopped fennel, sea salt, pepper, and olive oil. Finely chop up the tomato pulp that was set aside (from emptying the tomatoes earlier) and add to the mixture without too much of the juice.
- 2. Carefully fill the tomatoes with the mixture, put the lids on loosely, and drizzle lightly with olive oil. Bake in a 350 degree oven for 30 minutes. ** You can also add 2 tbsp. of good quality parmesan cheese to the mixture you fill the tomatoes with for additional flavor**
- 3. Fresh QUINOA SALAD with fennel: after filling the tomatoes, you should have some mixture left over. Add to this the lime juice, baby tomatoes, fennel greens, more chopped dill, and a dash of extra virgin olive oil. Serve as a quinoa salad!
- French style tomatoes farcies with grass fed beef
- 1. Cut the tops off the tomatoes, then carefully empty the insides with the help of a small paring knife and a small spoon (be careful not to pierce them). Save the softer pulp and juices from the insides in a bowl. Allow the empty tomatoes to drain, and keep their lids near them.
- 2. In a heavy pot heat 1 tbsp. olive oil, sauté the minced garlic and onions in the oil until softened and golden, then add and brown the beef with sea salt & pepper to taste. Break up the beef pieces with a wooden spoon or spatula. Chop up about 1/2 of the tomato pulp and add it with some of the juices to the browned beef and cook until the liquid is absorbed. Turn off the heat, let the mixture cool slightly, then add all of the finely chopped herbs and mix well.
- 3. Add about 3 tbsp. of good quality bread crumbs and combine well. Taste for salt, and adjust.
- 4. With a spoon carefully fill the tomatoes with the mixture all the way to the top and cover loosely with their lids. Place tomatoes tightly in a baking dish, drizzle lightly with olive oil, and bake in a 350 degree oven for about 40-45 minutes-up to an hour.

364. Warm Quinoa, Collard Greens, And Squash Salad

Serving: Serves 2 | Prep: | Cook: |Ready in:

Ingredients

- 1 acorn squash
- 1 cup dry quinoa
- 1/2 medium red onion
- 5 garlic cloves
- 1 green bell pepper
- 3 cups chopped collard greens
- 2 1/2 cups vegetable broth
- 1 tablespoon sea salt
- 1 tablespoon freshly ground black pepper
- 1 tablespoon coconut oil
- 1 teaspoon olive oil
- 1 tablespoon freshly chopped parsley

Direction

- Slice squash in half, remove pulp and seeds.
- Coat with olive oil, and half the salt and pepper.
- Roast on parchment-lined baking sheet at 450 for about 40 minutes until soft.
- Meanwhile, rinse and drain quinoa, cook in 2 cups of vegetable broth for about 15 minutes.
- Chop garlic, onion, and pepper- sauté with remaining salt and pepper in coconut oil until soft.
- Cook greens in 1/2 cup vegetable broth until just wilted- about 12 minutes.
- Peel and cube roasted squash.
- Combine all ingredients, including fresh parsley. Serve warm.

365. {Veg & GF} Quinoa & Pomegranate Tabbouleh Salad

Serving: Serves 2 | Prep: 0hours20mins | Cook: 0hours15mins | Ready in:

Ingredients

- 1/2 cup Quinoa
- 10 Small Rosa Tomatoes
- 1/4 Cucumber
- 1/2 Lemon
- 3 tablespoons Olive Oil
- 1 handful Pomegrante Seeds
- 1 bunch Fresh Italian Parsley
- 15 Mint Leaves
- Salt and Pepper to Taste

Direction

- Boil your Quinoa as per the instructions on the packet. Once cooked, chill in a bowl in fridge
- Dice your tomatoes and cucumber & wash your parsley and mint and chop finely
- Add all of the above into the cooled Quinoa and then add in the juice of half a lemon, 15ml of olive oil, salt and pepper to taste and finally your pomegranate seeds
- Serve and enjoy! Should keep for 2 days in an airtight container

Index

A

Ale 43,138

Almond 3,4,8,13,14,36,40,41,107,147,158,190,200

Apple 3,4,6,14,15,17,22,23,36,57,96,105,109,126,173,187

Apricot 6,7,142,158

Artichoke 8,33,203

Asparagus 3,7,16,26,30,76,167

Avocado 3,4,5,6,7,16,18,23,26,32,41,46,63,66,71,73,84,99,100,136,137,151,154,159,172,177

B

Bacon 4,5,51,91,114

Bagel 4,53,54

Baking 16,17,19,105,106,158

Balsamic vinegar 141

Banana 3,4,22,42

Basil 3,4,5,6,7,19,25,66,74,78,89,90,91,128,129,150,164,178,182,183,187

Beans 3,6,9,13,26,58,102,147

Beef 8,208

Beer 143

Berry 3,6,37,147

Black beans 102

Black pepper 58,74

Blackberry 5,107

Blueberry 3,26,40

Bran 173

Bread 3,4,22,55,78

Broccoli 3,4,6,18,19,29,39,75,78,138,153

Broth 7,58,119,167,168,176

Brown sugar 9

Brussels sprouts 53,92,188

Buns 143

Burger 3,5,6,7,8,9,18,24,88,102,103,124,143,145,183,193

Butter 3,4,6,7,8,9,13,17,20,29,32,47,48,138,139,158,159,178,187,190,196

C

Cake 4,5,7,8,9,43,53,54,55,60,92,158,185

Calvados 173

Cannellini beans 110

Caramel 3,6,10,16,103,137

Cardamom 17

Carrot 3,4,6,7,10,18,19,26,34,39,51,102,106,126,154

Cashew 4,52

Cauliflower 3,5,6,31,81,101,140

Cava 125

Celery 12,102,106,123

Champ 14

Chard 3,5,6,8,11,31,100,101,140,145,191

Chayote 3,32

Cheddar 3,4,19,31,33,49,78

Cheese 4,5,6,7,8,19,33,34,63,66,73,78,101,105,114,116,138,142,161,174,178,197,198,203

Cherry 3,4,5,6,8,23,33,48,68,73,87,109,146,148,180,208

Chestnut 5,91

Chicken 3,4,5,6,7,8,33,34,39,41,45,58,77,89,137,143,148,168,176,196,205

Chickpea 4,5,6,19,45,79,80,83,124,127,143,147

Chilli 97

Chipotle 3,23,34,91,172

Chips 43,105,124

Chives 97

Chocolate 3,4,5,6,9,26,35,43,48,49,55,92,104,105,149

Chorizo 6,132

Cinnamon 3,6,13,14,15,17,36,40,45,105,116,126,139,179,190

Cloves 12,13,23,40,45,78,97,161,164,165,187

Cocoa powder 9

Coconut 3,5,7,8,9,13,32,33,34,37,38,39,42,43,104,105,107,167,190

Collar 3,8,27,209

Coriander 13,119,153,196

Coulis 8,189

Couscous 4,5,8,56,105,189

Crab 7,180

Crackers 3,35

Cranberry 4,5,41,73,87,105

Cream 4,18,42,43

Crisps 5,106

Crumble 3,14,67,96,154,157,197

Cucumber 5,6,26,50,72,82,98,109,123,126,144,210

Cumin 4,26,45,46,63,142,153,179,191,196

Curly kale 72

Currants 6,12,114,196

Curry 4,5,8,45,47,48,64,112,193

Custard 4,42

D

Date 4,6,8,42,135,200

Dijon mustard 53,63,74,84,116,129,138,162,176,194

Dill 98,126

Dried apricots 157

Dried cherries 45,198

E

Edam 4,6,52,128,129,143,144

Egg 4,5,6,7,8,17,19,47,58,61,63,65,78,82,98,100,106,118,156,1 57,158,178,191,204,206

English muffin 20

English mustard 133

F

Falafel 6,127

Fat 33,34,175,193

Fennel 6,7,129,130,167

Feta 3,4,6,7,8,25,29,33,41,57,62,67,73,105,109,115,118,148,156,167,191,192,196,197

Fig 7,160

Fish 135

Flour 4,6,16,19,55,102,105,106,107,127,158

Fruit 3,5,7,8,36,83,173,193

G

Garlic 4,6,7,12,13,19,33,34,45,58,78,89,96,97,102,105,106,109,118,137,142,148,153,157

Gin 3,5,6,7,13,37,39,55,91,99,119,177

Gouda 161

Grain 5,93

Grapes 6,88,117

Guacamole 4,64

H

Halloumi 6,145,146

Ham 9

Harissa 4,5,7,65,80,84,180

Hazelnut 7,160

Heart 8,33,203

Herbs 4,5,8,57,78,79,97,185,191

Honey 5,7,9,17,97,105,107,143,147,154,159,168

J

Jus 21,23,72,104,139

K

Kale 3,4,5,6,7,8,18,22,52,71,72,73,85,110,114,118,125,131,133,151,153,160,164,180,200,204

Ketchup 6,124

Kidney 3,26

Kohlrabi 50

L

Lamb 3,27

Leek 6,7,63,115,133,172

Lemon 3,4,5,6,33,39,46,50,51,72,73,74,75,76,83,96,98,99,109,112,117,124,125,128,129,137,143,148,159,162,187,197,198,210

Lentils 7,87,155

Lettuce 4,5,24,66,94,105,109

Lime 3,5,6,7,26,32,35,97,110,117,119,137,146,168,177,187

M

Macadamia 3,32,192

Manchego 167

Mandarin 8,204

Mango 5,99

Maple syrup 19,36,74,160,190

Mayonnaise 185

Meat 3,6,20,21,148

Milk 3,9,13,33,40,107,147

Millet 4,5,66,81

Mince 32,33,34,39,87,108,161

Mint 4,6,73,114,115,124,126,128,129,138,139,146,187,210

Miso 4,5,7,52,81,82,156

Molasses 6,8,146,208

Mozzarella 33

Muffins 3,4,6,16,49,118,126

Mushroom 3,5,6,7,8,21,84,85,102,113,124,137,150,151,183,196,200,207

Mustard 4,22,43,102,142

N

Nectarine 5,86

Nut 3,5,6,25,40,72,87,88,99,100,102,117,170,175

O

Oatmeal 5,9,78,102,126

Oats 3,5,28,88,147

Oil 5,7,9,12,14,17,23,26,33,34,43,46,50,58,63,72,73,89,97,98,99,100,101,102,103,105,107,114,122,124,125,131,153,157,159,179,180,182,197,210

Okra 5,89

Olive 5,12,17,23,26,31,39,45,50,54,58,63,67,72,73,74,76,79,82,89,97,98,99,100,102,103,109,112,114,124,125,131,134,137,142,143,153,157,159,179,187,188,196,197,205,210

Onion 3,4,6,7,12,13,16,19,33,34,42,45,47,97,102,106,114,119,123,126,129,131,137,141,153,179,180,182,191

Orange 4,5,6,12,14,52,90,91,115,137,158,196

Oregano 89,113,179

P

Paella 11

Paneer 4,46

Paprika 179,191

Parfait 3,37

Parmesan 52,54,96,128,132,140,165,179

Parsley 3,4,7,26,33,35,50,62,78,106,107,123,126,157,210

Pasta 4,51

Peach 3,5,6,7,14,34,97,124,153

Peanuts 6,13,146

Pear 4,6,8,55,56,141,147,189

Peas 4,7,8,46,51,74,153,156,179,207

Pecan 17,196

Pecorino 67

Peel 32,36,39,48,50,72,86,90,100,127,143,152,156,168,173,176,209

Pepper 3,4,5,6,8,13,17,19,33,34,50,56,57,58,62,63,78,79,80,83,91,97,100,102,107,110,114,119,120,121,124,126,150,153,165,179,188,190,210

Pesto 4,5,7,75,89,95,110,164,165,176

Pickle 5,6,96,124,129,130

Pie 4,42,66

Pineapple 4,64

Pistachio 3,6,7,19,114,153,154

Pizza 3,5,8,30,113,198

Plum 5,6,34,107,135

Pomegranate 4,8,69,114,159,194,208,210

Pork 3,5,20,97,98

Port 31,130,183

Potato 5,6,7,8,100,106,140,161,176,183,184

Pulse 18,44,61,75,110,133,148

Pumpkin 3,6,35,138

Q

Quinoa 1,3,4,5,6,7,8,9,10,11,12,13,14,15,16,17,18,19,20,21,22,23,24,25,26,27,28,29,30,31,32,33,34,35,36,37,38,39,40,41,42,43,44,45,46,47,48,49,50,51,52,53,54,55,56,57,58,60,61,62,63,64,65,66,67,68,69,70,71,72,73,74,75,76,77,78,79,80,81,82,83,84,85,86,87,88,89,90,91,92,93,94,95,96,97,98,99,100,101,102,103,104,105,106,107,108,109,110,111,112,113,114,115,116,117,118,119,120,121,122,123,124,125,126,127,128,129,130,131,132,133,134,135,136,137,138,139,140,141,142,143,144,145,146,147,148,149,150,151,152,153,154,155,156,157,158,159,160,161,162,163,164,165,167,168,169,170,171,172,173,174,175,176,177,178,179,180,181,182,183,184,185,186,187,188,189,190,191,192,193,194,195,196,197,198,199,200,201,202,203,204,205,206,207,208,209,210

R

Radish 5,6,50,100,123,137

Raisins 3,6,11,12,17,117,179

Raita 112

Red lentil 91

Red onion 23,109

Red wine 87

Rice 3,4,5,6,40,56,66,93,98,106,108,118,133

Rosemary 7,158

S

Sage 3,8,11,12,197

Salad 3,4,5,6,7,8,10,12,13,14,15,17,18,22,23,25,26,30,34,35,41,46,50,52,54,58,59,62,63,65,67,69,71,72,73,75,76,79,81,83,84,86,87,90,91,94,99,100,103,104,105,109,114,115,116,117,119,126,128,129,130,132,136,137,144,146,147,148,151,152,153,154,155,156,157,158,159,160,161,167,168,169,170,172,177,178,180,181,182,183,184,186,187,191,195,198,201,204,208,209,210

Salmon 4,5,6,7,53,88,132,155

Salsa 4,6,11,60,118,174

Salt 9,17,19,21,23,26,27,31,33,36,42,43,45,46,47,49,50,54,58,62,63,67,72,73,88,91,94,97,100,102,105,107,110,112,113,114,117,118,119,122,124,125,126,127,129,132,134,137,140,142,143,147,150,153,157,159,161,164,165,168,180,182,187,191,192,193,197,198,210

Sausage 6,8,98,122,140,188

Scallop 7,164

Sea salt 44,74,79,148,156,190,205

Seasoning 21,33,34,53,54,55

Seeds 3,4,6,28,35,51,74,114,138,147,210

Sesame seeds 165

Shallot 9,50,87,102,137

Soda 16,105

Sorrel 7,176

Soup 3,4,5,6,7,8,40,42,45,84,85,119,168,190

Spinach 3,4,5,6,7,8,13,14,21,26,33,34,46,63,78,100,116,119,126,156,176,192

Squash 3,4,5,6,7,8,10,11,12,13,17,20,47,48,49,50,58,81,122,124,138,139,159,160,173,198,209

Steak 4,7,65,177

Stew 3,13,179

Stock 119,193

Strawberry 5,7,91,178

Stuffing 6,121,122,124,151

Sugar 17,40,43,73,105,158

Sunflower seed 187

Swiss chard 11,191

Syrup 3,37,179

T

Tabasco 127

Taco 6,7,8,149,151,172,174,175,185

Tahini 5,8,80,103,109,125,201

Tangerine 6,116

Tapioca 106

Tarragon 7,178

Tea 207

Teriyaki 4,52

Thyme 6,7,142,154

Tilapia 5,83

Toffee 4,42

Tofu 3,6,7,8,15,116,156,174,194

Tomato 3,4,5,6,7,8,13,26,33,34,41,46,57,66,68,73,89,90,99,100,102,107,108,113,115,143,148,154,164,167,179,180,189,190,191,192,208,210

Turkey 3,8,21,193

Turmeric 46

V

Vegan 8,55,193,194

Vegetable stock 157,164,165

Vegetables 3,4,5,7,8,25,58,76,119,130,139,162,204,205,206

Vegetarian 4,8,61,195,208,209

Vinegar 19,26,198

W

Waffles 170

Walnut 3,4,6,8,11,12,22,23,50,61,112,142,165,197,198

Watermelon 8,198

Wine 8,12,14,26,205

Worcestershire sauce 88,177

Wraps 4,5,66,109

Z

Zest 8,12,50,88,126,201

Conclusion

Thank you again for downloading this book!

I hope you enjoyed reading about my book!

If you enjoyed this book, please take the time to share your thoughts and post a review on Amazon. It'd be greatly appreciated!

Write me an honest review about the book – I truly value your opinion and thoughts and I will incorporate them into my next book, which is already underway.

Thank you!

If you have any questions, **feel free to contact at:** author@slushierecipes.com

Doris Lamont

slushierecipes.com

Made in the USA
Columbia, SC
01 January 2025